AF848487

100350411

Stereotactic and Image Directed Surgery of Brain Tumours

For Churchill Livingstone
Publisher: Michael Parkinson
Project editor: Dilys Jones
Copy editor: Rich Cutler
Production controller: Lesley Small
Sales promotion executive: Caroline Boyd

Stereotactic and Image Directed Surgery of Brain Tumours

Edited by

David G. T. Thomas MA FRCP FRCS
Professor of Neurosurgery, National Hospital
for Nervous Diseases, London, UK

CHURCHILL LIVINGSTONE
EDINBURGH LONDON MADRID MELBOURNE NEW YORK AND TOKYO 1993

10035041l
616.99281059
STE xx

CHURCHILL LIVINGSTONE
Medical Division of Longman Group UK Limited

Distributed in the United States of America by Churchill Livingstone Inc., 650 Avenue of the Americas, New York, N. Y. 10011, and by associated companies, branches and representatives throughout the world.

© Longman Group UK Limited 1993

All rights reserved. No part of this publication may be reproduced, stored in a retrieval system, or transmitted in any form or by any means, electronic, mechanical, photocopying, recording or otherwise, without either the prior permission of the publishers (Churchill Livingstone, Robert Stevenson House, 1–3 Baxter's Place, Leith Walk, Edinburgh EH1 3AF), or a licence permitting restricted copying in the United Kingdom issued by the Copyright Licensing Agency Ltd, 90 Tottenham Court Road, London, W1P 9HE.

First published 1993

ISBN 0-443-04445-7

British Library of Cataloguing in Publication Data
A catalogue record for this book is available from the British Library.

Library of Congress Cataloging in Publication Data
Stereotactic and image directed surgery of brain tumours/edited by D. G. T. Thomas.
p. cm.
Includes bibliographical references and index.
ISBN 0-443-04445-7
1. Brain—Tumors—Surgery. 2. Stereoencephalotomy. 3. Brain—Biopsy. I. Thomas, D. G. T. (David Glyndor Treharne)
[DNLM: 1. Brain Neoplasms—surgery. 2. Diagnostic Imaging. 3. Stereotaxic Techniques. WL 368 I31]
RD663.I46 1993
616.99' 281059—dc20
DNLM/DLC
for Library of Congress 92–49428
CIP

Printed and bound in Great Britain by
Butler & Tanner Ltd, Frome and London

The publisher's policy is to use **paper manufactured from sustainable forests**

Contents

Contributors

M. J. Apuzzo MD
Edwin M. Todd/Trent H. Wells Jnr Professor, Department of Neurological Surgery, University of Southern California, School of Medicine; Director of Neurosurgery, Kenneth R. Norris Jnr Cancer Hospital and Research Institute, Los Angeles, California, USA

Michael Brada BSc MB ChB MRCP FRCR
Senior Lecturer and Consultant in Radiotherapy and Oncology, Head of Neuro-oncology Unit, Institute of Cancer Research and Royal Marsden Hospital, London, UK

R. Bradford BSc MD FRCS
Consultant Neurosurgeon, The Royal Free Hospital and School of Medicine, London, UK

Parakrama T. Chandrasoma MD
Associate Professor of Pathology, Chief of Anatomic Pathology, Los Angeles County-University of Southern California Medical Center, Los Angeles, USA

Chi-Shing Zee MD
Associate Professor of Radiology, USC School of Medicines, Los Angeles, USA

Lawrence S. Chin MD
Clinical Instructor, Department of Neurological Surgery, University of Southern California School of Medicine, Los Angeles, California, USA

D. L. Collins MEng
Graduate Student, Biomedical Engineering, Montreal Neurological Institute, McGill University, Montreal, Canada

John L. Darling MSc PhD
Senior Lecturer in Neuro-oncology, Gough Cooper Department of Neurological Surgery, Institute of Neurology, London, UK

Patrick A. Finlay BSc PhD CEng MIMechE MIEE
Managing Director, Armstrong Projects Ltd., Beaconsfield, UK

John D. Graham BSc MRCP FRCR
Consultant in Clinical Oncology, Bristol Oncology Centre, Bristol, UK

Philip H. Gutin MD
Professor of Neurological Surgery and Radiation Oncology, University of California School of Medicine, San Francisco, USA

Christopher J. Henri MSc
Graduate Student, Biomedical Engineering, Montreal Neurological Institute, McGill University, Montreal, Quebec, Canada

Patrick J. Kelly MD
Professor of Neurological Surgery, Mayo Clinic and Mayo Medical School, Rochester, Minnesota, USA

N. D. Kitchen FRCS
Research Registrar, Gough Cooper Department of Neurological Surgery, Institute of Neurology, London, UK

John Koivukangas MD PhD
Assistant Professor, Department of Neurosurgery, University of Oulu, Oulu, Finland; Visiting Professor, Department of Neurosurgery, University of Minnesota, Minneapolis, USA

Douglas Kondziolka MD MSc FRCS(C)
Assistant Professor of Neurological Surgery, Presbyterian University Hospital, University of Pittsburgh School of Medicine, Pittsburgh, USA

Louis Lemieux PhD
Research Fellow, Department of Clinical Neurology, Institute of Neurology, London and Department of Medical Physics, Royal Postgraduate Medical School, Hammersmith Hospital, London, UK

M. L. Levy MD
Clinical Instructor, Department of Neurological Surgery, USC School of Medicine, Los Angeles, USA

L. Dade Lunsford MD
Professor of Neurological Surgery, Radiology and Radiation Oncology, University of Pittsburgh, School of Medicine, Pittsburgh; Director, Specialized Neurosurgical Center, University of Pittsburgh Medical Center, Pittsburgh, USA

Ch. B. Ostertag MD
Professor, Abteilung Stereotaktische Neurochirurgie, Neurochirurgische Universitatsklinik, Freiburg, Germany

Malcolm P. Pell MB BS FRACS
Consultant Neurosurgeon, St Vincent's Clinic, New South Wales, Australia

T. M. Peters PhD FCCPM
Associate Professor, Department of Neurology and Neurosurgery and Departments of Radiology, Biomedical Engineering and Medical Physics, Montreal Neurological Institute, McGill University, Montreal, Canada

Craig Rabb MD
Clinical Instructor, Department of Neurological Surgery, University of Southern California, Los Angeles, USA

Robert M. Redfern MB BS FRCS
Consultant Neurosurgeon, Morriston Hospital, Swansea, UK

Tamas Revesz MD MRCPath
Senior Lecturer in Neuropathology, Department of Neuropathology, Institute of Neurology, London; Honorary Consultant at the National Hospital for Neurology and Neurosurgery, London, UK

Francesco Scaravilli MD PhD FRCPath
Professor, Department of Neuropathology, Institute of Neurology, London, UK

Penny K. Sneed MD
Assistant Professor, Department of Radiation Oncology, University of California, San Francisco, California, USA

David G. T. Thomas MA MB BChir FRCP(Glas) FRCSEd
Professor of Neurosurgery, the National Hospital for Neurology and Neurosurgery, London, UK

R. Wootton PhD DSc
Professor and Director of Medical Physics, Royal Postgraduate Medical School, Hammersmith Hospital, London, UK

Preface

The last decade has seen the widespread application of CT scanning and MR imaging, which were invented in the 1970s, to image directed surgery of brain tumours. Formerly, stereotactic methods were based on more invasive neuroradiological methods, which were highly complex and more hazardous. In surgery in general minimally invasive methods are gaining ground because they are associated with less morbidity and by shortening hospital stay they save money. Image directed surgery of brain tumours offers these contributions in neurosurgery. At present only a minority of neurosurgeons are trained and technically equipped to employ such techniques. This volume is intended to bring an increased awareness of these methods and their diverse applications. Research and development in image processing is creating frameless stereotactic systems, which, coupled with robotic instrumentation, should make it possible for more neurosurgeons, without requiring additional years of training, to achieve better results in the operative surgical management of brain tumours. In this effort to improve treatment neurosurgeons are currently supported by colleagues in radiotherapy and oncology. It is likely that in future, as well as the currently used interstitial radiotherapy and chemotherapy, novel methods of treatment of intrinsic brain tumours will require image directed application of gene therapy and of biological response modifiers. Such new therapeutic methods will be based largely on current basic science investigations in the field of neuro-oncology. Much of this research itself is dependent upon image directed surgery to provide material for study. Thus, the evolving techniques of this branch of neurosurgery are increasingly central to the modern management of brain tumours.

London, 1993 D. G. T. Thomas

Acknowledgements

I would like to acknowledge the technical editorial assistance which I have received from Dr H. A. C. Cockburn and from Mrs J. Urquhart, as well as the secretarial support from Miss H. Gossling and Mrs B. Gallagher. The forbearance of the contributors, not least in the question of grammatical and spelling usages or differences on the two sides of the Atlantic Ocean are also gratefully acknowledged.

D. G. T. Thomas

1. Historical perspective

R. M. Redfern

INTRODUCTION

Image directed stereotactic surgery of brain tumours differs fundamentally from functional stereotactic surgery used in treatment of movement disorders. In the latter, anatomical atlases are generally used to predict the location of a selected subcortical target in relation to relatively fixed deep seated landmarks, mainly in the region of the third ventricle, whereas, by contrast, the investigation and surgical treatment of the former necessitates radiological demonstration of the lesion. This difference arises because tumours (and arteriovenous malformations (AVMs) and epileptogenic foci) do not occur at specific sites whose location can be accurately predicted solely on clinical grounds. Thus, with the exception of AVMs, which may be demonstrated by angiography, treatment of structural lesions by stereotactic surgery has in general had to await the availability of high resolution images derived from computerized tomography (CT) or magnetic resonance imaging (MRI) scanners. When linked to stereotactic systems such scanners now facilitate accurate location of intracranial targets relative to extracranial coordinates. However, although these techniques have only flourished in the last 15 years or so, the foundations of such surgery, and indeed of neurosurgery itself, are rooted in the 19th century and earlier.

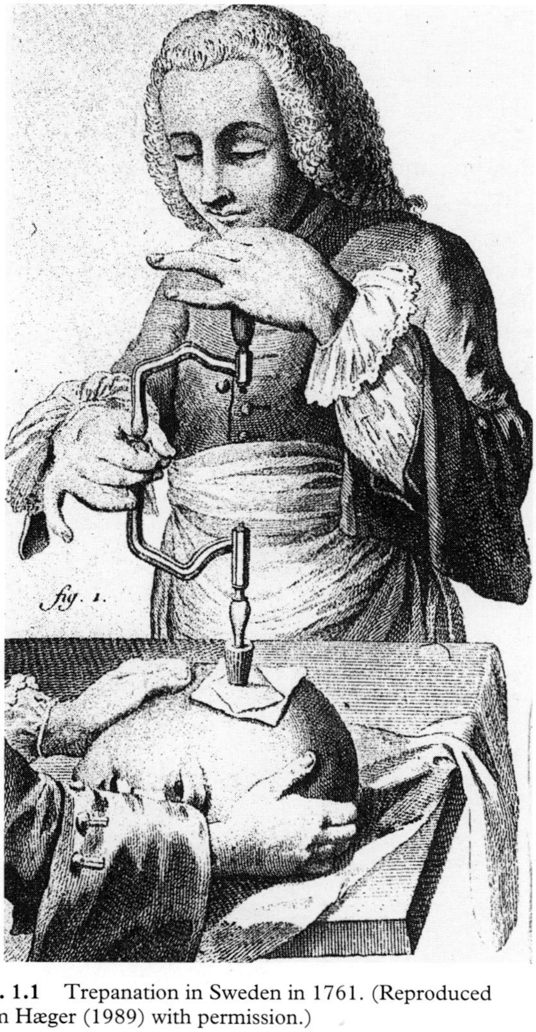

Fig. 1.1 Trepanation in Sweden in 1761. (Reproduced from Hæger (1989) with permission.)

ORIGINS OF NEUROLOGICAL SURGERY

The oldest, albeit crude, method of locating intracranial targets is skull trepanation, a procedure which has been practised in modern Europe for over two centuries (Fig. 1.1) although archaeological evidence suggests that both ritual and therapeutic trepanation, possibly for relief of symptoms following trauma, was performed across Europe and in Peru as early as 3000 BC. Some of these skulls exhibit callus formation, indicating prolonged survival of the 'patient'. More remarkably still, Hæger (1989) records that Soviet archaeologists working along the Dnieper river in the 1960s found trepanned skulls dating back to the Middle Stone Age, 12 000 years ago. Thus, target directed procedures in neurosurgery are not new!

In 300 BC Erasistratos, in Alexandria, recognized the intellectual function of the brain (an idea later shared by Galen who held it to be the seat of intelligence, movement and sensation), but not until understanding of its functional organization occurred could neurology develop, and thence a rational approach to the surgical treatment of tumours and other lesions. Religious constraints throughout the Middle Ages prevented progress until, in the 17th century, Descartes pronounced that the soul resides in the pineal gland to which sensory messages were sent and whence information was passed to the muscles. In the late 18th century Gall introduced phrenology (Fig. 1.2), which was based on the idea that the brain comprised areas representing a moral or mental activity; although the theory proved to be erroneous, his original premise — that there existed a functional organization of the cerebral cortex — was valid. The proposal by the Italian anatomist Rolando that the cerebral hemispheres controlled motor functions, and the work of the British neurologist Hughlings Jackson, who, from studying patients with certain types of epileptic seizures, postulated that the brain was divided into coordinated centres, subsequently gave credibility to the idea of somatotopic organization of motor areas. Later, two German physiologists, Fritsch and Hitzig, observed that electrical stimulation of the brain in dogs and monkeys evoked distinct muscular movements and suggested a topographical arrangement of muscle groups within the motor cortex; their findings were extended by Ferrier, who, from further experiments in monkeys, proposed a map of the functional organization of the human brain.

A more precise identification of areas involved in motor control resulted from the work of Sherrington (1906). The first study of the human motor cortex, in patients undergoing brain

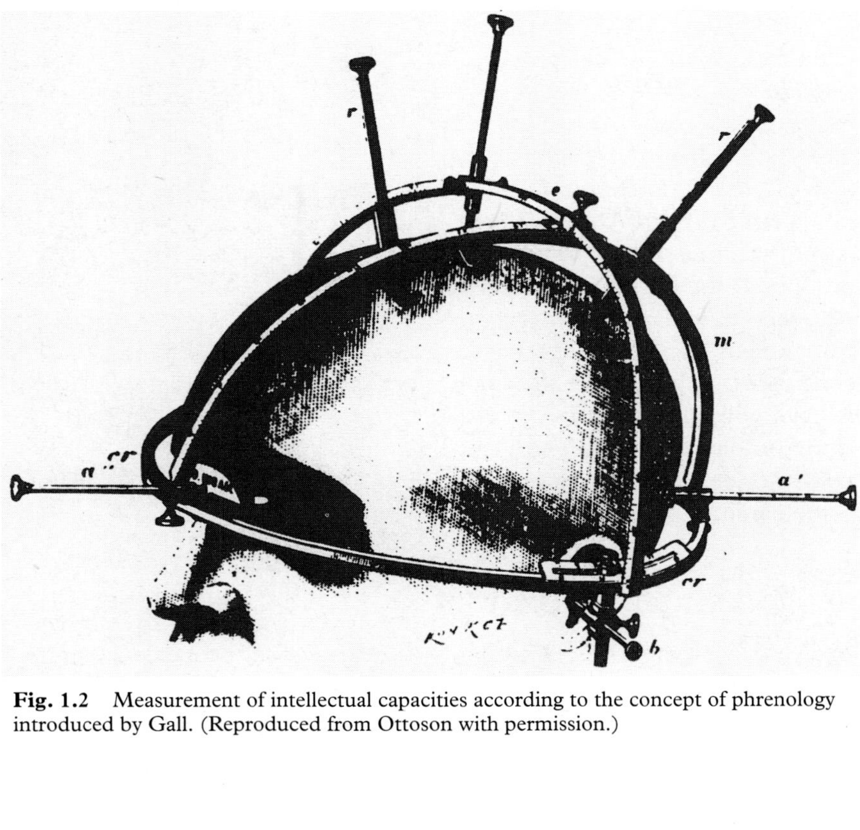

Fig. 1.2 Measurement of intellectual capacities according to the concept of phrenology introduced by Gall. (Reproduced from Ottoson with permission.)

surgery, was made by Foerster, who, in 1925, found that electrical stimulation of the precentral gyrus evoked discrete movements of muscles on the contralateral side of the body. Foerster's work was subsequently confirmed and extended by Wilder Penfield and others in the 1930s (Penfield & Boldrey 1937, Ottoson 1983).

Although the site of a structural abnormality within the central nervous system (CNS) could thus now be predicted on clinical grounds, the localization of such a lesion at operation was dependent on indirect radiological methods (encephalography, ventriculography or angiography) and on wide exposure of the lesion by craniotomy; surgery for small deeply situated lesions clearly necessitated the development of refined and more accurate techniques.

ORIGINS OF STEREOTACTIC SURGERY

> Tools used by the surgeon must be adapted to the task and where the human brain is concerned they cannot be too refined.
>
> Lars Leksell

The first stereotactic system intended for the study of human cerebral anatomy probably derives from the University of Utrecht (Harting

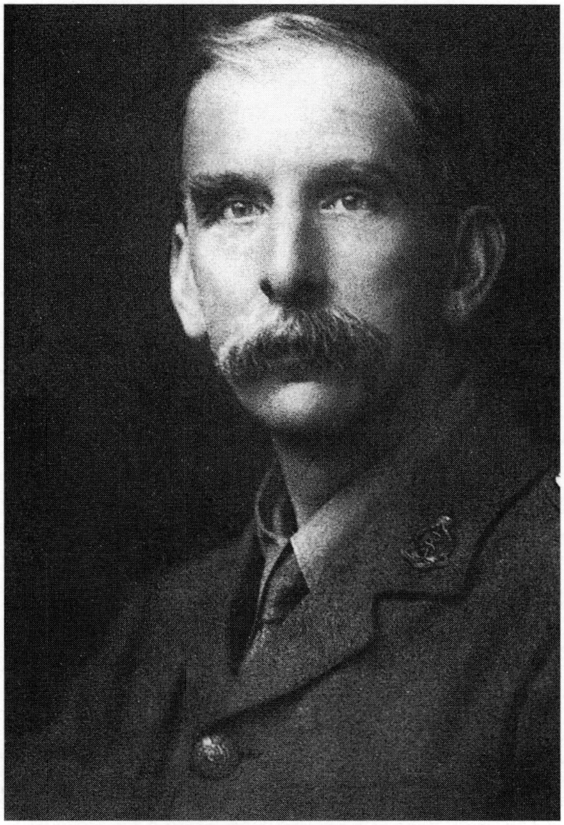

Fig. 1.4 Sir Victor Horsley. (Courtesy of P. Stanworth.)

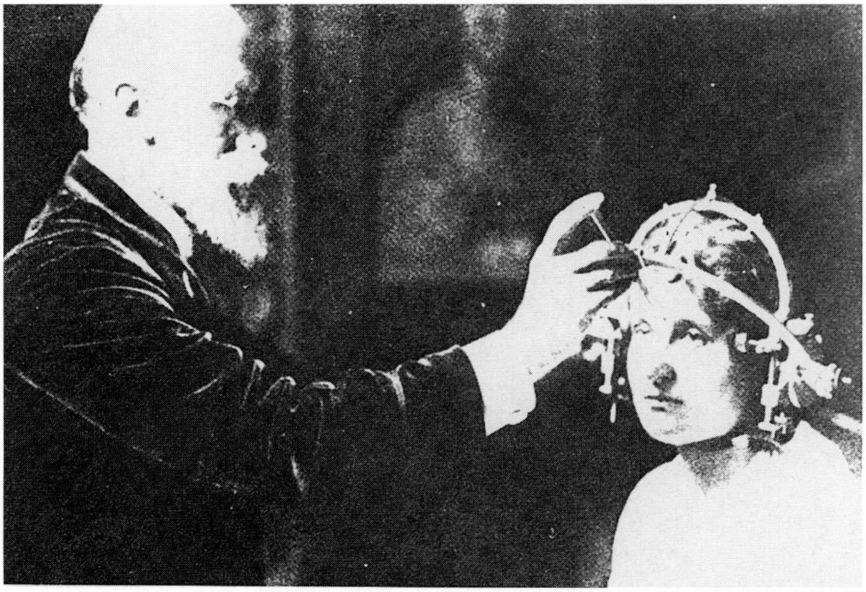

Fig. 1.3 Zernow's surface measuring apparatus ('encephalometer'). (Reproduced from Kandel & Schavinsky (1972) with permission.)

1861), and Spiegel (1970) has drawn attention to the use of guided instruments for animal experimentation by Dittmar and Woroschiloff in the 1870s. In 1889 Professor Zernov, an anatomist at Moscow University, introduced his 'encephalometer' (Fig. 1.3), for locating surface anatomical landmarks in the brain, which was later successfully used on three patients by Altuchov (Kandel & Schavinsky 1972) and by Rossolimo (1895), who used a modified version

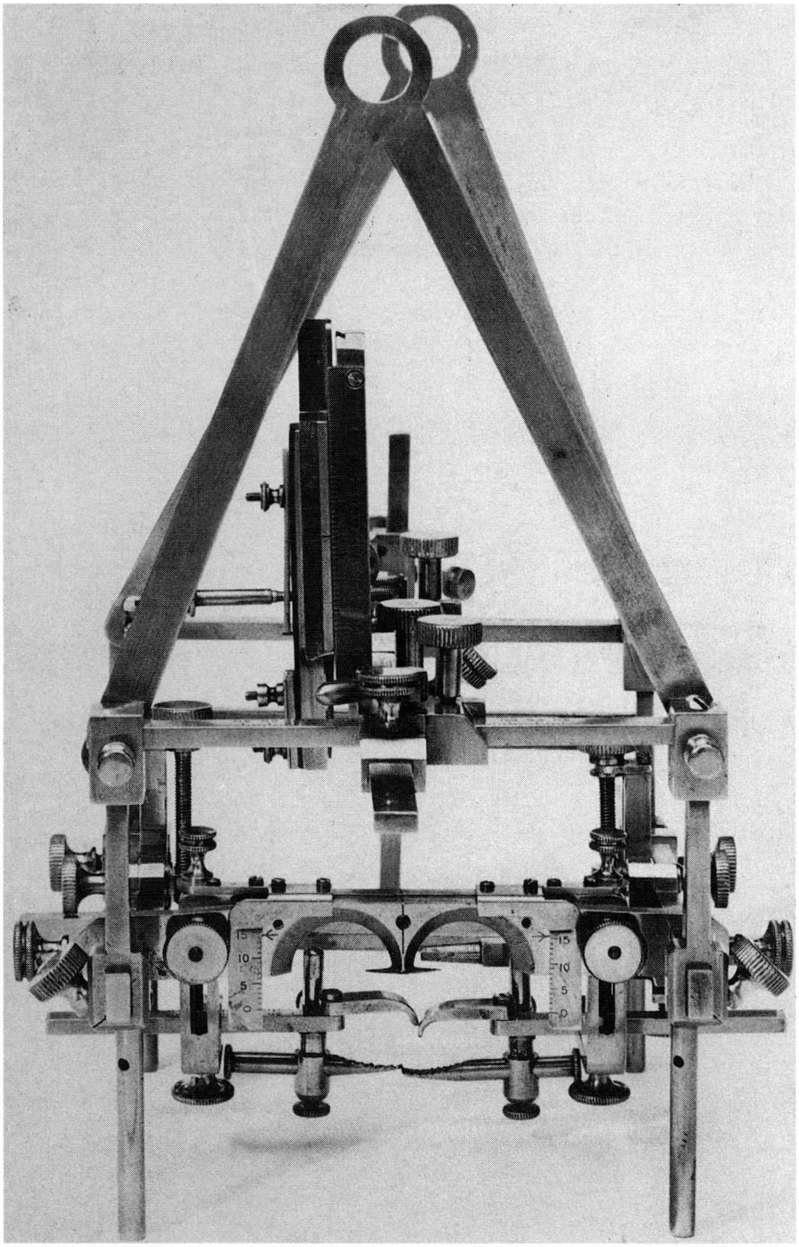

a

Fig. 1.5 The original Horsley–Clarke stereotactic apparatus viewed from **a** in front and **b** above. (Reproduced from Redfern (1989) with permission from *The British Journal of Neurosurgery* and the Trustees of The Science Museum, London.)

of the instrument to drain a lesion which was probably a cystic glioma (Iizuka 1975).

In 1906, during their investigation of cerebellar structure and function in Macaque monkeys, Sir Victor Horsley (Fig. 1.4) and Richard Clarke found that to facilitate production of reproducible lesions deep within the cerebellum it was necessary to construct an instrument specifically for this purpose (Fig. 1.5) (Clarke & Horsley 1906, Horsley & Clarke 1908). Clarke (1920) later modified the instrument and ultimately devised an equatorial system with an angled aiming arc which facilitated the introduction of a needle (or electrode) through almost any point on the calvarial surface (Fig. 1.6); despite obvious advantages in experimental study of the CNS conferred by this instrument and its predecessor, neither was much utilized until the 1930s (Ingram et al 1932).

In 1918, Aubrey Mussen (Fig. 1.7a), a Canadian neurologist, designed a stereotaxic instrument (Fig. 1.7b) for use in man in conjunction with an atlas of the human brain. Mussen further proposed that it might prove possible to locate an abnormal area by detecting a change in electrical resistance compared to surrounding brain. Unfortunately, however, he was unable to persuade any neurosurgeon to use the instrument so that its potential was never realized (Picard et al 1983).

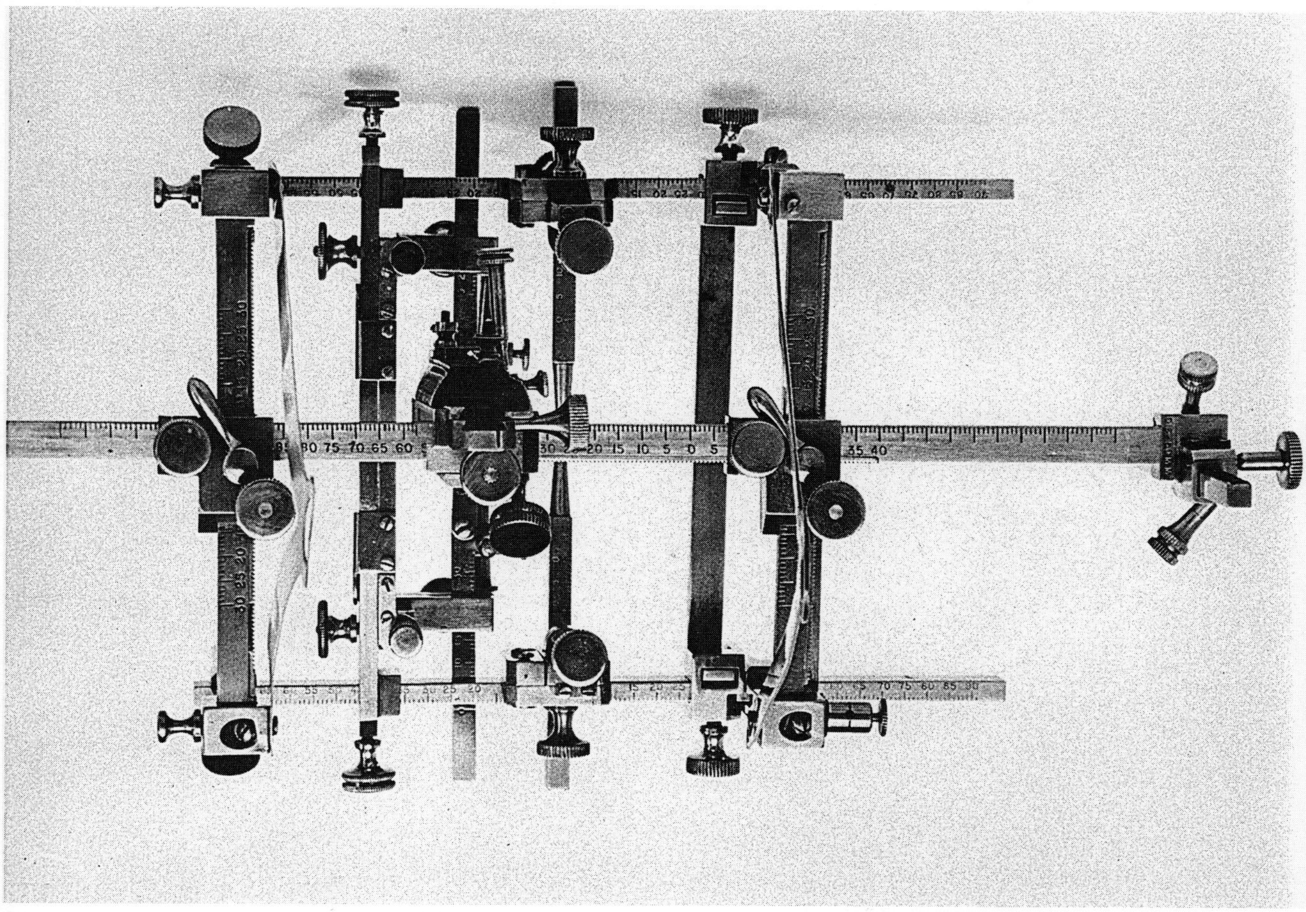

b

Fig. 1.5 *Contd*

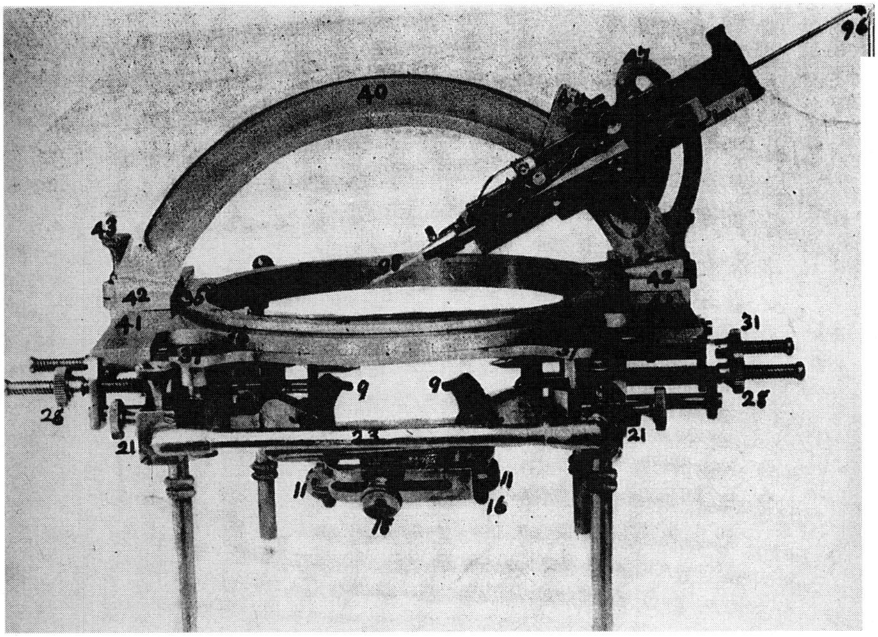

Fig. 1.6 The modified Horsley–Clarke apparatus with equatorial system. (Reproduced from Redfern (1989) with permission from *The British Journal of Neurosurgery* and The Trustees of The Science Museum, London.)

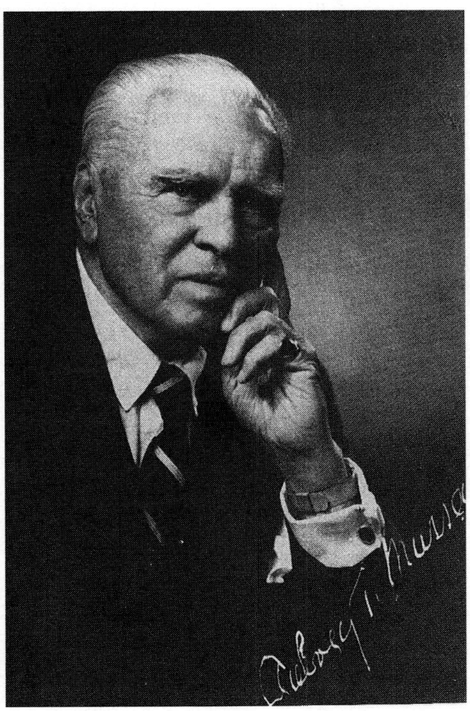

a

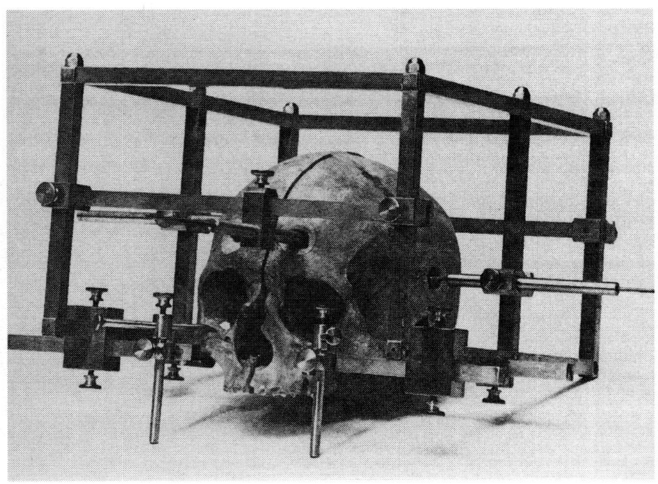

b

Fig. 1.7 **a** Dr Aubrey T. Mussen and **b** the first human stereotactic apparatus, designed by Mussen. (Reproduced from Picard et al (1983) with permission from *The Journal of Neurosurgery*.)

Thus, although Kirschner (1933) reported the use of a stereotaxic system for treatment of tic douloureux which utilized fixed (external) landmarks around the skull base, it was not until 1947, with the introduction of the technique of Spiegel (Fig. 1.8) and Wycis, that the wider potential of a human application of stereotactic surgery was realized. Although the instrument which Spiegel and Wycis introduced (Fig. 1.9) was primarily intended for functional disorders, it is evident that they were also mindful of its potential in the management of brain tumours (Spiegel et al 1947).

The possibility of offering surgical treatment to many patients with movement disorders soon led to the introduction of numerous stereotactic

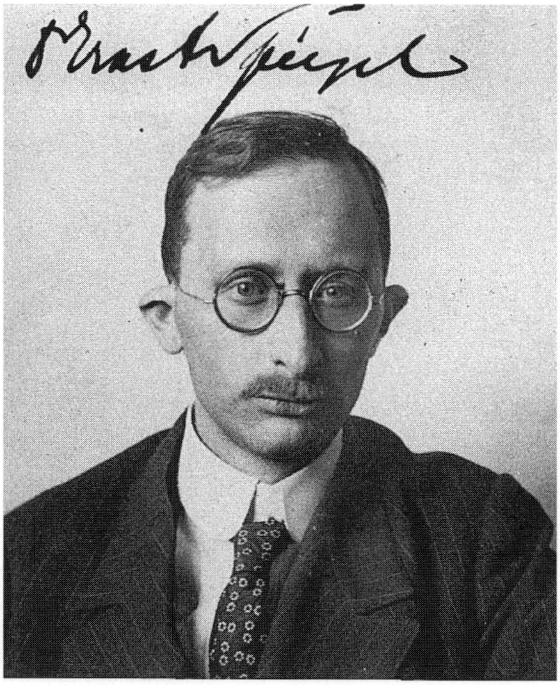

Fig. 1.8 Dr Ernest A. Spiegel.

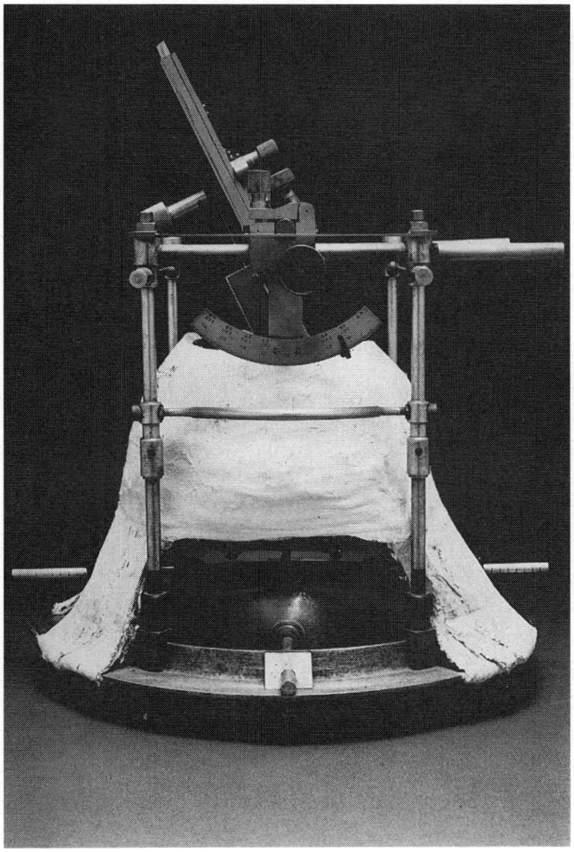

Fig. 1.9 The Spiegel–Wycis stereotaxic apparatus. (Reproduced from Redfern (1989) with permission from *The British Journal of Neurosurgery* and The National Museum of American History, Smithsonian Institution, Washington, DC.)

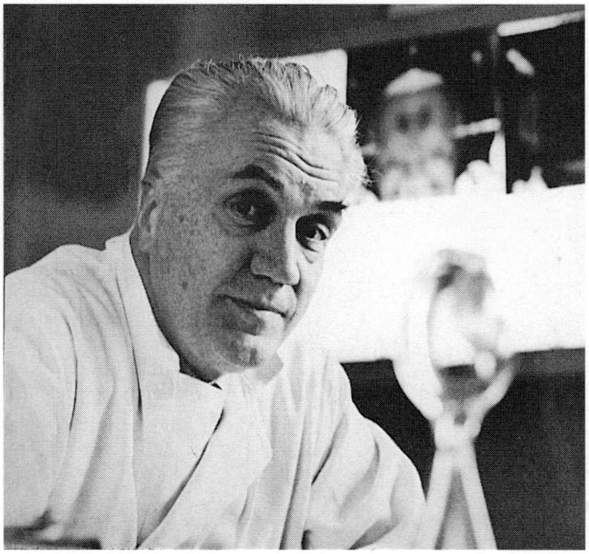

Fig. 1.10 Professor Lars Leksell. (Courtesy of Elekta Instrument AB, Stockholm.)

instruments (Redfern 1989), many of which rapidly became obsolete. Some, however, and particularly those designed by Lars Leksell in Stockholm (Fig. 1.10) and by Riechert and Mundinger in Freiburg, survive in modified form and have been adapted for use both in image guided and in functional procedures; later systems, such as the Brown–Roberts–Wells (BRW) frame (Radionics, Burlington, Massachusetts, USA) and that developed by Hitchcock in the UK, have also become increasingly popular.

Whereas CT and MRI guided stereotaxy have become the mainstay of image guided techniques, intraoperative ultrasound has also proved to be of value.

ULTRASOUND IN NEUROSURGERY

Very high frequency sound waves, 'ultrasound', produce echoes when reflected from the interfaces between tissues of different characteristics, but during passage the intensity of the emitted signal is attenuated both by the distance travelled and by the tissue through which the signal passes; attempts have been made with varying degrees of success to exploit this phenomenon in disease states.

Jefferson & Hill (1966) attribute the first medical application of the attenuation of sound waves by the body to d'Arsonval (1886), who investigated the potential of the body to modify transmitted sound signals in the chest. However, although underwater echo sounding for maritime use was introduced in 1918 and ultrasound was used to detect flaws in metal casting in the 1930s (Jefferson & Hill 1966), it was not until the 1950s that ultrasound was first applied in man. French et al (1951) devised a technique through the opened skull to detect cerebral tumours at autopsy, and Wild & Reid (1953) subsequently reported the in vivo localization of a brain tumour at operation. However, as reviewed by Jefferson & Hill (1966), the repeated failure to establish a reliable technique led the US Atomic Energy Commission to officially abandon further attempts to develop diagnostic ultrasound in 1955.

Ironically, in Sweden in the same year Leksell (1955a) devised an ultrasonic method of detecting displacement of midline structures which he termed 'echo-encephalography'. The method was subsequently further developed and popularized so that, until the introduction of CT scanning, it was frequently employed for assessment of intracranial complications in head injured patients.

Although safe and inexpensive, its application is limited by loss of signal which occurs during passage through the skull so that little energy reaches the brain. Thus, whereas diagnostic ultrasound has become an invaluable investigative tool in other specialties, in neurosurgical practice it now has only three main applications. Firstly, Doppler techniques are used to determine blood flow characteristics in extracranial or intracranial vessels. Secondly, an ultrasound probe applied over the anterior fontanelle may be used as a reliable, non-invasive means of detecting large intracranial abnormalities, such as subdural fluid, hydrocephalus or intracerebral haematomas, in neonates and infants. Thirdly, techniques have been developed which utilize an ultrasound probe, placed on the brain surface via a burr hole or at craniotomy (Fig. 1.11a), to locate intracerebral haematomas or tumours (Fig. 1.11b,c); by obviating the need for application of a stereotactic frame, such techniques may still be of value in some cases of brain tumour biopsy (Rubin et al 1980) and ventricular cannulation (Chandler et al 1982).

An inherent problem with ultrasound biopsy of tumours is the limited manoeuvrability due to the need to position the lesion within the midline of the arc of scanning, which is relatively narrow; however, by making an accurate depth correction, which allows for incident angles away from the centre of the arc, and by attaching a simple adaptor to the needle guide used for the procedure, targets off the centre of the arc can readily be reached, thereby increasing the usefulness of the technique (Hamlyn 1990). Furthermore, after taking a biopsy the needle track to the lesion can usually be seen, thus confirming correct placement of the needle (Fig. 1.12). The technique demands interpretational

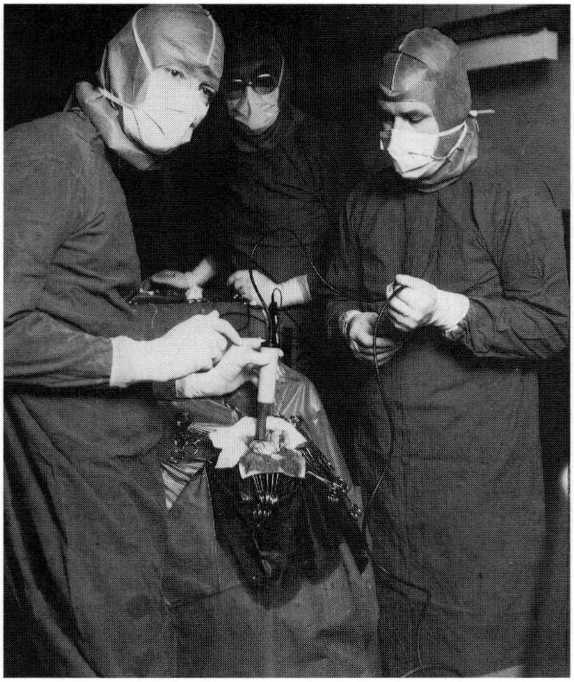

a

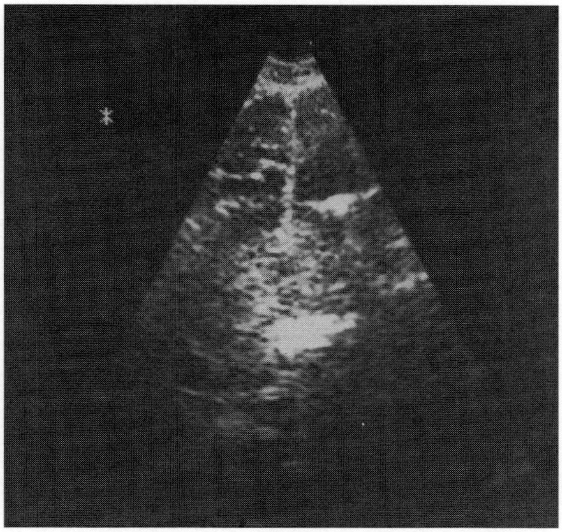

Fig. 1.12 Operative ultrasound scan demonstrating needle track down to target after biopsy of Grade III/IV glioma. (Courtesy of P. Hamlyn.)

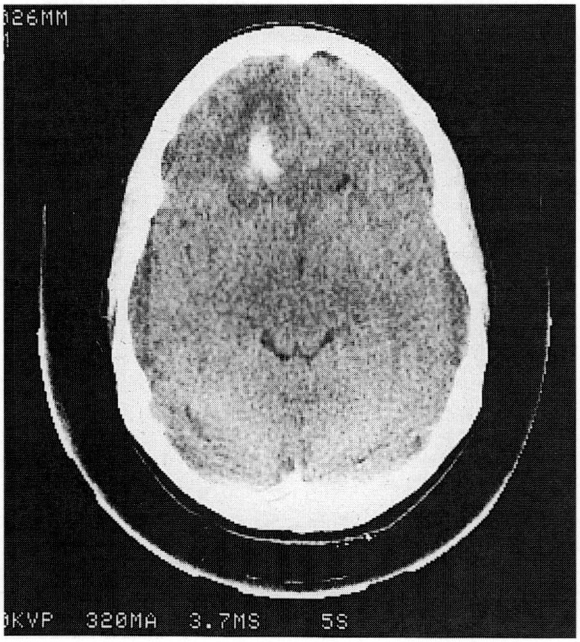

b

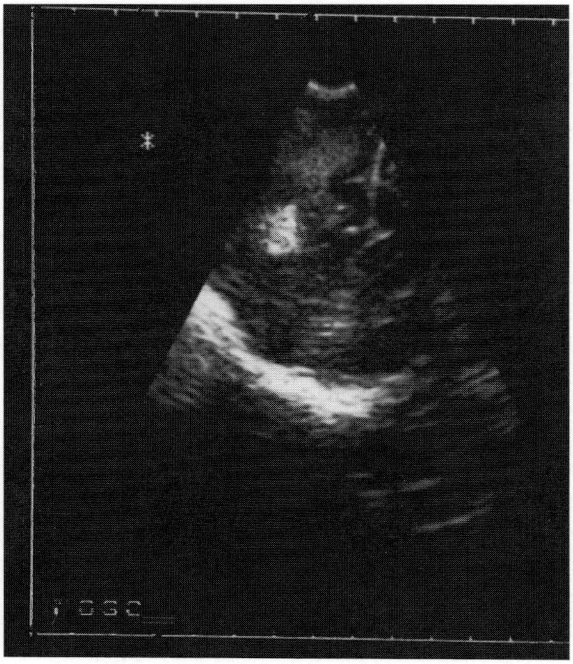

c

Fig. 1.11 **a** The Brüel and Kjær neurosurgical ultrasound system in use at open operation and **b** preoperative CT scan and **c** operative ultrasound scan of a frontal glioma showing the echodense tumour against the lower margin of the falx. (Courtesy of Mr David Williams, Brüel & Kjær (**a**), and P. Hamlyn (**b** & **c**).)

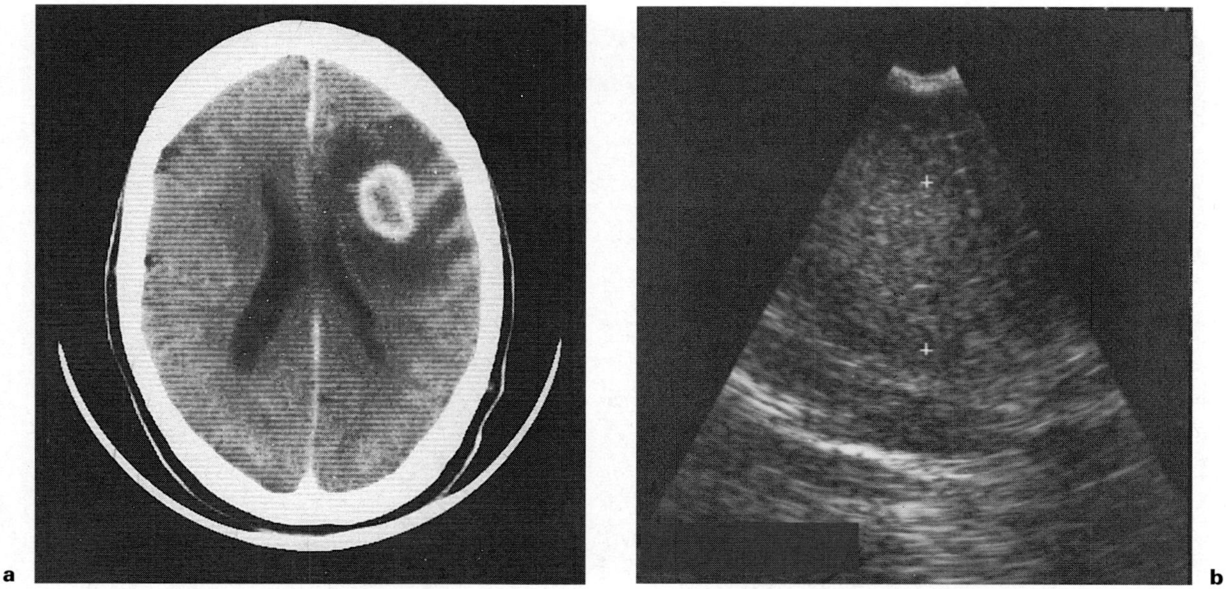

Fig. 1.13 **a** Preoperative CT scan and **b** operative ultrasound scan of a frontal metastasis demonstrating difficulty sometimes encountered in identification of targets using ultrasound. On the ultrasound scan the limits of the tumour are marked (+). (Courtesy of P. Hamlyn.)

expertise since some lesions which are clearly demonstrated using CT may be difficult to identify with ultrasound (Fig. 1.13).

CT AND MRI GUIDED STEREOTACTIC SURGERY

Stereotactic instruments

Many modern stereotactic systems employ the ‘concentric arc’ principle whereby a movable arc or gantry (bow) is used to define an imaginary sphere in space; the arc is so positioned on a rigid frame that its geometric centre coincides with the chosen target point. Since the radius of a sphere is constant, an exploring probe passed at right angles to any tangent to the arc must then pass through its centre and thus, at a known depth, to the target point; instruments which operate on this principle include the frames of Leksell, Hitchcock and Weiss. In systems in which the patient’s head (attached to the base frame) is moved within the arc-radius frame (rather than the arc being moved around the head) the term ‘focal point’ is used; such a method is employed in the Todd–Wells stereotactic system.

Other systems operate on the ‘polar coordinate’ principle in which, having located the target point radiographically, its coordinates are calculated from the needle depth and from the angles of incidence in two perpendicular planes; this principle is used in Cooper’s stereotactic system, in the McCaul frame (Fig. 1.14a,b), and in early models of the Riechert–Mundinger system.

Another group of polar coordinate systems additionally incorporate a ‘phantom’ device. A mechanical ‘dummy run’ is first performed in which the target is ‘set up’ within the phantom frame from radiologically determined coordinates, such that with the bow positioned on the phantom the needle tip is positioned at the target point. After removing the needle, but with the same coordinates still applied to the bow, the bow is repositioned on the ‘working’ frame attached to the patient and the procedure is performed. The BRW and Cosman–Roberts–Wells (CRW) systems and the later Riechert–

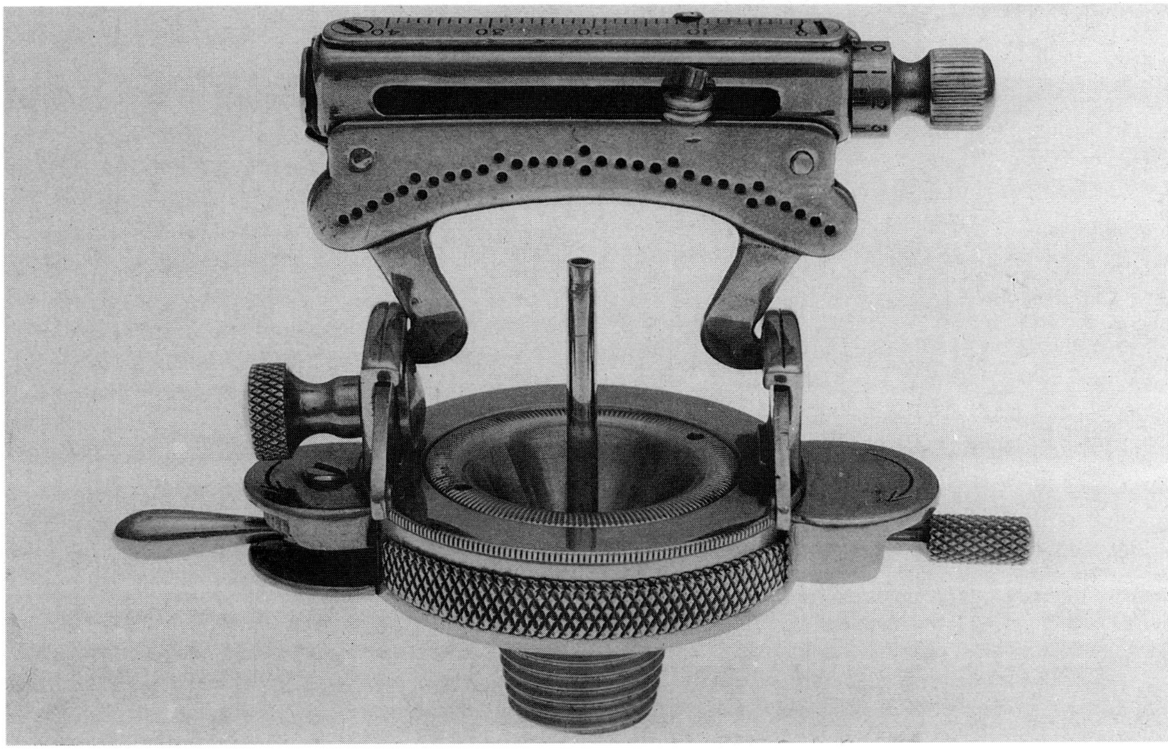

a

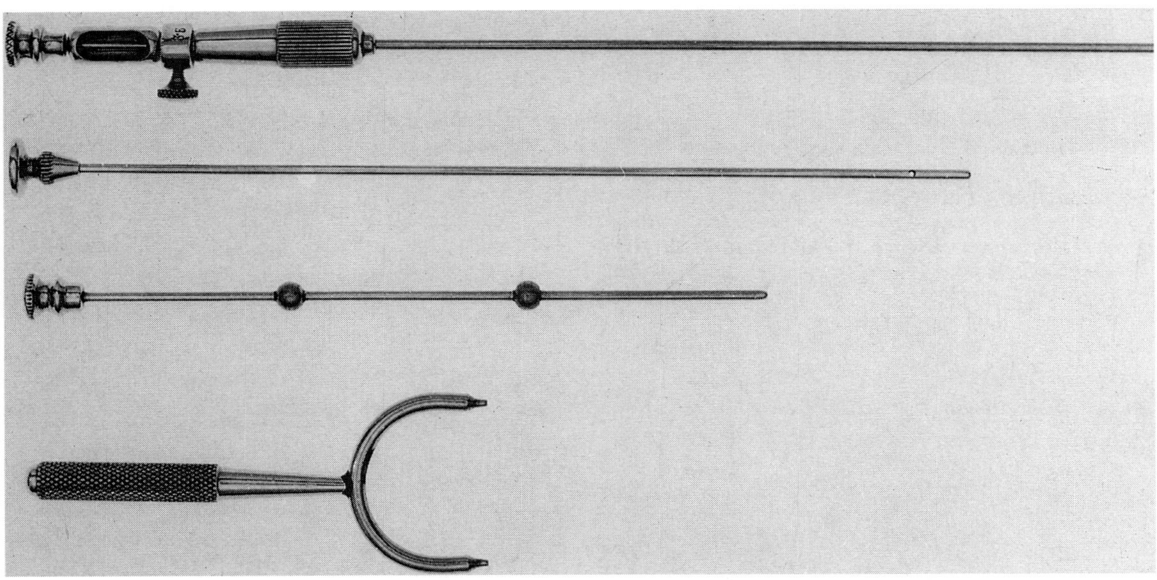

b

Fig. 1.14 A 'polar coordinate' system: **a** the McCaul frame and **b** its accessories for adjustment of the aiming device and introduction of ^{90}Y seeds during stereotactic subcaudate tractotomy, as currently used by J R Bartlett. A 'phantom-type' system: **c** the Riechert–Mundinger system, showing method of calculation of electrode trajectory and (below) a diagrammatic representation for alternative mathematical calculation of target coordinates. (Courtesy of J R Bartlett (**a** and **b**) and F Mundinger (**c**).)

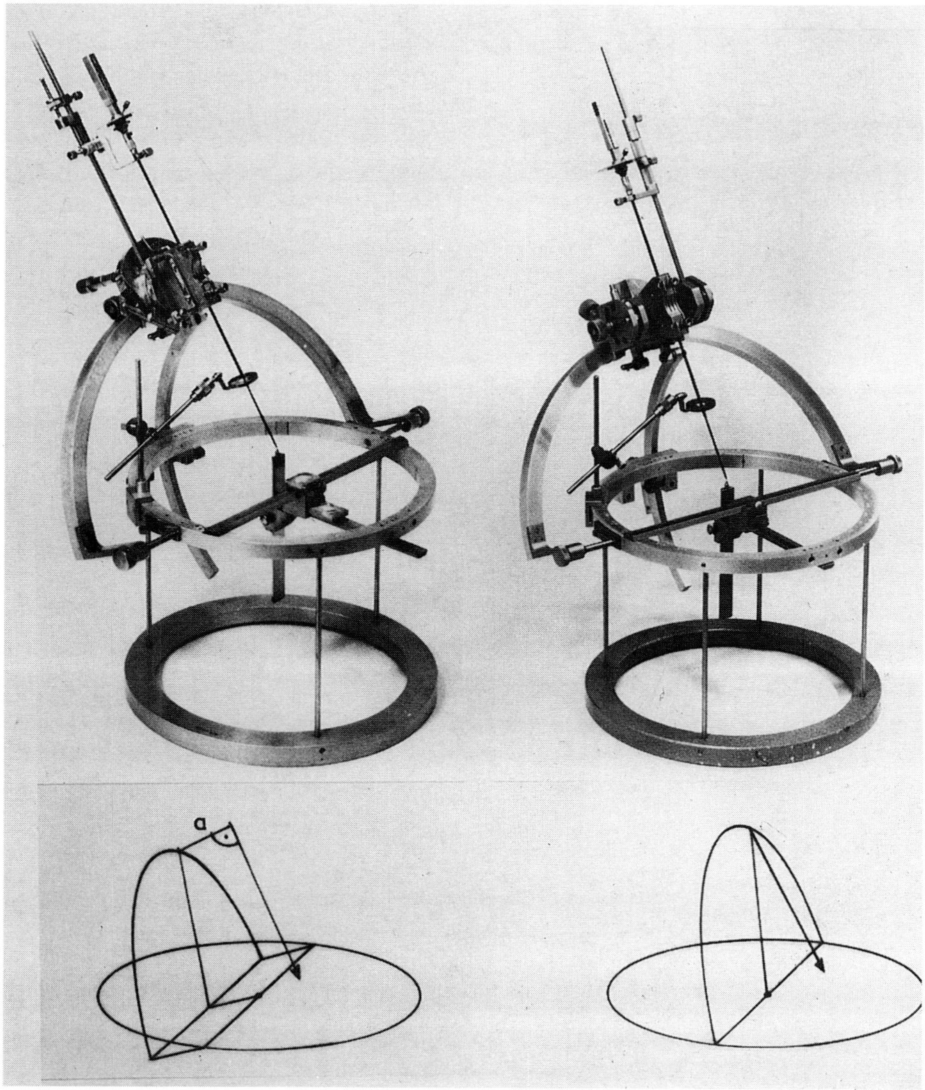

c

Fig. 1.14 *Contd*

Mundinger frame (Fig. 1.14c) employ this phantom method.

The Leksell frame

Although of great historical significance, the original stereotactic method of Spiegel and Wycis was by modern standards somewhat cumbersome. Using information derived from ventriculography, it was necessary to undertake a mathematical determination of the three dimensional coordinates of the chosen target point and then to calculate the direction from the needle holder to the target by trigonometry.

The more rational concentric method was developed in Stockholm by Leksell (1949), who introduced a stereotactic system consisting of an outer, adjustable semicircular frame bearing a movable needle carrier and mounted on an inner frame firmly fixed to the skull (Fig. 1.15a); using radiological control, and by carefully adjusting the apparatus, a target point at the geometric

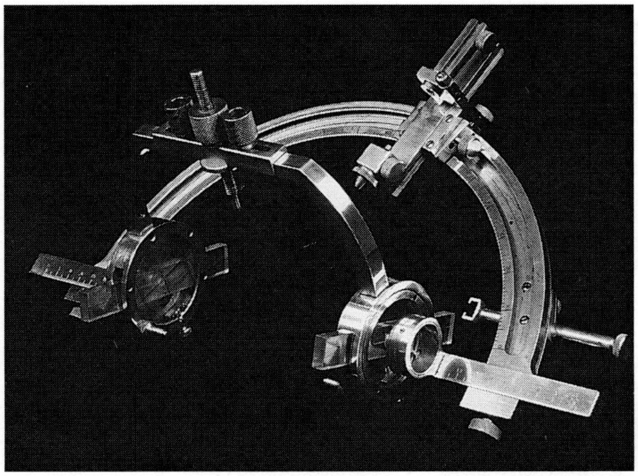

a

centre of the system could be reached; before undertaking the operative procedure the site of the needle tip was checked by lateral and anteroposterior radiographs.

Later, and particularly when used for stereotactic radiosurgery (see the section on the gamma knife), Leksell found that a heavier construction than his original instrument was required;

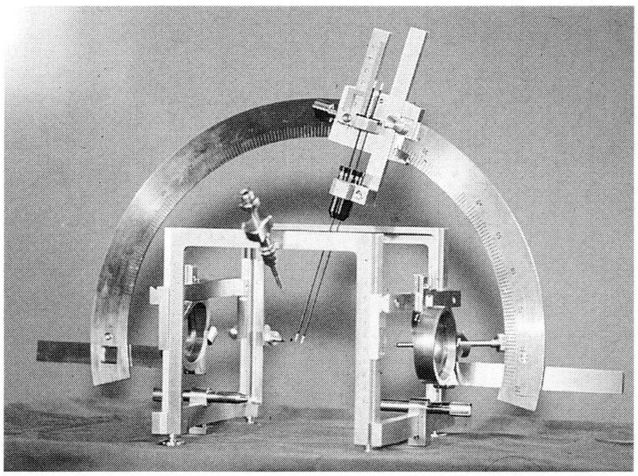

b

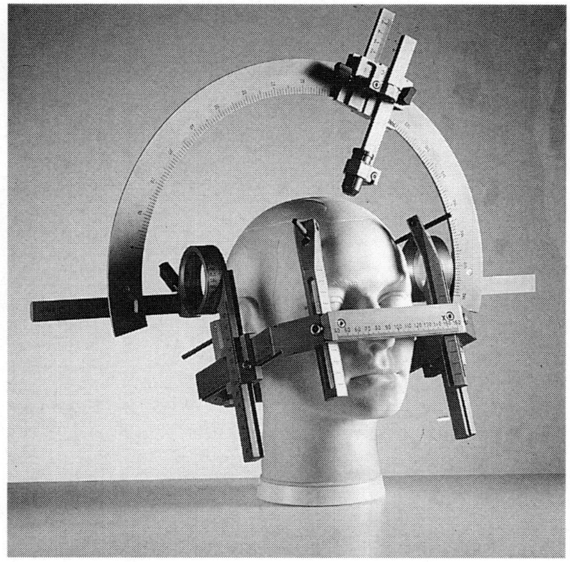

d

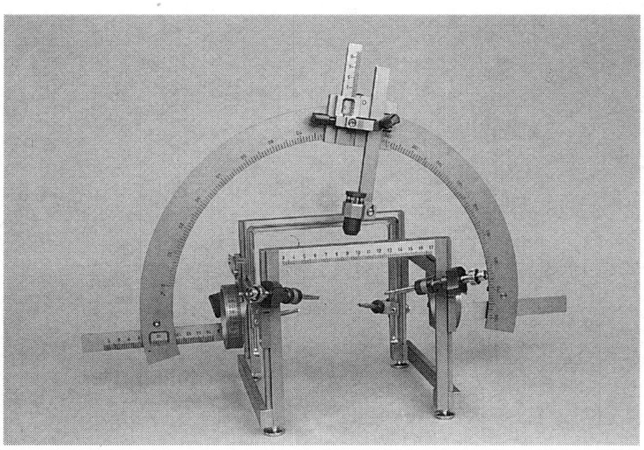

c

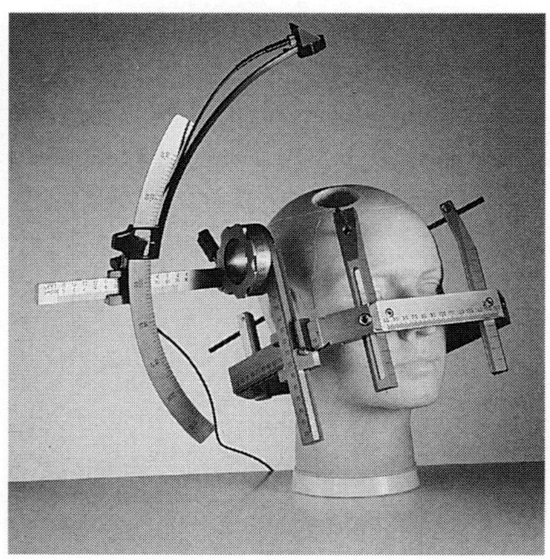

e

Fig. 1.15 **a** The original Leksell frame. **b** The modified Leksell frame, showing adjustable side bars, but still maintaining the concentric-type design. Subsequent modifications allowed use initially with **c** CT and later with **d** CT or MRI (15.4). **e** The Steiner–Lindquist Microsurgical Guide, incorporates a non-invasive laser beam, for use in open microsurgical procedures. (Courtesy of Elekta Instrument AB, Stockholm.)

accordingly, various modifications were introduced (Leksell 1955b). A square inner frame was constructed from aluminium bars, with a pitch rack cut into their outer faces which carried removable side bars; these side bars also carried a rack which carried the axis rods of the outer, semicircular frame (bow). The outer frame now comprised one of two types, either a heavier arc capable of carrying an X-ray tube (for stereotactic radiosurgery) or ultrasonic generator (for delivery of focused ultrasound), or a lighter bow and electrode carrier (for open stereotactic procedures) (Fig. 1.15b).

Leksell's early instruments relied on air ventriculography or encephalography for delineation of the target but the system has been

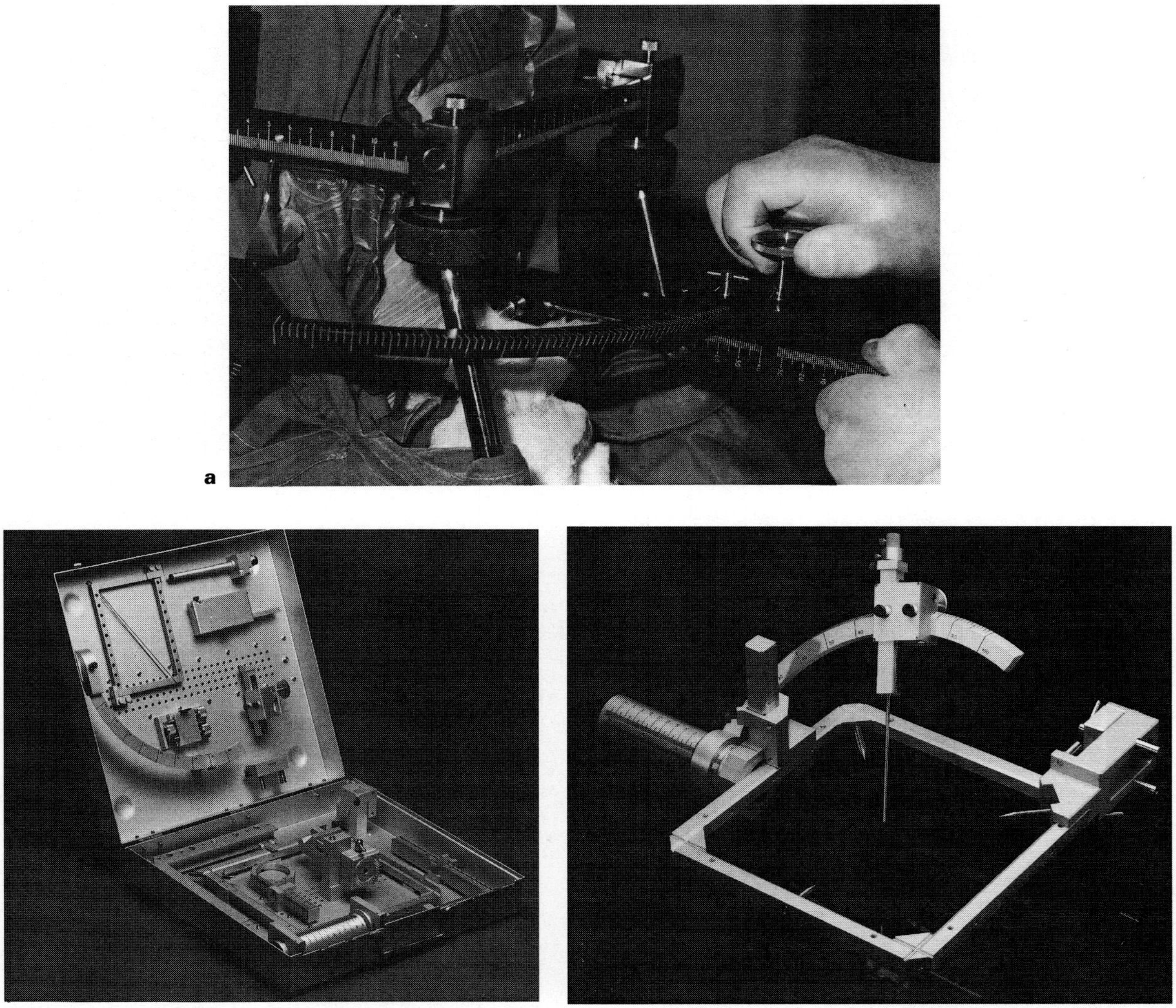

a b c

Fig. 1.16 **a** The Hitchcock stereotactic system showing the original frame (16.1); **b** the current system in its carrying/sterilizing case; **c** the assembled system with base ring, carrying arc and needle carrier; **d** the frame attached to the operating table via a Mayfield mount; and **e** the CT mount (shown here on a GE 8800 CT scanner). (Courtesy of D. Pitman and with permission from E R Hitchcock.)

progressively modified for use with CT or MRI. The CT compatible Leksell D frame (Fig. 1.15c), having first been adapted for use with MRI (Leksell et al 1985), was later fitted with a new fixation frame, the G frame, which, by virtue of low fixation points, now also facilitates open stereotactic procedures (Leksell et al 1987) (Fig. 1.15d); dedicated software permits computer calculation of target coordinates, and procedures such as stereotactic craniotomy are simplified by use of a laser guide (Fig. 1.15e).

The Hitchcock system

Although now mainly used during intracranial procedures, this instrument arose from the need for a stereotactic instrument suitable for use in the spine. Commenting on the success of percutaneous spinothalamic tractotomy even with the then currently available instruments, Hitchcock (1969) suggested that with better target siting, and with more reliable fixation and lesion making, it should be possible to improve results still further. To this end he introduced a new stereotactic frame (Fig. 1.16a), consisting of a rigid metal alloy hollow square frame, attached to the skull by three fixation points and incorporating a 'sliding fixture' posteriorly which allowed vertical and lateral adjustment of the electrode carrier; preoperative teleradiography was used to determine the position of the odontoid process, of importance in defining the coordinates of the target. The selection of the target point was based upon observations made during earlier studies in which high cervical spinothalamic tractotomy had been undertaken by other methods (Hitchcock 1967, Hitchcock & Leece 1967).

The instrument may be employed for all stereotactic posterior fossa and intracranial procedures, and has been modified for use with angiography, CT or MRI (Fig. 1.16b–e). Its simplicity of design facilitates 'open' procedures, such as stereotactic craniotomy, and also, as with the Leksell system, makes it a suitable instrument for training — an attribute often sadly overlooked by the designers of some surgical instruments. Other recent additions include a stereotactic CT scan interface device (SCID) designed for follow-up of tumours which, although less precise, permits out-patient and repeat scanning without the need for frame repositioning with pins

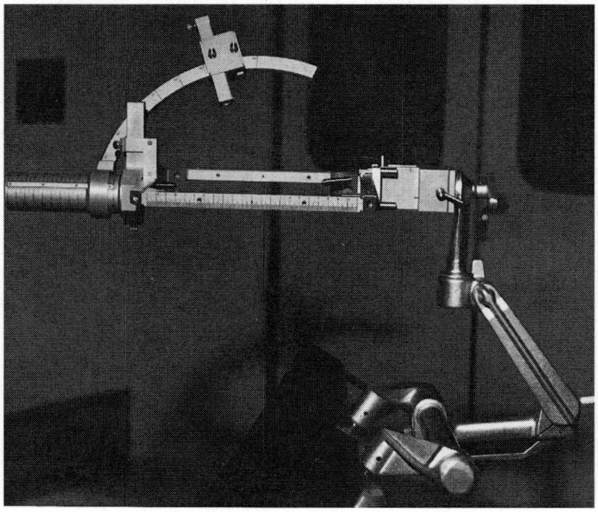

d

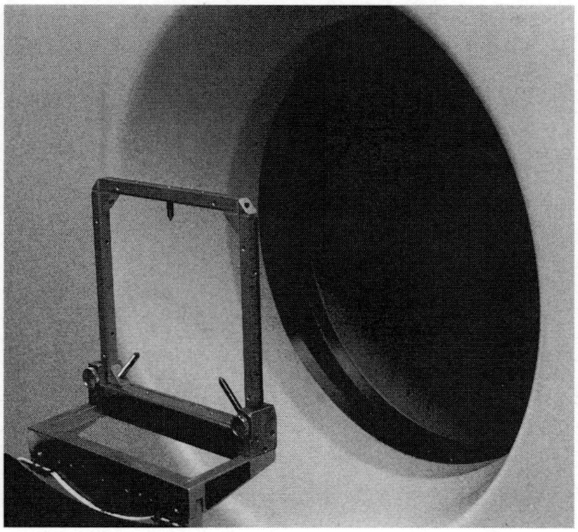

e

Fig. 1.16 *Contd*

(Hitchcock 1988), and a repeat fixation kit which allows re-utilization of previous points of fixation of the frame thus, in some circumstances, obviating the need for repeat CT scanning. The system has also been adapted for use with a linear accelerator (Hitchcock et al 1989a).

The Riechert–Mundinger system

This Cartesian based system, initially devised in Freiburg in 1950 by Riechert & Wolff (1953), was later modified by Riechert & Mundinger (1955). The system includes a circular base ring, fixed to the patient and to the operating table, to which attaches a removable target bow which carries an adjustable electrode holder. In earlier models, after determination of target coordinates by ventriculography, it was necessary to calculate the various angles of incidence of the electrode and its depth of insertion; the later introduction of a mechanical phantom device (of identical dimensions to the base ring) greatly simplified this stage of the procedure (Fig. 1.14b), although when used for functional procedures with conventional ventriculography an X-ray enlargement factor had still to be considered.

Despite its complexity, the high degree of accuracy (< 1 mm) and improved design of accessories has facilitated successful use of the instrument in over 10 000 stereotactic operations

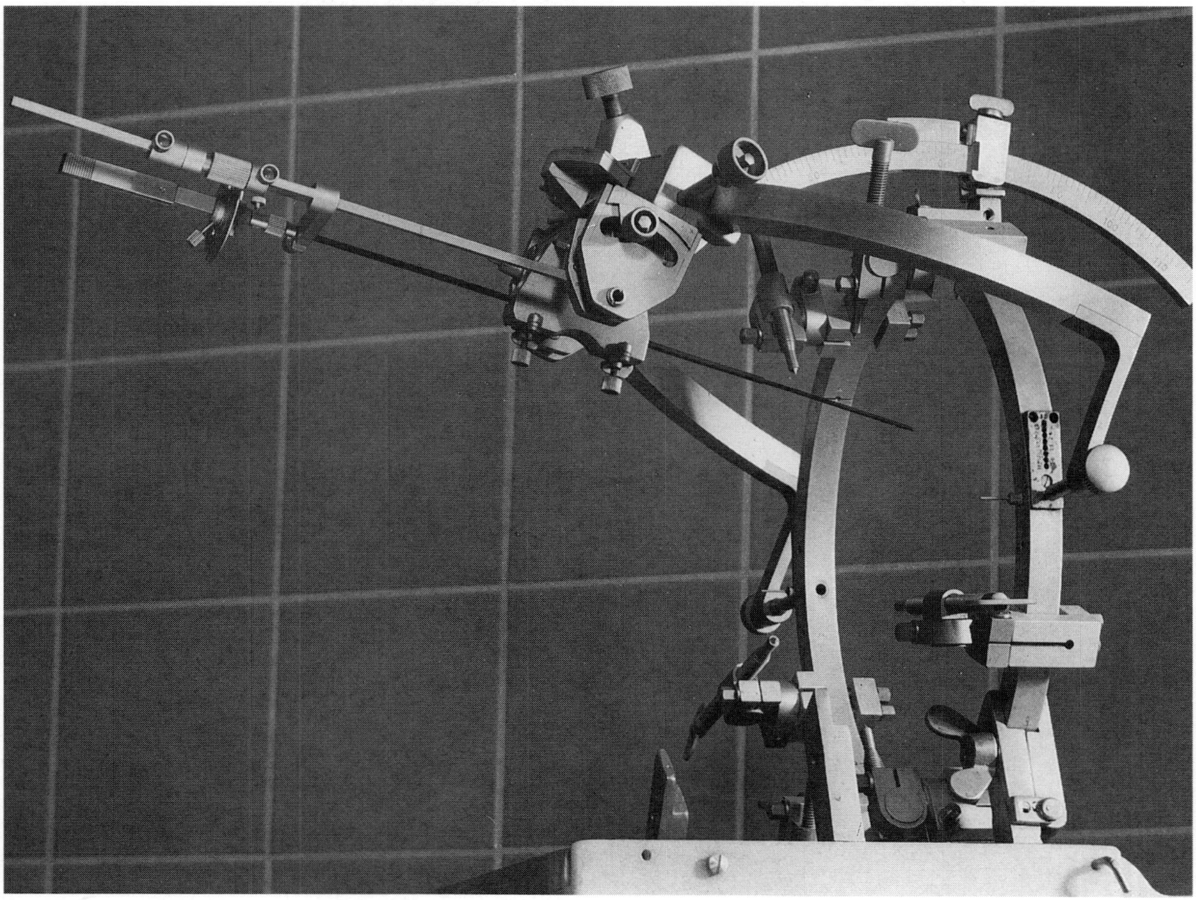

a

Fig. 1.17 **a** Riechert–Mundinger system showing the electrode in its holder on the aiming arc, mounted on the base ring and **b** adaptation of the system for CT integration. (Courtesy of F Mundinger.)

over a 40 year period, including 1488 biopsies between 1965 and 1987 (Mundinger, 1988). The introduction, in 1970, of dedicated software for computer calculation of target coordinates, thus allowing multiple lesion making or biopsies via a single burr hole (Birg & Mundinger 1973), and later integration with CT (Birg & Mundinger 1982, Mundinger & Birg 1984) and MRI (Birg et al 1985) have secured its continuing successful application (Fig. 1.17).

The Todd–Wells and COMPASS systems

In 1959, Schaltenbrand constructed a complex stereotactic system designed so as to allow a target point to be brought to the focal point of the frame (Schaltenbrand 1975). The Todd–Wells stereotactic frame, introduced in 1972 (Todd 1972), represents a much simplified application of the focal point principal, and consists of a base ring, attached to the patient,

b

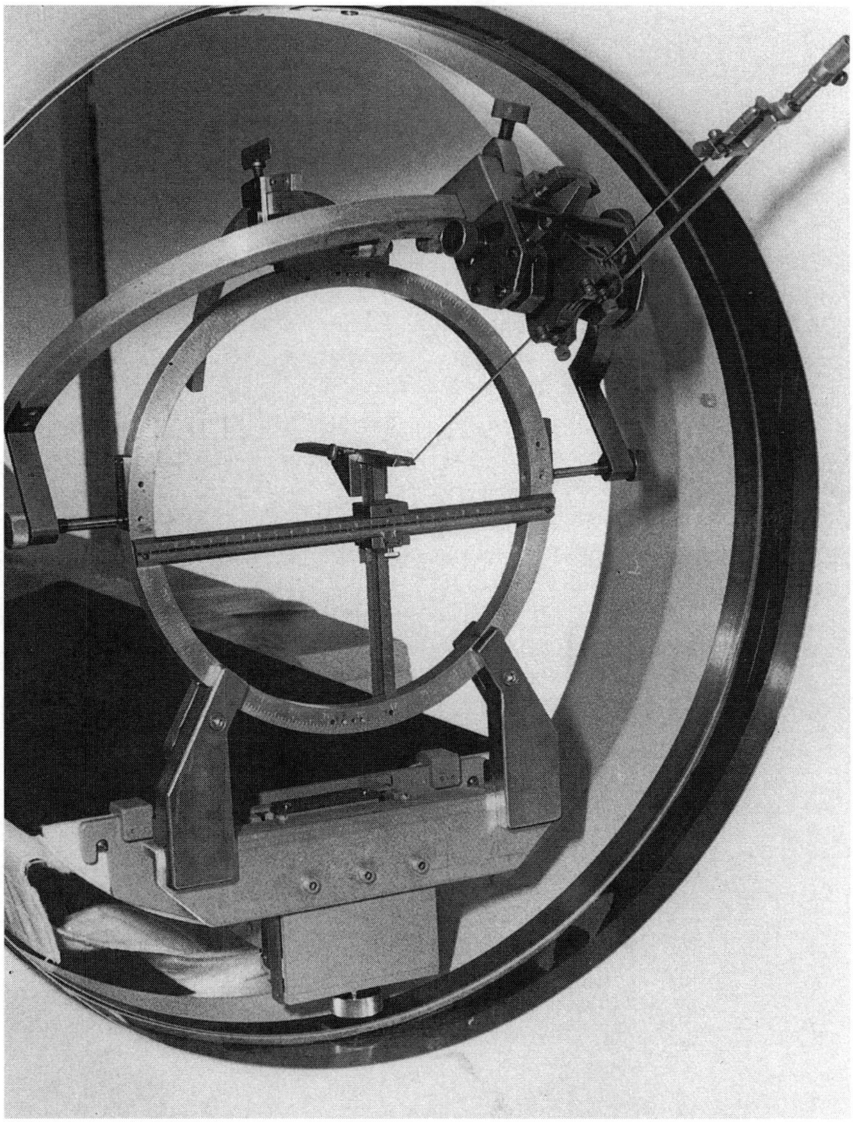

Fig. 1.17 *Contd*

which may be rotated in three planes within a second, arc-radius frame so that the target point and the focal point of the arc-radius frame coincide. By virtue of the facility not only for access to a target from an infinite number of spherical radii but also to allow procedures with the frame inverted on the patient's head, the system found a wide range of applications, including functional procedures, intracranial foreign body removal and transsphenoidal hypophysectomy; it was also adapted for extracranial use, for example in removal of foreign bodies from the limbs. Mullan et al (1965), who had occasionally observed spontaneous occlusion of intracranial aneurysms, undertook preliminary animal studies and then described a method of inducing electrothrombosis in aneurysms using a fine electrode; to overcome the somewhat haphazard nature of the earlier freehand approach Todd (1972) later proposed a stereotactic method of electrode placement. A further ingenious, although by present standards hazardous, stereotactic approach to the problem of aneurysms — the placement of ferromagnetic seeds within the aneurysmal fundus as a means of inducing thrombosis — was also proposed by Todd as a suitable application of his system. Although a highly engineered precision instrument, its ascendancy was curtailed by the necessity to construct systems compatible with CT. However, the COMPASS stereotactic system, the physical geometry of which is based on the Todd–Wells system, has become currently the most advanced instrument for image based lesion excision (see Ch. 6 for details).

The BRW and CRW systems

Unlike other stereotactic systems which have been modified for use with CT or MRI, the BRW stereotaxic system (Radionics), a polar coordinate system, was designed specifically for integration with modern imaging techniques (Brown 1979a,b, Brown et al 1980), with an accuracy of about 1 mm (Roberts & Brown 1980). It has been widely popularized since its introduction barely 10 years ago and, although most frequently used in conjunction with CT or MRI directed targeting, and procedures involving ventriculography may also be undertaken using a phantom device.

The system comprises a circular head ring assembly, which attaches to the patient, and a removable localizer assembly (either for CT or for MRI) which fixes to this basal ring during imaging. After determining target coordinates with dedicated computer software (or by use of an arc system placed on the phantom device) the arc system is positioned on the head ring assembly. Advantages conferred by the low fixation of the base ring, as with the Hitchcock and Riechert–Mundinger systems, and the Leksell G frame, include the facility to approach selected targets through virtually any point over the calvarium and to perform open stereotactic procedures. In addition to a wide range of accessories, the availability of a positron emission tomography (PET) head ring assembly adds a new dimension to the system.

The most significant recent development of the system, however, is the combination of the focal point principal of the original Todd–Wells instrument with the BRW system. The resultant CRW system (Fig. 1.18) greatly simplifies the

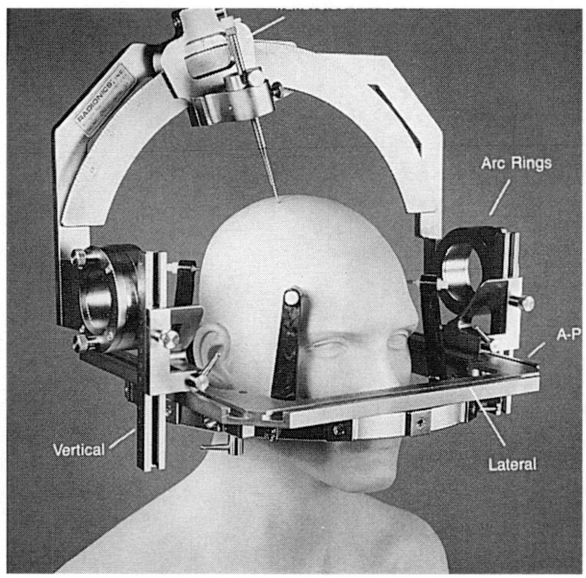

Fig. 1.18 CRW system showing the base ring, arc system and biopsy guide. (Courtesy of E. Cosman.)

procedure for setting up the target point at the focal point of the arc, whilst still maintaining the versatility of the BRW system in respect of selection of point of entry and trajectory.

Both the BRW and CRW systems may be used with a non-invasive relocatable localizer system based on the upper jaw, devised by Gill, Thomas and Cosman (GTC localizer, Radionics).

Adaptation of existing stereotactic instruments

Whilst all the commercial stereotactic systems mentioned above are instruments of high precision and great versatility, they nonetheless have one problem in common, namely that they are all expensive. In an era in which, at least in the UK, health care is becoming increasingly dominated by economic considerations, there has thus been a tendency for neurosurgeons wishing to offer a stereotactic service either to adapt older instruments or to design custom built equipment for use in conjunction with CT and MRI. Several examples of such systems (Bell et al 1989, Dervin & Miles 1989) have recently been reported to have proved satisfactory in practice and no doubt other similar instruments will continue to find favour. However, whilst not intending to decry the endeavour or ingenuity of the protagonists of such equipment, it should be borne in mind that the use of non-commercial instruments may be difficult to defend in the event of litigation. In consideration of the cost of medical lawsuits, and following the introduction of Crown indemnity in the UK, this factor may be used as an argument for procuring local funding for a commercially recognized instrument.

Current and future applications of image guided surgery

Stereotactic biopsy and stereotactic craniotomy

The therapy of gliomas necessitates careful histological assessment but, despite the widespread preoperative use of steroids since the late 1960s, and even after the introduction of CT scanning in the 1970s, biopsy of intracranial masses remained a fairly hazardous technique until stereotactic surgery became popularized. The performance of a 'freehand' procedure could be a daunting prospect for both surgeon and patient. In addition to the chance of 'missing' the target — with the increased risk of complications resulting from multiple 'blind' passes of a brain cannula — there was also the possibility that an unrepresentative tissue sample might be obtained or that some other misadventure might occur, for example, the inadvertent drainage of a cerebral abscess into the ventricular system.

For such reasons the application of the stereotactic technique to the management of intracranial mass lesions represents a great surgical advance so that it is probably not now acceptable for any but the largest lesions to be approached other than stereotactically or by an ultrasound technique; indeed, the literature now abounds with many accounts of the successful application of both CT and MRI guided techniques for biopsy of supratentorial mass lesions (Ostertag et al 1980, Thomas et al 1984, 1986, Apuzzo et al 1987). Furthermore, relatively inaccessible lesions, particularly in the brain stem, which could hitherto only with safety be approached by an open technique, may now be readily biopsied stereotactically (Coffey & Lunsford 1985, Hood et al 1986, Thomas et al 1988).

Not only is stereotactic biopsy accompanied by a low morbidity and mortality (2.2 and 0.9%, respectively, in nearly 4000 reported cases; Neal & Apuzzo 1989), but it has also proved to be a reliable method of obtaining accurate histological samples of intracranial tumours, essential in current therapy and in the design and evaluation of new treatment modalities for such neoplasms. For example, in a series of 292 patients with mass lesions of the brain, Thomas & Nouby (1989) obtained a positive diagnosis in 271 (92.8%), with no diagnosis in only 21 cases (7.2%); complications occurred within the first week in 14 cases (4.7%), including one death (0.3%). Others have also reported a positive diagnostic yield in over 90% of cases (Apuzzo & Sabshin 1983, Lunsford & Martinez 1984, Mundinger & Birg 1984, Ostertag 1988). In order to allow subsequent location of the biopsy site Mundinger & Birg

(1984) mark the target point with a fine silver wire (0.1 mm in diameter).

In addition to its diagnostic role, stereotactic biopsy may also be used as the primary therapy for various conditions, including aspiration of cystic tumours, cerebral abscesses or intracerebral haematomas. In this latter context, the development of instruments designed specifically for the task, such as the Backlund haematoma evacuator (Backlund & Holst 1978), has considerably increased the scope of the procedure.

Excision of deep seated lesions is facilitated by stereotactic craniotomy, which combines the advantage of good visualization afforded by open craniotomy with the precision of stereotaxy, thereby reducing the risk of damage to surrounding tissue and lower morbidity and mortality. Where the diagnosis is known preoperatively the craniotomy (or trephine) site may be planned after stereotactic calculation of tumour coordinates. Alternatively, it may be necessary to perform a preliminary stereotactic biopsy to distinguish between a tumour and an abscess; if a tumour is demonstrated the stereotactic frame is left in situ and the system is used to select a safe trajectory and suitable exposure. After opening the dura the approach to the lesion is established using the stereotactic system and the tumour is resected. Whilst CT and MRI assisted stereotaxy have been of fundamental importance in advancing the scope of stereotactic craniotomy, the method has nonetheless been practised for over 35 years in some centres (see Riechert 1980b).

Clearly, stereotactic systems which have a low profile, such as the Hitchcock, CRW, Riechert–Mundinger or Leksell G frame, facilitate the performance of craniotomies. Although the method does not require the use of additional, sophisticated (and expensive) equipment, problems with exposure of a lesion at some depth may be eased by the use of a device which maintains the patency of the track. For this reason a number of such systems have been devised, usually involving the use a tubular retractor advanced down the track to the lesion (Sheldon et al 1980, Kelly et al 1986a, Kelly 1988, Hitchcock et al 1989b). The tumour may then be resected by conventional techniques or by use of computer controlled laser excision (Kelly et al 1986a).

Discussing the problem both of establishing a sterile field with a stereotactic frame in position and also of movement of the target following the introduction of air into the head, Torrens (1989) suggested the use of a fine catheter inserted to the target site at a preliminary CT guided stereotactic biopsy and then cut off flush with the brain surface before closure of the burr hole. A subsequent craniotomy, without the encumbrance of a stereotactic frame, would allow the tube (which moves with the brain) to be followed to the tumour.

Interstitial and intracavity irradiation

The use of external beam X-irradiation may be accompanied by problems relating to skin exposure and damage to surrounding structures. To circumvent such problems and to permit administration of greater doses to the tumour attempts have been made to focus the source of irradiation on the target alone (see the section on the gamma knife), or to place radioisotopes within the lesion either interstitially or in the cavity following tumour resection.

Interstitial radiation therapy itself dates back to the 1920s when Tönnis unsuccessfully attempted to treat gliomas in three patients by placing a paraffin plug charged with radium in the tumour cavity after aspiration (Mundinger 1966). In the 1930s there followed further unsuccessful attempts by Rawling, Cushing and others to use similar techniques (Mundinger 1966) so that it was not until the early 1950s that the effectiveness of radioisotopes was established when Riechert and Mundinger made a series of reports of stereotactic delivery of radioisotopes to irradiate the pituitary body and various brain tumours (Riechert 1980a) and Wycis et al (1954) reported the successful treatment of a cystic craniopharyngioma by stereotactic injection of phosphorus-32 (^{32}P).

The differing physical properties of the available radioisotopes (half-life and type of emission) allow their use to be tailored to the site, size and histological nature of the lesion. For deeply situated or cystic lesions, isotopes with predominantly or wholly beta emission (penetration up to a few millimetres) such as ^{32}P may be used whereas, for larger, solid tumours where deeper penetration is required, isotopes which emit gamma rays (with penetration similar to X-rays) such as cobalt-60 (^{60}Co), tantalum-182 (^{182}Ta) or iridium-192 (^{192}Ir) have been employed. ^{60}Co, which has a half-life of 5.3 years and must therefore be removed from the tissue to avoid late radionecrosis, was first used by Becker & Scheer (1952) in the form of beads threaded on a string, a technique adopted by Klar (1954) for treatment of gliomas. ^{182}Ta, which emits both beta and gamma rays, with a half-life of 111 days, has also been used for treatment of cerebral gliomas, the isotope being removed after a few days.

When seeds of radiogold (^{198}Au), a radioisotope with mixed emission (beta and gamma), were used in the treatment of gliomas the prolonged irradiation time allowed migration from the injection site to occur and the method was found to be unsatisfactory (Sachs 1954). Mundinger and Riechert used suspensions of ^{198}Au extensively throughout the 1950s but, because of failure of the method to destroy the tumour margins, later abandoned the isotope in favour of ^{182}Ta (Mundinger 1966). However, the use of any gamma emitting radioisotope in this fashion placed the operator at considerable risk from the cumulative effect of exposure during the latter part of the operation so that alternative strategies were sought.

With larger tumours Riechert and Mundinger placed opaque wires, and later inactive tantalum powder, to delineate the size and site of the tumour bed (Riechert 1980a) and performed postoperative irradiation with ^{60}Co needles which were left in situ until 40–45Gy had been delivered to the tumour margins. From 1960 onwards Mundinger changed from ^{182}Ta to ^{192}Ir, another predominantly gamma emitting isotope with a shorter half-life (74 days) and much lower energy than ^{60}Co (0.3 MeV as opposed to 1.15 MeV), and designed a special apparatus (the GammaMed system) which minimized the risk to the operator by employing a remote method involving stereotactic placement of a cannula into the tumour through which the isotope was delivered.

Drake et al (1963) reported their results of treatment of three glioblastomas with caesium-137 (^{137}Cs); the survival time averaged 7 months, the patients dying not from residual tumour but from the combined effects of damage to the basal ganglia and raised intracranial pressure due to radionecrosis. Mundinger (1966) suggests that excision of the necrotic tissue might have prolonged survival but felt that, for technical reasons relating to containment of the isotope, ^{137}Cs was more suited for teletherapy units rather than for interstitial application.

Riechert (1980) has outlined the results of the use of radioisotopes in the treatment of gliomas. Whereas the overall survival rate was increased by 35% in glioblastomas, it was found that the results were greatly improved if the average focal dose to the tumour exceeded 100Gy. By comparison with patients only treated surgically, those also receiving postoperative irradiation with radioisotopes had a 95% probability of prolonged survival. The improved technical design of the GammaMed system, which allows delivery of the complete radiation dose within a few minutes, has further improved the results; in 173 patients with gliomas treated postoperatively with radioisotopes between 1964 and 1969 the average survival time was up to three times longer than in those patients treated only by surgery. In Freiburg, between 1952 and 1987, over 1600 patients with gliomas were treated with radioisotopes (Mundinger 1988), the best results being obtained in those with frontal or parieto-occipital lesions.

For tumours such as craniopharyngiomas, which frequently have a largely cystic component and for which operative morbidity and mortality may be high, the use of local radiation therapy offers many advantages. The instillation of intracavity radioisotopes was proposed by Leksell in 1951 (Leksell & Liden 1951), and between 1960 and 1980 Leksell and Backlund treated over 100 patients with craniopharyngiomas, using radiosurgery for solid lesions and intracavity radioisotopes for cystic tumours (Lunsford 1989). Others, including Kobayashi et al (1981) and Strauss et al (1982), have also reported the successful use of radioisotopes in the treatment of cystic craniopharyngiomas. Yttrium-90 (^{90}Y) or ^{32}P are usually chosen by virtue of their beta emission (limited penetration) and short half-life (2.5 and 14 days, respectively). Advances in the variety of available treatment methods now allows management to be tailored to the individual lesion such that a combination of treatments may be indicated, including surgical decompression, stereotactic radiosurgery (see the section on the gamma knife) for inoperable solid tumour, and intracavity instillation of radioisotopes for any cystic component (Lunsford 1989). Such a diverse approach may also be appropriate for other intracranial neoplasms.

The gamma knife

Whereas previously neural destruction had been undertaken using a needle and by electrolysis or electrocoagulation (Horsley & Clarke 1908, Spiegel et al 1947), Leksell realized that it should be 'feasible to replace the needle by narrow beams of radiant energy directed at the target' (Leksell 1951). The method of cross-irradiation of the target which he initially suggested utilized his original frame in the following fashion. The needle guide was replaced by a tube, connected to an X-ray tube fitted with a collimator; the beam was then aimed at the target which, by repositioning the tube at multiple sites over the convexity of the skull, could thus receive the full (fractionated) dose whilst surrounding tissue was subjected to much smaller doses.

As discussed above (see the section on the Leksell frame), Leksell made various modifications to his original instrument in order to undertake stereotactic radiosurgery with X-irradiation (Leksell 1955b) and was encouraged by the results of a psychosurgical operation (Leksell et al 1955). In an earlier publication he had considered the possibility of using gamma irradiation for lesioning (Leksell 1951) but, although experimental and clinical studies attested to the potential efficacy of this source (Larsson et al 1963), he found that the delivery system, a synchrocyclotron, was unsuitable for routine neurosurgical use (Leksell 1968).

From this need to combine a workable source of gamma irradiation with an accurate stereotactic method, the first ^{60}Co gamma unit (the 'gamma knife') evolved, being installed in Stockholm in 1968. The system consisted of a shielded hemispherical central body containing 179 beam sources of ^{60}Co, focused via individual collimator tubes on to the centre of the hemisphere. An inner collimator helmet, attached through the stereotactic frame to an operating table, allowed precise placement of the target point at the focal centre of the irradiated field.

The first reported cases treated with the gamma unit were two patients with intractable pain from metastatic carcinoma, who successfully underwent stereotactic radiolesions of the centre median. Although the irradiation itself took over 2 hours and was performed under general anaesthetic, in neither case was any operative difficulty encountered (Leksell 1968). Leksell (1971) subsequently reported on the satisfactory long-term follow-up (18 years) after application of the technique in the treatment of two patients with trigeminal neuralgia, and in other patients with intractable pain (Steiner et al 1980).

Having established the efficacy of gamma knife surgery, various restraints on its wider application remained. These included the cost of the equipment, the availability of physicists to undertake the dosimetric calculations and, in respect of treating small neoplasms, the necessity to be able to accurately locate the target within the stereotactic system. The first two problems are theoretically not insurmountable, but the third had to await developments in neuroimaging before the method could be applied other than in functional neurosurgery.

The diagnostic revolution which followed the introduction of CT in the 1970s led to modification (including the incorporation of 201 ^{60}Co sources and a variety of helmets allowing the delivery of four different beam sizes) and wider application of the gamma unit to treatment of intracranial tumours and AVMs. Following their earlier reports of successful stereotactic radiosurgery for acoustic neuromas (Norén & Leksell 1979, Norén et al 1983), a later series of 115 cases was equally encouraging. Of 91 unilateral tumours, 49% progressively decreased in size,

42% exhibited arrested tumour growth, and only 9% were unaffected by treatment; for the 24 bilateral tumours corresponding results were, respectively, 25, 42 and 33%; 15% of patients exhibited a transient facial paresis with no cases of lasting facial paralysis; there was no mortality in either group of patients (Leksell 1987). Lunsford et al (1989) have recorded similar success in the treatment of acoustic neuromas, in terms both of arrested tumour growth and of low morbidity.

In managing AVMs the neurosurgeon often faces the dilemma as to whether to subject the patient to the immediate risk of surgical morbidity or to the deferred risks of rebleeding. However, recurrent haemorrhage from AVMs tends to occur at longer intervals than with aneurysms (Shaw 1987) which may partly account for success in their treatment with stereotactic radiosurgery. Irradiation causes only slow obliteration of the feeding vessels and fistula and yet, despite the theoretical risk of a long latency period before obliteration of the fistula, only 5% of 550 cases treated in the Karolinska Institute up to 1987 rebled during this period; total (86.5%) or partial obliteration (11.5%) was observed in the vast majority of 104 cases followed up for 2 years (Leksell 1987). The incidence of delayed radiation necrosis was 3%, the risk being greatest with a large irradiated field, so that for AVMs with a diameter of over 3 cm only the feeding vessels are treated.

The success of the gamma unit in Stockholm has led to new instruments being installed at centres in the UK (Sheffield), the USA (Pittsburgh and Chicago) and elsewhere. Furthermore, in addition to the conditions discussed above, the technique has now been successfully used for various other tumours, including pituitary adenomas, meningiomas, craniopharyngiomas and solitary brain metastases (Coffey 1990).

Because of the considerable capital cost of establishing gamma knife equipment, consideration has been given to the possibility of modifying existing and more conventional radiation therapy equipment. In one such theoretical solution it was proposed to exploit the facility of a linear accelerator to rotate around a fixed point — the target (Heifetz et al 1983). Circumventing the problem of irradiation of surrounding tissues would pose somewhat greater technical difficulties than with the gamma knife but, by arranging the centre of rotation of the couch (on which the patient lies during therapy) such that it coincides with the axis of rotation of the linear accelerator, it was envisaged that it would be possible to deliver the radiation at various angles of inclination to the patient's head, thereby keeping excessive surrounding exposure to a minimum. Other workers, including Hartmann et al (1985), who used a modified Riechert– Mundinger frame, Colombo et al (1985) and Hitchcock et al (1989a), have subsequently demonstrated the feasibility of such techniques both experimentally and in clinical studies in man, in the management of AVMs and of benign and malignant tumours. To avoid confusion with the results of gamma knife therapy, Leksell (1987) suggests that the technique be termed 'single high dose stereotactic radiation therapy' or, when fractionated, 'stereotactic radiation therapy'.

The use of a stereotactically focused external source of irradiation, with a gamma unit or a linear accelerator (linac) system, represents a major advance in the management of many intracranial conditions. Whereas in functional disorders an obvious drawback of such systems is the inability to undertake temporary lesioning (see Redfern 1989), in the management of tumours and AVMs, although some delay occurs before elimination of the target structure commences, the absence of risk of intracranial haemorrhage and infection offers considerable advantages over other methods of treatment.

Interstitial hyperthermia of brain tumours

An important biological feature of gliomas is their tendency to produce local invasion without distant spread, a property which led to the rationale for aggressive local treatment with radioisotope implantation (brachytherapy, as outlined above). Attempts have also been made to exploit the locally invasive property of gliomas by studying the effect of temperature changes in the vicinity of the tumour.

Treatment by local cooling was attempted by Rowbotham et al (1959), who administered liquid nitrogen to the surface of human gliomas to induce freezing; although cryogenic surgery was soon introduced for production of temporary and permanent lesions in functional neurosurgery (Cooper 1962), the method was not found suitable for tumour therapy.

Conversely, hyperthermia, which has a significant oncolytic effect (Salcman & Samaras 1981, Hahn 1982), is non-toxic and potentiates the effect of radiation therapy (Hofer et al 1976) and chemotherapy (Marmor 1979, Hahn 1982), remains a possible adjunct to glioma therapy.

In 1971 the first study of the effect of interstitial hyperthermia therapy in gliomas was undertaken by Sutton (1971), who combined treatment with intravenous 5-fluoruracil. Others have employed a variety of techniques with mildly encouraging results, limited response being observed in up to 80% of cases (Winter et al 1985, Marchosky et al 1988).

A current clinical trial aims to investigate the combined effect of hyperthermia with brachytherapy in management of grade III/IV gliomas (Roberts et al 1986). After biopsy, microwave antennae introduced via stereotactically positioned interstitial catheters are used to induce a temperature of 42–43°C for 60 minutes at the tumour margins. The antennae are then replaced by ^{192}Ir seeds such that 20 Gy is delivered over 3–9 days. A second hyperthermia treatment is undertaken before the catheters are finally removed. The treatment has been shown to be technically feasible and reasonably well tolerated, but preliminary results are not spectacular. Of the first six patients entered into the study, five died within 16 months (range, 1.5–16 months; average time from treatment to death, 9.5 months), the sixth being alive at 10 months.

In order to avoid morbidity from damage to surrounding structures, precise temperature control and accurate placement of the heat source and radioisotopes are of paramount importance if such treatment is to find a role in the management of malignant gliomas. Much further study is thus required before its widespread use can be advocated. If it proves to be efficacious then reinvestigation of previously studied techniques of heat production, such as induction of stereotactically positioned interstitial ferromagnetic seeds (Walker & Burton 1966) or focused ultrasound (Meyers et al 1957), may prove suitable alternatives to the use of stereotactically implanted catheters (Shimm et al 1988).

CONCLUSION

Extensive investigations of stereotactic surgical techniques, primarily in the treatment of movement disorders, has led to a wide variety of instruments and experience. Adaptation of this experience and modification of some instruments to accommodate recent high definition imaging systems has resulted in the development of a number of extremely sophisticated, yet adaptable, stereotactic systems. Such systems now allow much safer and effective investigation and treatment of many neurological conditions to be undertaken and it is the current range of image guided surgery for brain tumours with which this book is concerned.

But what of the future? In 1986 Kelly and coworkers described a method of selectively resecting the amygdala and hippocampus, in patients with medically intractable partial complex temporal lobe epilepsy, which first involved three dimensional reconstruction of digitized coronal images of these structures obtained with a low field strength MRI unit (Kelly et al 1986b). The resection was undertaken through a 4 cm temporo-occipital trephine using a laser beam which was stereotactically guided in accordance with information derived from the three dimensional reconstruction.

In this technique the laser is computer monitored and directed by linkage to the stereotactic system but nonetheless remains under the control of the neurosurgeon. Recent developments in the field of robotics, however, suggest that it may ultimately be possible to dispense with the stereotactic frame and undertake certain procedures solely in accordance with image derived data. Using a Unimation Puma 200 robot, interfaced with a CT scanner and with a probe guide as its end effector, Kwoh et al (1988) have developed a technique for undertaking brain tumour biopsy without the use of a stereotactic frame. To be semantic it could be argued that their CT scanner is effectively a large stereotactic frame, as the head of the patient is firmly attached to its couch and target coordinates are relayed from it directly to the robot. Nonetheless, the system does facilitate positioning of the probe guide in such a way as to allow a given target to be approached via a burr hole at any point over the calvarium with both speed and accuracy (submillimetre with calibration). Its first clinical test was in April 1985 when, after the robot had first been calibrated, the system was successfully used to undertake a biopsy of an intrinsic brain tumour in a 52-year-old man. Kwoh et al (1988) suggest that such robots might also be used for radioisotope placement in brachytherapy and electrode placement for deep brain stimulation.

Progress in the field of robotics is considered in more detail elsewhere. Although the stereotactic investigation and treatment of intracranial neoplasms now relies increasingly on precision instruments and diagnostic imaging systems, the role of the neurosurgeon remains central. Improved results, however, will ultimately depend on the design of new treatment protocols resulting from the greater understanding of the biological behaviour of brain tumours which is afforded by image guided techniques.

REFERENCES

Apuzzo M L M, Sabshin J K 1983 Computed tomographic guidance stereotaxis in the management of intracranial mass lesions. Neurosurgery 12: 277–285

Apuzzo M L M, Chandrasoma P T, Cohen D, Zee C S, Zelman V 1987 Computer imaging stereotaxy: experience and perspective related to 500 procedures applied to brain masses. Neurosurgery 20: 930–937

Backlund E-O, Holst H von 1978 Controlled subtotal evacuation of intracerebral haematomas by stereotactic technique. Surgical Neurology 9: 99–101

Becker J, Scheer K E 1952 Strahlentherapeutische Anwendung von radioaktivem Kobalt In Form vom Perlen. Strahlentherapie 86: 540–547

Bell B A, Howard R, McKenzie A I, Marsh H T, Uttley D 1989 A low cost system for performing CT stereotaxic brain biopsy. British Journal of Neurosurgery 3: 561–568

Birg W, Mundinger F 1973 Computer calculations of target parameters for a stereotactic apparatus. Acta Neurochirurgica 29: 123–129

Birg W, Mundinger F 1982 Direct target point determination for stereotactic brain operations from CT data and the calculation of setting parameters for polar-coordinate stereotactic devices. Applied Neurophysiology 45: 387–395

Birg W, Mundinger F, Mohadjer M, Weigel K, Fuermaier R 1985 X-ray and magnetic resonance stereotaxy for functional and nonfunctional neurosurgery. Applied Neurophysiology 48: 22–29

Brown R A 1979a A computerized tomography–computer graphics approach to stereotaxic localization. Journal of Neurosurgery 50: 715–720

Brown R A 1979b A stereotactic head frame for use with CT body scanners. Investigative Radiology 14: 300

Brown R A, Roberts T S, Osborn A G 1980 Stereotaxic frame and computer software for CT-directed neurosurgical localization. Investigative Radiology 15: 308–312

Chandler W F, Knake J E, McGillicuddy J E, Lillehei K O, Silver T M 1982 Intraoperative use of real-time ultrasonography in neurosurgery. Journal of Neurosurgery 57: 157–163

Clarke R H 1920 The Johns Hopkins Hospital reports (special volume) part I: investigation of the central nervous system: methods and instruments. The Lord Baltimore Press, Baltimore, pp 1–120

Clarke R H, Horsley V 1906 On a method of investigating the deep ganglia and tracts of the central nervous system (cerebellum). British Medical Journal ii: 1799–1800

Coffey R J 1990 Personal communication

Coffey R J, Lunsford L D 1985 Stereotactic surgery for mass lesions of the midbrain and pons. Neurosurgery 17: 12–18

Colombo F, Benedetti A, Pozza A, Arango R C, Chierego G, Marchetti C 1985 Stereotactic radiosurgery utilizing a linear accelerator. Applied Neurophysiology 48: 133–145

Cooper I S 1962 A cryogenic method for physiologic inhibition and production of lesions in the brain. Journal of Neurosurgery 19: 853–855

Cushing H 1935 Intrakranielle Hirntumoren. Springer, Berlin

d'Arsonval A 1886 Sur un appareil destiné à mesurer la conductibilité des tissus vivants par le son. Comptes Rendus de la Societé de Biologie 3: 103–104

Dervin J E, Miles J B 1989 A simple system for image directed stereotaxis. British Journal of Neurosurgery 3: 569–574

Drake C G, Pfalzner P M, Linell E A (1963) Intracavity irradiation of malignant brain tumours. Journal of Neurosurgery 20: 428–434

French L A, Wild J J, Neal D 1951 The experimental application of ultrasonics to the localization of brain tumors. Preliminary report. Journal of Neurosurgery 8: 198–203

Haeger K 1989 The illustrated history of surgery. Harold Starke, London

Hahn G M 1982 Hyperthermia and cancer. Plenum Press, New York

Hamlyn P J 1990 Personal communication
Harting P 1861 Le képhalographe: nouvel instrument destiné à déterminer la figure et les dimensions du crane ou de la tête humaine. University of Utrecht, Utrecht
Hartmann G H, Schlegel W, Sturm V, Kober B, Pastyr O, Lorenz W J 1985 Cerebral radiation surgery using moving field irradiation at a linear accelerator facility. International Journal of Radiation, Oncology, Biology, Physics 11: 1185–1192
Heifetz M D, Wexler M, Thompson R 1983 Single-beam radiotherapy knife: a practical theoretical model. Journal of Neurosurgery 60: 814–818
Hitchcock E 1967 Hypothermic subarachnoid irrigation for intractable pain. Lancet i: 1133–1135
Hitchcock E R 1969 Stereotaxic spinal surgery: a preliminary report. Journal of Neurosurgery 31: 386–392
Hitchcock E 1988 The Hitchcock system. In: Lunsford L D (ed) Modern stereotactic neurosurgery. Martinus Nijhoff, Boston, pp 47–61
Hitchcock E, Leece B 1967 Somatotopic representation of the respiratory pathways in the cervical cord of man. Journal of Neurosurgery 27: 320–329
Hitchcock E, Kitchen G, Dalton E, Pope B 1989a Stereotactic LINAC radiosurgery. British Journal of Neurosurgery 3: 305–312
Hitchcock E R, Issa A M A, Sotelo M G 1989b Stereotactic excision of deeply seated intracranial mass lesions. British Journal of Neurosurgery 3: 313–320
Hofer K G, Choppin D A, Hofer M G 1976 Effect of hyperthermia on the radiosensitivity of normal and malignant cells in mice. Cancer 38: 279–287
Hood T W, Gebarski S S, McKeever P E, Venes J L 1986 Stereotaxic biopsy of lesions of the brain stem. Journal of Neurosurgery 65: 172–176
Horsley V, Clarke R H 1908 The structure and functions of the cerebellum examined by a new method. Brain 31: 45–124
Iizuka J 1975 Development of a stereotaxic endoscopy of the ventricular system. Confinia Neurologica 37:141–149
Ingram W R, Ranson S W, Hannett F I, Zeiss F R, Terwilliger E H 1932 Results of stimulation of the tegmentum with the Horsley–Clarke stereotaxic instrument. Archives of Neurology and Psychiatry 28: 513–541
Jefferson A, Hill A I 1966 Echo-encephalography. In: Krayenbühl H, Maspes P E, Sweet W H (eds) Progress in neurological surgery, vol 1. Karger, Basel, pp 64–93
Kandel E I, Schavinsky Y V 1972 Stereotaxic apparatus and operations in Russia in the 19th century. Journal of Neurosurgery 37: 407–411
Kelly P J 1988 Volumetric stereotaxis and computer-assisted stereotactic resection of subcortical lesions. In: Lunsford L D (ed) Modern stereotactic neurosurgery. Martinus Nijhoff, Boston, pp 169–184
Kelly P J, Kall B A, Goerss S 1986a Computer-assisted stereotaxic laser resection of intra-axial brain neoplasms. Journal of Neurosurgery 64: 427–439
Kelly P J, Sharborough F W, Kall B A, Goerss S J 1986b MRI based computer-assisted stereotactic resection of hippocampus and amygdala in patients with temporal lobe epilepsy. Paper presented at the 7th Meeting of the European Society for Stereotactic and Functional Neurosurgery, Birmingham, 5–7 June 1986
Kirschner M 1933 Die Punktionstechnik und die Elektrokoagulation des Ganglion Gasseri. Über «gezielte» Operationen. Archiv der Klinische für Chirurgie 176: 581–620
Klar E 1954 Eine kombinierte chirurgisch-radiologische Behandlung beim Glioblastoma multiforme mit radioaktivem Kobalt Co 60. Langenbecks Archiv für Klinische Chirurgie 280: 55–65
Kobayashi T, Kageyama N, Ohara K 1981 Internal irradiation for cystic craniopharyngioma. Journal of Neurosurgery 55: 896–903
Kwoh Y S, Hou J, Jonckheere E A, Hayati S 1988 A robot with improved absolute positioning accuracy for CT guided stereotactic brain surgery. IEEE Transactions on Biomedical Engineering 35: 153–160
Larsson B, Leksell L, Rexed B 1963 The use of high energy protons for cerebral surgery in man. Acta Chirurgica Scandinavica 125: 1–7
Leksell D 1987 Stereotactic radiosurgery: present status and future trends. Neurological Research 9: 60–68
Leksell L 1949 A stereotaxic apparatus for intracerebral surgery. Acta Chirurgica Scandinavica 99: 229–233
Leksell L 1951 The stereotaxic method and radiosurgery of the brain. Acta Chirurgica Scandinavica 102: 316–319
Leksell L 1955a Echo-encephalography. 1. Detection of intracranial complications following head injury. Acta Chirurgica Scandinavica 110: 255–259
Leksell L 1955b Further note on a stereotaxic instrument for man. Kungl Fysiografiska Sällskapets I Lind Förhandlingar 25: 138–141
Leksell L 1968 Cerebral radiosurgery. 1. Gammathalamotomy in two cases of intractable pain. Acta Chirurgica Scandinavica 134: 585–595
Leksell 1971 Stereotaxic radiosurgery in trigeminal neuralgia. Acta Chirurgica Scandinavica 137: 311–314
Leksell L, Liden K 1951 A therapeutic trial with radioactive isotopes in cystic brain tumours. In: Radioisotope techniques: medical and physical applications, vol 1, HMSO, London
Leksell L, Herner T, Liden K 1955 Stereotaxic radiosurgery of the brain. Report of a case. Kungl Fysiografiska Sällskapets I Lind Förhandlingar 25: 1–10
Leksell L, Leksell D, Schwebel J 1985 Stereotaxis and nuclear magnetic resonance. Journal of Neurology Neurosurgery and Psychiatry 48: 14–18
Leksell L, Lindquist C, Adler J R, Leksell D, Jernberg B, Steiner L 1987 A new fixation device for the Leksell stereotaxic system. Journal of Neurosurgery 66: 626–629
Lunsford L D 1989 Stereotactic treatment of craniopharyngioma: intracavity irradiation and radiosurgery. Contemporary Neurosurgery 11: 1–6
Lunsford L D, Martinez A J 1984 Stereotactic exploration of the brain in the era of computed tomography. Surgical Neurology 22: 222–230
Lunsford L D, Flickinger J, Lindner G, Maitz A 1989 Stereotactic radiosurgery of the brain using the first United States 201 cobalt-60 source gamma knife. Neurosurgery 24: 151–159
Marchosky J A, Moran C, Fearnot N 1988 Volumetric interstitial hyperthermia: phase 1 clinical study. Abstract from the 8th Annual Meeting of the North American Hyperthermia Group, Philadelphia
Marmor J B 1979 Interactions of hyperthermia and chemotherapy in animals. Cancer Research 39: 2269–2276

Meyers R, Fry W J, Fry F J, Dreyer L L, Schultz D F, Noyes R F 1959 Early experiences with ultrasonic irradiation of the pallidofugal and nigral complexes in hyperkinetic and hypertonic disorders. Journal of Neurosurgery 16: 32–54

Mullan S, Raimondi A J, Dobben G, Vailati G, Hekmatpanah J 1965 Electrically induced thrombosis in intracranial aneurysms. Journal of Neurosurgery 22: 539–547.

Mundinger F 1966 The treatment of brain tumour with radioisotopes. In: Krayenbühl H, Maspes P E, Sweet W H (eds) Progress in neurological surgery, vol 1. Karger, Basel, pp 202–257

Mundinger F, 1988 Personal communication

Mundinger F, Birg W 1984 CT-stereotaxy in the clinical routine. Neurosurgical Review 7: 219–224

Neal J H, Apuzzo M L J 1989 History, instrumentation, and utility of stereotactic surgery. In: Chandrasoma P T, Apuzzo M L J (eds) Stereotactic brain biopsy. Igaku-Shoin, New York, pp 1–21

Norén G, Leksell L 1979 Stereotactic treatment of acoustic tumours. In: Szikla G (ed) Stereotactic cerebral irradiation. Elsevier/North-Holland, Amsterdam, pp 241–244

Norén G, Arndt J, Hindmarsh T 1983 Stereotactic radiosurgery in cases of acoustic neurinoma: Further experiences. Neurosurgery 13: 12-22

Ostertag C B 1988 Reliability of stereotactic brain tumour biopsy. In: Lunsford L D (ed) Modern stereotactic neurosurgery. Martinus Nijhoff, Boston, pp 129-136

Ostertag C B, Mennel H D, Kiessling M 1980 Stereotactic biopsy of brain tumours. Surgical Neurology 14: 275-283

Ottoson D 1983 Physiology of the nervous system. Macmillan, London

Penfield W, Boldrey E 1937 Somatic motor and sensory representation in the cerebral cortex of man as studied by electrical stimulation. Brain 60: 389-443

Picard C, Olivier A, Bertrand G 1983 The first human stereotaxic apparatus: the contribution of Aubrey Mussen to the field of stereotaxis. Journal of Neurosurgery 59: 673-676

Rawling B L 1932 A contribution to the surgery of the pituitary region. British Journal of Surgery 19: 68-77

Redfern R M 1989 History of stereotactic surgery for Parkinson's disease. British Journal of Neurosurgery 3: 271-304

Riechert T 1980a Methods of stereotactic irradiation with isotopes (without hypophysis). In: Riechert T (ed) Stereotactic brain operations. Hans Huber, Bern, pp 73-82

Riechert T 1980b The combined open-stereotactic operation. In: Riechert T (ed) Stereotactic brain operations. Hans Huber, Bern, pp 83-117

Riechert T, Mundinger F 1985 Beschreibung und Andwendung eines Zielgerätes für stereotaktische Hirnoperationen (II. Modell). Acta Neurochirurgica (suppl) 3: 308-337

Riechert T, Wolff M 1953 Die technische Durchführung von gezielten Hirnoperationen. Archiv für Psychiatrie und Zeitschrift Neurologie 190: 297-316

Roberts D W, Coughlin C T, Wong T Z, Fratkin J D, Douple E B, Strohbehn J W 1986 Interstitial hyperthermia and iridium brachytherapy in treatment of malignant glioma: a phase I clinical trial. Journal of Neurosurgery 64: 581-587

Roberts T S, Brown R 1980 Technical and clinical aspects of CT-directed stereotaxis. Applied Neurophysiology 43: 170-171

Rossolimo G 1895 Zur Symptomatologie und chirurgischen Behandlung einer eigentumlichen Grosshirncyste Deutsche Zeitschrift für Nervenheilkunde 6: 76-94

Rowbotham G F, Haigh A L, Leslie W G 1959 Cooling cannula for use in treatment of cerebral neoplasm. Lancet i: 12-15

Rubin J M, Mirfakhraee M, Duda E E, Dohrmann G J, Brown F 1980 Intraoperative ultrasound examination of the brain. Radiology 137: 831-832

Sachs E 1954 The treatment of glioblastomas with radium. Journal of Neurosurgery 11: 119-121

Salcman M, Samaras G M 1981 Hyperthermia for brain tumours: biophysical rationale. Neurosurgery 9: 327-335

Schaltenbrand G 1975 Personal observations on the development of stereotaxy. Confinia Neurologica 37: 410-416

Shaw M D M 1987 Vascular malformations of the brain. In: Miller J D (ed) Northfield's surgery of the central nervous system, 2nd ed. Blackwell Scientific, Edinburgh, pp 440-471

Sheldon C, McGann G, Jacques S, Lutes J R, Frazier R E, Kartz R, Kuki R 1980 Development of a computerized microstereotaxic method for localisation and removal of minute CNS lesions under direct 3-D vision. Journal of Neurosurgery 52: 21-27

Sherrington C S 1906 The integrative action of the nervous system. Yale University Press, New Haven

Shimm D, Hynynen K, Guthkelch A N, Aristiabel S, Fleischer A, Roemer R 1988 Scanned focused ultrasound hyperthermia for intracranial neoplasm. Abstract from the eighth annual meeting of the North American Hyperthermia Group, Philadelphia

Spiegel E A 1970 The influence of stereoencephalotomy on the physiology of the human subcortex. Progress in Neurology and Psychiatry 25: 55-77

Spiegel E A, Wycis H T, Marks M, Lee A J 1947 Stereotaxic apparatus for operations on the human brain. Science 106: 349-350

Steiner L, Forster D, Leksell L, Meyerson B A, Boethius J 1980 Gammathalamotomy in intractable pain. Acta Neurochirurgica 52: 173-184

Strauss L Sturm V, Georgi P, Schlegel W, Ostertag H, Clorius J H, van Kaick G 1982 Radioisotope therapy of cystic craniopharyngiomas. International Journal of Radiation, Biology, Oncology, Physics 8: 1581-1585

Sutton C H 1971 Tumour hyperthermia in the treatment of malignant gliomas of the brain. Transactions of the American Neurological Association 96: 195-199

Thomas D G T, Nouby R M 1989 Experience in 300 cases of CT-directed stereotactic surgery for lesion biopsy and aspiration of haematoma. British Journal of Neurosurgery 3: 321-326

Thomas D G T, Anderson R E, du Boulay G H 1984 CT-guided stereotactic neurosurgery: experience in 24 cases with a new stereotactic system. Journal of Neurology, Neurosurgery and Psychiatry 14: 9-16

Thomas D G T, Davis C H, Ingram S, Olney J S, Bydder G M, Young I R 1986 Stereotaxic biopsy of the brain under MR imaging control. American Journal of Radiology 7: 161-163

Thomas D G T, Bradford R, Gill S, Davis C H 1988

Computer-directed stereotactic biopsy of intrinsic brain stem lesions. British Journal of Neurosurgery 2: 235-240

Todd E M 1972 Stereotaxy: procedural aspects. (Personal project in the Master of Liberal Arts Program, University of Southern California.) Trent Wells Inc, California

Torrens M 1989 Editorial comment. In: Hitchcock E R, Issa A M A, Sotelo M G 1989b Stereotactic excision of deeply situated intracranial mass lesions. British Journal of Neurosurgery 3: 313-320

Walker A E, Burton C V 1966 Radiofrequency telethermocoagulation. Journal of the American Medical Association 197: 700-4

Wild J J, Reid J M 1953 The effects of biological tissues on 15-ms pulsed ultrasound. Journal of the Acoustical Society of America 25: 270-280

Winter A, Laing J, Paglione R, Sterzer F 1985 Microwave hyperthermia for brain tumours. Neurosurgery 17: 387–399

Wycis H T, Robbins R, Spiegel-Adolf M, Meszaros J, Spiegel E A 1954 Studies in stereoencephalotomy. III. Treatment of a cystic craniopharyngioma by injection of radioactive P^{32}. Confinia Neurologica 14: 193-202

2. Tissue culture of stereotactic biopsy material

J. L. Darling

INTRODUCTION

The relative therapeutic resistance of many brain tumours is an area which requires further biological investigation in order to improve their prognosis. With regard to malignant glioma, the mechanisms of radiation and drug resistance and how these might be circumvented are an area of active research interest. Specific questions about hormonal responsiveness in meningioma, radiation sensitivity in low grade astrocytoma and craniopharyngioma and the reasons for treatment failure in radiation sensitive tumours like medulloblastoma need to be addressed. In order to carry out these studies, there is a need for representative short term cultures and cell lines which will provide relevant clinical information. Stereotactic neurosurgical techniques are of considerable importance in providing tissue diagnoses in many cases inaccessible to conventional neurosurgical procedures. However, the small size of the biopsy has provided not only problems of histopathological interpretation for the neuropathologist but also for the basic scientist who requires tumour material for scientific study. The purpose of this review is to detail the methods used to produce short term cell cultures and cell lines from small stereotactic biopsies and to examine the advantages and disadvantages of each of these methods.

COLLECTION AND HANDLING OF BIOPSY MATERIAL

Conventional resection techniques provide at least 100 mg of tumour tissue, while stereotactic biopsy techniques provide only 10–15 mg. At The National Hospitals for Neurology and Neurosurgery, stereotactic biopsy samples are usually taken with a side cutting Sedan cannula which produces a biopsy 10 mm long and 1 mm in diameter. Unless the sample can be processed immediately after removal, it is imperative that it be kept moist. Samples should be aseptically transferred to a biopsy collection medium, comprising of Ham's F-10 or F-12 medium, buffered with 20 mM 4-(2-hydroxyethyl)-1-piperazine ethanesulphonic acid (HEPES) and supplemented with 200 units/ml of penicillin, 200 μg/ml streptomycin, 100 μg/ml of kanamycin or gentamycin and 2.5 μg/ml of amphotericin B (Fungizone, Flow Laboratories, Irvine, UK). The biopsy collection medium contains penicillin and streptomycin at double the normal strength used in complete growth medium together with the addition of high concentrations of the aminoglycoside antibiotics kanamycin or gentamycin and the antifungal polyene antibiotic amphotericin B. Kanamycin and gentamycin are useful against streptomycin resistant enterobacteria including *Proteus* species, and bacteria which are naturally resistant to neomycin and kanamycin may remain sensitive to gentamycin.

If tissue is collected and cannot be processed immediately, it should be stored in 15–20 ml of biopsy collection medium at 4°C. If the ratio of biopsy collection medium to tissue is kept high, ensuring that the tissue is well oxygenated, viability appears to be maintained for long periods of time even at ambient temperatures. The success rate for samples which have been taken 24–48 hours before processing is no different than for samples prepared for cell culture immediately after removal. Occasional samples which have been delayed for up to a week in the postal system have also been successfully cultured.

CULTURE METHODS FOR SMALL NEUROSURGICAL BIOPSIES

Enzymatic disaggregation methods

Enzymatic disaggregation is the traditional approach for producing near single cell suspensions from tissue samples for cell culture studies. Although mechanical disaggregation has been advocated, either by repeated vigorous pipetting, rapid passage through small bore hypodermic needles or by forcing the tissue samples through a fine stainless steel mesh, this usually results in a reduction in the viability of the cells. When enzymatic disaggregation has been used for stereotactic biopsies the yield of cells is low, of the order of 2–5 $\times$ 10^5 cells per biopsy. In a series of consecutive samples taken from seven patients with malignant glioma, we were unable to produce viable cultures following digestion with crude bacterial collagenase preparations (grade 1A, Sigma Chemical Company, Poole, Dorset, UK) while the normal success rate using this technique on resection specimens is of the order of 80–90%. Presumably this is due to the small number of viable tumour cells in stereotactic biopsies which have difficulty growing when plated at low cell densities. We therefore explored the use of explants as an alternative to enzymatic disaggregation for stereotactic biopsies.

Coverslip explant culture for small surgical biopsies

There have been a number of other studies which have used explanted biopsy material to grow short term cultures from human brain tumours. In order for these to be successful, it is essential that the small tumour fragments are anchored firmly to the growth substratum. We have modified a method originally developed for skin biopsies (Warren and de la Cruz 1972) for small biopsy samples taken during stereotactic neurosurgical operations (Thomas et al 1984). The method is illustrated diagrammatically in Fig. 2.1 and the detailed protocol is given below:

1. Biopsies are washed in biopsy collection medium.
2. Using a sterile 1 ml pipette, two small spots

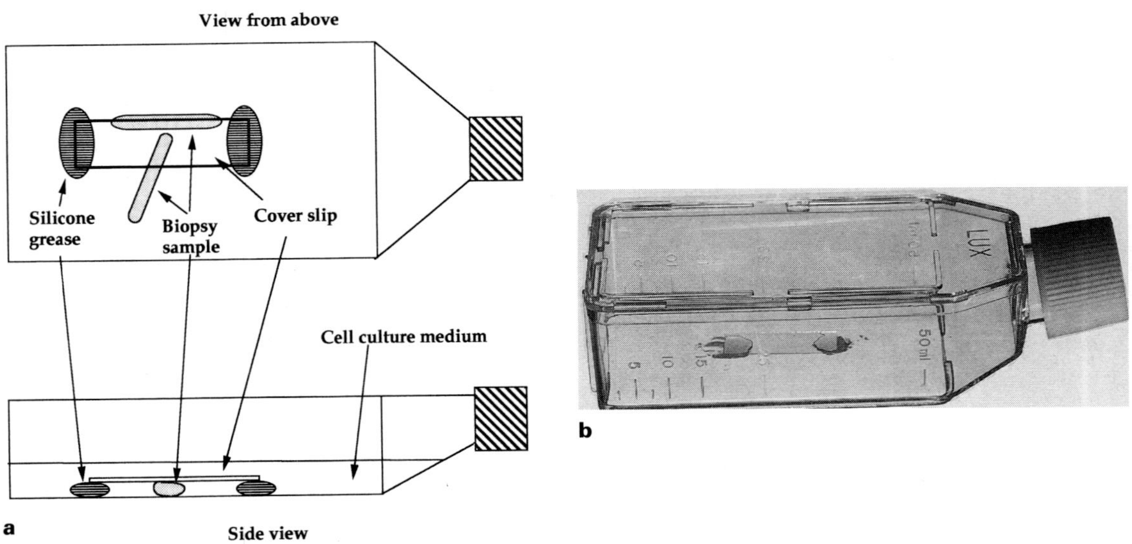

Fig. 2.1 **a** Schematic illustration of the stereotactic biopsy using the coverslip explant technique. The diagram shows two alternative positions for biopsy samples. **b** An example of a cell culture flask with a coverslip in position (reproduced with permission from Thomas et al 1984).

of sterile silicone grease (Edwards high vacuum grease) are placed approximately 1 cm apart on the base of a 25 cm^2 plastic cell culture flask. The grease is sterilized by autoclaving in a glass Bijou bottle. Using a sterile pair of forceps, the tumour fragment is placed between the spots of silicone grease in a drop of biopsy collection medium.

3. A sterile glass coverslip (9 × 22 mm, No. 1 thickness, Chance Propper, Smethwick, Warley, UK) is placed over the biopsy and spots of silicone grease, and the coverslip pressed down using sterile forceps until the biopsy sample is held firmly down against the plastic surface and the coverslip is firmly anchored by the silicone grease. Care must be taken to ensure that the biopsy is half under the coverslip and half out of the coverslip.

4. Complete growth medium (5 ml; see below) is then added carefully down the side of the flask, taking care not to dislodge the coverslip or explant. The flask is then incubated at 37°C. After 24–48 hours of incubation, a further volume of growth medium can be added to give a total volume of 10 ml per flask. When there are signs of significant cell proliferation from the biopsy (Fig. 2.2), the coverslip and remains of the biopsy can be removed with sterile forceps and the cultures refed with fresh complete growth medium.

5. When a large area of cells has developed, the cultures can be passaged in the normal manner into larger culture flasks.

Other explant methods

Cell adhesion may be accomplished in other ways, including the simple expedient of allowing the tumour fragments to dry slightly to the plastic flask. Tumour samples are minced into approximately 1 mm^3 fragments and placed on the growth surface of culture flasks in a very small volume of culture medium. Adherence is effected by incubating the flask for 15–20 minutes with the flask growth surface oriented normally, or by inverting the flask so that the growth surface is uppermost and placing it in a well humidified incubator at 37°C for 30 minutes before the careful addition of culture medium (Cravioto 1986, Jacobsen et al 1987). Once there are signs of cell proliferation, the volume of culture medium can be increased progressively over a period of 1–2 weeks.

CELL CULTURE MATERIALS AND TECHNIQUES

Culture media

A wide range of culture media have been used to produce primary cultures of human brain tumours (for a review see Darling 1991), ranging from simple defined media like Eagle's minimal essential medium to more complex formulations like Dulbecco's modification of Eagle's medium (DMEM) or Ham's F-10 and F-12. Most of these media have been supplemented with extra glutamine and, occasionally, non-essential amino acids. Although both horse and human sera have been used as supplements to these defined media, most workers have used 10–20% v/v fetal calf serum (FCS) as an adequate supplement for primary cultures of human brain tumours. In the author's experience, new born calf serum is incapable of supporting the growth of human brain tumour cells, although other workers have found it satisfactory (Haynes and Weller 1978, Benediktsson et al 1983). Batch testing of sera is mandatory as there is considerable variation between batches in their ability to support the growth of brain tumour cells. For general culture work, it is unnecessary to heat inactivate the serum before use.

Refeeding cultures

Cultures produced from explanted stereotactic biopsies do not usually require refeeding during the first 5–7 days of incubation. Occasionally, if there is a particularly large number of red blood cells the culture can be washed gently with 10 ml of Hanks' balanced salt solution (BSS) to remove them. Thereafter cultures should be refed every 2–3 days although some cultures that are slow growing will need feeding less often than this. To feed the cultures, remove the old media by suction and add fresh complete growth medium gently to the flask, taking care not to displace the explants. In general, 25 cm^2 flasks require 10 ml of medium.

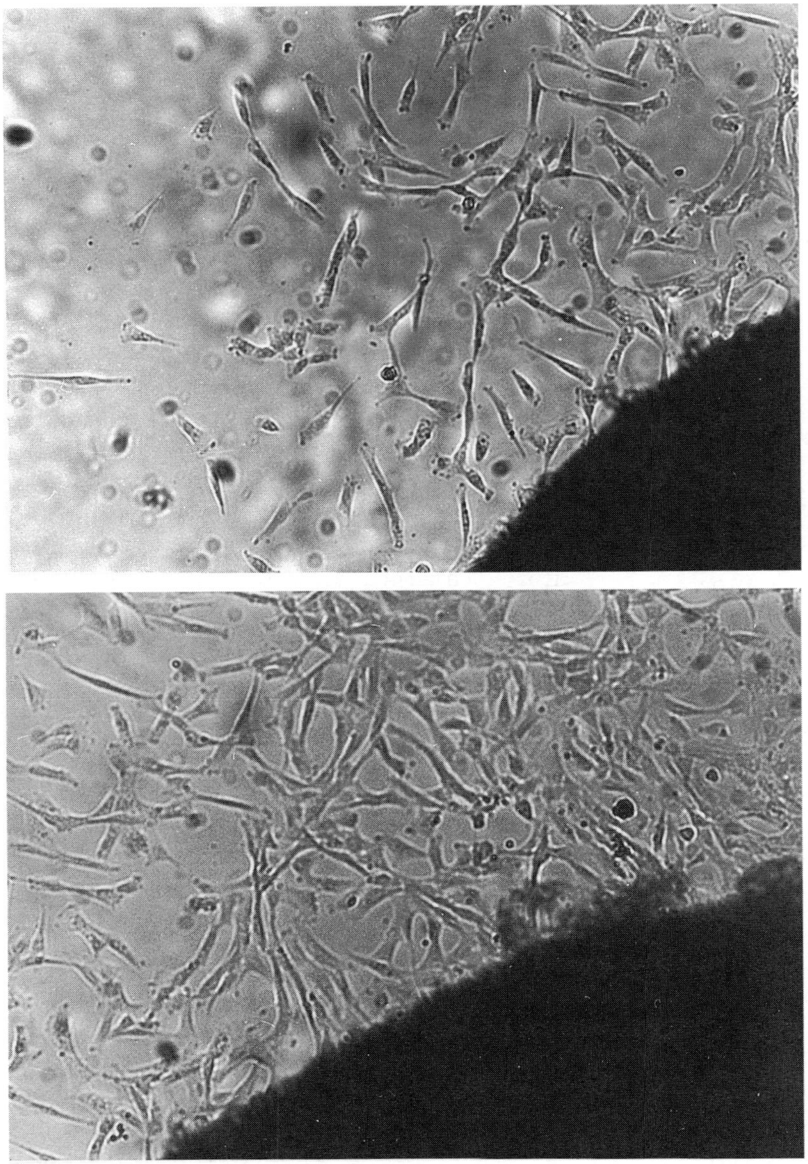

a

b

Fig. 2.2 Coverslip explant cultures from a malignant (grade IV) astrocytoma: **a** 3 days in culture; **b** 7 days in culture

Passaging cultures

In order to passage cells, the spent medium is removed and the cells washed twice with 10 ml of Hanks' BSS. If, whilst washing the monolayer, the residue of the original biopsy is detached it should be discarded. The silicone grease is not affected by trypsin or the washes with Hanks' BSS. The monolayer is rinsed with 1 ml of trypsin solution (0.25% trypsin in Hanks' BSS with 0.5 gl^{-1} sodium bicarbonate and antibiotics, but without calcium, magnesium and phenol red, Flow Laboratories) and a further aliquot of 3 ml of trypsin is added and the flask incubated for between 5 and 10 minutes, or until the cells begin to detach from the plastic surface. At this point, 7 ml of complete growth medium is added to each flask. The cell suspension is then transferred to a sterile universal container and centrifuged for 5 minutes at 250*g*. The supernatant is removed and the cells resuspended in 10 ml of fresh complete growth medium. The cells are counted and either prepared for cell freezing or further passage. It is the practice in the author's laboratory to passage the total contents of primary cultures from 25 cm^2 flasks into a 75 cm^2 flask (in effect, a 1:3 split). If larger cell numbers are required a further passage of the contents of the 75 cm^2 flask into one or two 175 cm^2 flasks is performed.

Occasionally, cells which migrate out of the biopsy explant and begin to proliferate do not form a monolayer which evenly covers the bottom of the flask but pile up patchily, reaching several cell thicknesses in places. When this occurs, the culture should be trypsinized and either passaged into several further flasks or, if there are insufficient cells for this, they should be replated into a single fresh cell culture flask.

Cell freezing

Cultures should be selected for freezing when they are in the mid to late exponential growth phase. Cell recovery with cells in the plateau phase is often less than when cells are frozen during exponential growth. The cells are detached with trypsin, a cell count is carried out and the cells recentrifuged to remove the supernatant. The cell pellet is gently resuspended in a 10% v/v solution of dimethyl sulphoxide (DMSO) (Sigma Chemical Company) in complete growth medium at a density of 1×10^6 cells/ml. Aliquots of 1 ml containing 1×10^6 cells are transferred into a freezing vial. The vial is sealed and placed immediately either in a foam expanded polystyrene box with a wall thickness of 15 mm which is placed in a –70°C freezer for at least 8 hours before transfer to the liquid phase of a liquid nitrogen freezer, or in a programmable controlled rate freezer (Planer Biomedical) set to produce a cooling rate of 1°C/min. Cultures are routinely frozen down between passage level 2 and 3. At this stage it is possible to freeze at least 3 million cells from most cultures of human malignant glioma. There have been anecdotal reports that glioma cells frozen in a solution of 10% v/v DMSO in undiluted FCS have a higher cell recovery upon thawing when compared to cultures frozen in 10% DMSO diluted with growth medium.

To revive cells from the liquid nitrogen bank, the vial is removed from the liquid phase and rapidly transferred to a covered plastic container containing water at 37°C, to avoid the possibility of entrained liquid nitrogen trapped within an incompletely sealed vial causing an explosion. Once the culture has thawed, the contents are removed aseptically from the vial and slowly diluted to 10 ml with fresh complete growth medium. This cell suspension can then be transferred to a 75 cm^2 flask and incubated overnight. The next day, the culture medium is removed and the cells refed. It is unnecessary, and indeed may impair cell viability, if the cell suspension is centrifuged to remove the residual DMSO before plating out the cells.

Mycoplasma screening using DNA staining

It is essential that all cultures taken from human tumours are examined to ensure that there is no evidence of mycoplasma infection before frozen stocks are prepared. This can most easily be carried out using a DNA staining technique based on Hoechst 33258 (Chen 1977). Detailed staining protocols are given by Hay (1986) and Freshney (1987).

CELL CULTURES FROM STEREOTACTIC BIOPSIES AS TOOLS IN EXPERIMENTAL NEURO-ONCOLOGY

The main advantage of cell culture is that it provides information about the dynamic properties of tumour cells in a way which conventional histology cannot. For example, although immunocytochemistry can demonstrate the expression of a growth factor receptor on a tumour cell, it cannot demonstrate if a particular cell is producing a growth factor or whether a growth factor is capable of affecting the growth of a cell. In this section several avenues of research will be outlined that are of potential clinical interest and in which stereotactic neurosurgical techniques are important in providing material for cell culture studies.

Tumour heterogeneity

The heterogeneous regional distribution of cells with particular genotypic and phenotypic properties have been comprehensively documented by many authors over the last decade. Malignant glioma is composed of multiple clonal subpopulations of cells thought to be derived from a single transformed cell. The genetic composition is heterogeneous as they have acquired further independent mutations during tumour progression and this genetic heterogeneity is reflected in their phenotypic heterogeneity. These cells differ in their sensitivity to cytotoxic drugs and perhaps radiation, as well as their ability to invade normal tissue, express certain antigens and to produce and respond to growth factors.

The advantages of using stereotactic biopsy material for cell culture studies is that samples are taken from sites within the tumour which are at a known location. It is known if the centre or the edge of the tumour has been sampled or if an area showing enhancement or other radiological feature has been sampled. Samples taken for tissue culture will be duplicates of those taken for histological analysis, which means that there can be a comparison between histological and cell culture results. In resection specimens the relationship between radiological location and any subsequent cell culture results is always lost and often histological samples may be taken for locations remote to the sample sent for cell culture.

There are, however, disadvantages to the use of small samples for cell culture. The question of sampling error becomes particularly important in studies which use stereotactic biopsy material as their starting point. There is a danger that a single small piece of tumour may be unrepresentative of the tumour or composed of necrotic tissue or normal brain (Fig. 2.3). If a large resection specimen is used as the starting material for initiating a culture, it is usually easy to see if it is largely necrotic or composed of normal brain. In addition, a resection specimen represents a substantial proportion of the tumour as a whole and the question of selective sampling becomes less important. The question of selective sampling may be circumvented by the use of multiple samples from a single tumour (Fig. 2.3).

Comparison of results before and after treatment in the same patient

The low rates of morbidity and/or mortality which are associated with stereotactic biopsy techniques enhance the likelihood of rebiopsy in patients with recurrent tumours. The primary neurosurgical reason for rebiopsy is to exclude the possibility of radiation necrosis. However, this provides the potential for comparing the cell biology and therapeutic sensitivity of primary and recurrent tumours in the same patient and to investigate whether therapy influences the cellular composition of recurrent tumours. Initial observations by Shapiro and her colleagues suggests that during chemotherapy and radiotherapy there is selection of a subpopulation of cells, present in small numbers at the time of diagnosis, which are intrinsically resistant to chemotherapy and irradiation in vitro and have a selective growth advantage as they display autocrine growth through the production of platelet derived growth factor (Shapiro et al 1991). The distribution of these resistant cells at the time of diagnosis could be mapped using multiple stereotactic biopsies and also what alterations occur in their distribution following tumour recurrence.

Measurement of chemosensitivity and radiosensitivity

The measurement of chemosensitivity and radiosensitivity is only possible using cultured cells and there is now a considerable body of data which suggests that there is a relationship between in vitro chemosensitivity and clinical outcome in patients with malignant glioma (Kornblith et al 1981, Thomas et al 1985). There are also data which suggest that there is a broad relationship between the radiotherapeutic sensitivity of tumours in situ and cell survival in vitro (Fertil and Malaise 1981, Deacon et al 1984). It is likely to be clinically important in the future to routinely measure parameters like radio- or chemosensitivity in order to optimize therapy. This will be even more important in malignant or benign tumours where surgical removal is not possible because of an unfavourable location, but where radiotherapy or chemotherapy may produce worthwhile benefit.

Stereotaxis is now of considerable therapeutic as well as diagnostic importance. The interstitial implantation of radioactive seeds has been investigated by a number of workers and although there is always detailed radiation planning

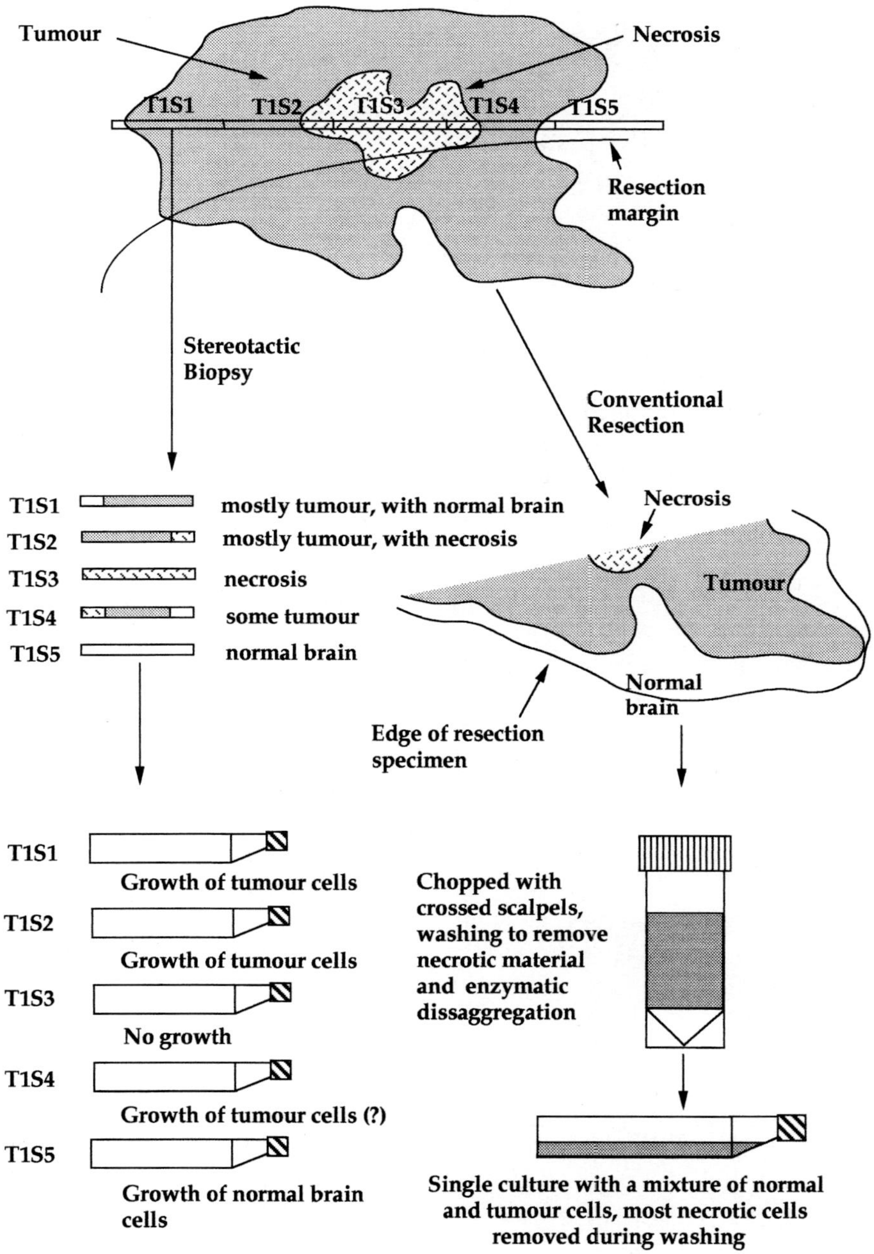

Fig. 2.3 An illustration of the different types of sampling error which may occur using small stereotactic biopsy samples. Samples taken stereotactically through a malignant glioma may be composed of normal brain around the edge of the tumour, tumour cells or necrotic material. As the exact biopsy site is known, it should be possible to correlate tissue culture findings with histology of duplicate samples taken at the same sampling site and with the radiological appearance of the tumour. There may be considerable variation in the properties of cultures derived from different stereotactic biopsies in the same patient. Resection specimens, however, have lost their radiological and histological orientation, and the culture will be a mixture of many different cell types.

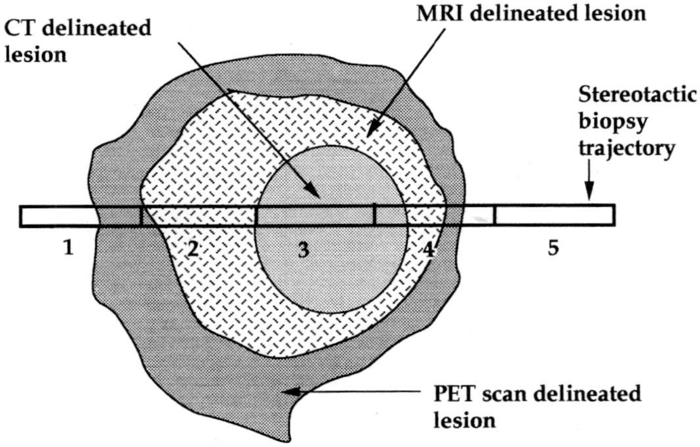

Fig. 2.4 A stereotactic biopsy trajectory though a malignant brain tumour in which the margins delineated by CT, MRI and PET have been superimposed. This trajectory should yield samples for in vitro study from different areas which can be used to determine the 'edge' of the tumour.

available so that doses are known at particular distances from a seed, there is little information on the radiobiology of cells in malignant glioma, particularly with regard to low dose effects and the role of repair in these cells. The combination of stereotactic biopsy and cell culture provides the framework for individualizing interstitial radiation treatment in the future.

Studies on the edge of the tumour

Neuroradiological imaging techniques like computerized tomography (CT), magnetic resonance imaging (MRI) or positron emission tomography (PET) rarely delineate the same tumour to the same extent (Fig. 2.4). A tumour which appears small on a CT scan may have a considerably larger apparent area when imaged using one of the other techniques. It is not clear which margin represents the true spread of tumour cells and which image should be considered the standard for planning neurosurgery or for radiotherapy. Using single stereotactic trajectories through brain tumours it has been possible to correlate conventional histology and expression of the proliferation associated antigen recognized by the monoclonal antibody Ki-67 (Gerdes et al 1984, Parkins et al 1991) with CT, MRI and PET scans and, whilst it was noted that most proliferating cells were confined to the CT image, there were often also significant numbers of cells outside it. There were never any proliferating cells outside the PET scan image (Thomas et al 1989). The application of cell culture techniques will allow studies to be carried out on the invasive properties, therapeutic sensitivity and molecular characteristics of cells isolated from regions delineated by different neuroradiological techniques and ultimately allow the elusive 'tumour edge' to be defined exactly.

ACKNOWLEDGEMENTS

The author is grateful for the technical assistance of Grazyna Lewandowicz, Sally Ashmore, Suzanne Clarke, Maria Hine and Bryn Watkins, who between them have carried out over 500 coverslip explants. The work in the author's laboratory is supported by the Brain Research Trust, Cancer Research Campaign and the Medical Research Council.

REFERENCES

Benediktsson G, Carlsson J, Nilsson S, Jakobsson P A, Ponten J 1983 The detachment, attachment and growth capacity of human glioma and glia cells in culture. Acta Pathologica, Microbiologica et Immunologica Scandinavica Section A 91: 291–296

Chen T R 1977 In situ detection of mycoplasma contamination in cell cultures by fluorescent Hoechst 33258 stain. Experimental Cell Research 104: 255

Cravioto H 1986 Human and experimental gliomas in tissue culture. Progress in Neuropathology 6: 165–188

Darling J L 1991 Brain. In: Masters J R W (ed) Human cancer in primary culture. Kluwer, Dordrecht p231–251

Deacon J M, Peckham M J, Steel G G 1984 The radioresponsiveness of human tumours and the initial slope of the cell survival curve. Radiotherapy and Oncology 2: 317–323

Fertil B, Malaise E P 1981 Inherent cellular radiosensitivity is a basic concept for human tumour radiotherapy. International Journal of Radiation, Oncology, Biology, Physics 7: 621–629

Freshney R I 1987 Culture of animal cells: a manual of basic technique. Alan R Liss, New York

Gerdes J, Lemke H, Baisch H, Wacker H H, Schwals O, Stein H 1984 Cell cycle analysis of a cell proliferation associated human nuclear antigens defined by the monoclonal antibody Ki-67. Journal of Immunology 133: 1710–1715

Hay R J 1986 Preservation and characterisation. In: Freshney R I (ed) Animal cell culture: a practical approach. IRL Press, Oxford, PP 71–112

Haynes L W, Weller R O 1978 The effects of cytochalasin B and colchicine on cell motility and ultrastructure in primary cultures of malignant gliomas. Acta Neuropathologica (Berlin) 44: 21–30

Jacobsen P F, Jenkyn D J, Papadimitriou J M 1987 Four permanent cell lines established from human malignant gliomas: three exhibiting striated muscle differentiation. Journal of Neuropathology and Experimental Neurology 46: 431–450

Kornblith P L, Smith B H, Leonard L A 1981 Response of cultured human brain tumours to nitrosoureas: correlation with clinical data. Cancer 47: 255–265

Parkins C S, Darling J L, Gill S S, Wilson C B, Revesz T, Thomas D G T 1991 Cell proliferation in serial biopsies through human malignant brain tumours: measurement using Ki-67 antibody labelling. British Journal of Neurosurgery 5: 289–298

Shapiro J R, Scheck A C, Mehta B M, Moots P L, Fiola M R 1991 Karyotype, drug resistance and growth factor production in malignant glioma. British Journal of Neurosurgery 5: 209 (abstract)

Thomas D G T, Darling J L, Watkins B A, Hine M C 1984 A simple method for the growth of cell cultures from small biopsies of brain tumours taken during CT-directed stereotactic procedures. Acta Neurochirurgica (suppl) 33: 177–181

Thomas D G T, Darling J L, Paul E A, Mott T J, Godlee J N, Tobias J S, Capra L, Collins C D, Mooney C, Bozek T, Finn G P, Arigbabu S O, Bullard D E, Shannon N, Freshney R I 1985 Assay of anticancer drugs in tissue culture: Prediction of relapse free interval in patients with malignant cerebral glioma using an in-vitro chemosensitivity assay. British Journal of Cancer 51: 525–532

Thomas D G T, Gill S S, Wilson C B, Darling J L, Parkins C S 1989 Use of a relocatable stereotactic frame to integrate PET and CT image: application in human malignant brain tumours. Stereotactic and Functional Neurosurgery 54–55: 388–392

Warren R J, de la Cruz C 1972 Fibroblasts from biopsies: an easier way Experimental Cell Research 71: 238

3. Stereotactic surgery: methods of CT and MRI directed biopsy

N. Kitchen R. Bradford D. G. T. Thomas

INTRODUCTION

The surgical management of primary malignant brain tumours is controversial (Whittle and Gregor 1991) and prognosis remains generally poor despite the widely differing treatment regimens employed, prompting some to advocate radiotherapy or symptomatic treatment empirically without a tissue diagnosis in patients with poor prognostic indicators (Sandeman et al 1990). We believe such diagnostic conservatism is unwarranted for two reasons. Firstly, although malignant glioma is the commonest pathological diagnosis following biopsy of a cerebral mass lesion, other neoplastic (e.g. low grade glioma, lymphoma, metastasis) and non-neoplastic lesions (e.g. abscess, infarct, arachnoid cyst) frequently occur with widely different implications for the patient. Secondly, only by histological confirmation of a malignant glioma can patients be properly entered into rational treatment programmes and new therapies evaluated. In the past the surgical biopsy of brain tumours had a reputation for being a hazardous and unreliable procedure. This should no longer be true today; computerized tomography (CT) and magnetic resonance imaging (MRI) directed stereotactic biopsies are accurate and safe procedures with an extremely high diagnostic rate combined with minimal associated mortality and morbidity. There is, therefore, no longer any excuse for the neurosurgeon failing to make a histological diagnosis.

Detection and localization of cerebral mass lesions are based on clinical and radiological evidence. Symptoms and signs of raised intracranial pressure, combined with focal loss of cerebral function detected clinically, have led the neurosurgeon to investigate further by, in turn, air ventriculography (described by Dandy in 1918), arteriography (introduced by Moniz in 1927) and, more recently, CT and MRI. Although, with CT and MRI, lesions can be directly visualized, diagnosis still depends on histological analysis of tissue obtained at surgical biopsy. Even with the sophisticated neuroimaging now available, diagnostic certainty cannot be guaranteed. Indeed, histology changes the preoperative diagnosis in 5–20% of cases despite the newest generation scanners (Tans & de Jongh 1978, Kendall et al 1979, Choksey et al 1989, Lunsford et al 1990). This makes pathological confirmation mandatory in order to dispel doubt in both the neurosurgeon and patient so that further management can proceed confidently. This is all the more important because of the life threatening nature of many of the conditions thus diagnosed.

Conventional stereotaxis had been in clinical use since 1947 (Spiegel & Wycis 1952) in the field of functional neurosurgery, utilizing intracranial landmarks defined by plain radiography (e.g. calcified pineal gland), air ventriculography (e.g. foramen of Monro) and angiography. Desired target sites were calculated from these reference points using standard stereotactic atlases which gave the required coordinates based on 'normal' anatomy. Clearly this could only give approximate values as the atlases were not directly related to the patient's brain, but rather to a number of 'normal' brains which were said to cover normal variation. Clinically, however, for functional work this method proved quite satisfactory and stereotaxy was widely used for this purpose. In contrast, the application of this method to the biopsy of intracranial mass lesions was largely precluded by the inevitable yet unpredictable distortion of the normal brain anatomy by the mass itself, which made accurate localization in stereotactic space difficult. Prior to the introduction of CT, therefore, most biopsies of cerebral mass lesions were performed freehand either via burr holes or, more commonly, following trephine or craniotomy as part of larger decompressive procedures which were considered safer. Certainly in early series, burr hole biopsies had a formidable mortality rate with figures as high as 27% (Hitchcock & Sato 1964) and 40% (Frankel & German 1958) being recorded. More radical surgery was paradoxically safer (4 and 5% mortality rates in the above two series) and thus aggressive surgical management prevailed (Roth & Elvidge 1960). However, by the 1970s the situation had changed markedly, largely as a result of the regular use of dexamethasone, which circumvented the need for urgent debulking surgery and allowed a more appropriate emphasis on radiotherapy after tumour biopsy. Marshall et al (1974) reported a mortality rate for burr hole biopsies of less than 5% with a positive diagnosis in 85–90% of cases.

Today, direct visualization of an intracerebral lesion using CT or MRI scanning combined with modern stereotactic techniques enables the neurosurgeon to correlate radiological findings within the patient's own three dimensional stereotactic space and thus reliably biopsy any target of choice to within 1 mm. Significantly, this has been associated with a reduction in mortality to less than 1% and a diagnostic accuracy consistently over 90% (Table 3.1). This ability to safely and reliably biopsy any lesion revealed on modern neuroimaging represents a considerable advance in the field of neuro-oncology, not only in the area of clinical diagnosis but also because of the information it provides regarding various scan appearances themselves.

CT DIRECTED STEREOTACTIC BIOPSY

Following the introduction of CT scanning in the early 1970s there was almost immediate recognition of the huge potential that lay in combining this new form of neuroimaging with stereotaxy. Numerous 'conventional' frames were modified for CT usage. These included the well established Leksell, Talairach, Mundinger–Reichert, Hitchcock and Todd–Wells systems. Several others were designed specifically for CT compatibility, including the popular

Table 3.1 Results from four large series on the clinical use of CT directed stereotactic biopsy

Series	Number of cases	Positive diagnosis (%)	Mortality (%)	Morbidity (%)
Apuzzo et al (1987)	500	95.6	0.2	1
Thomas & Nouby (1989)	300	92.8	0.3	2.7
Lunsford et al (1990)	395	93	0	?
Wild et al (1990)	200	90	1	1

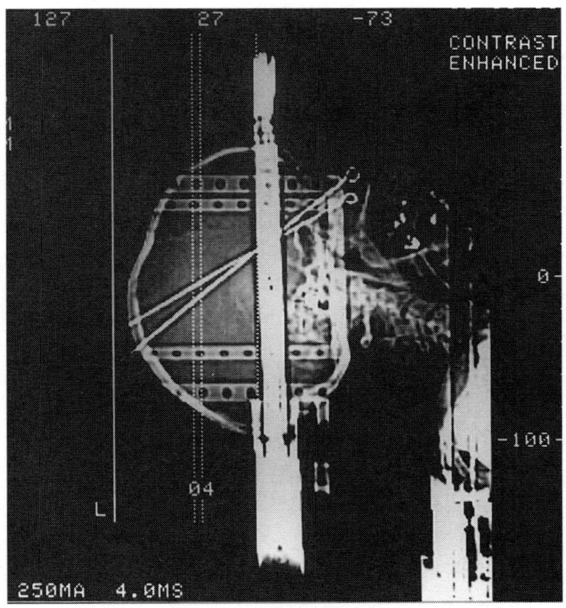

Fig. 3.1 Scout view taken during the CT scanning phase of stereotactic biopsy using the Hitchcock frame. The frame can be seen fixed in the scanner gantry. The +00° tilt confirms that the frame lies exactly in the same plane as a normal axial CT scan.

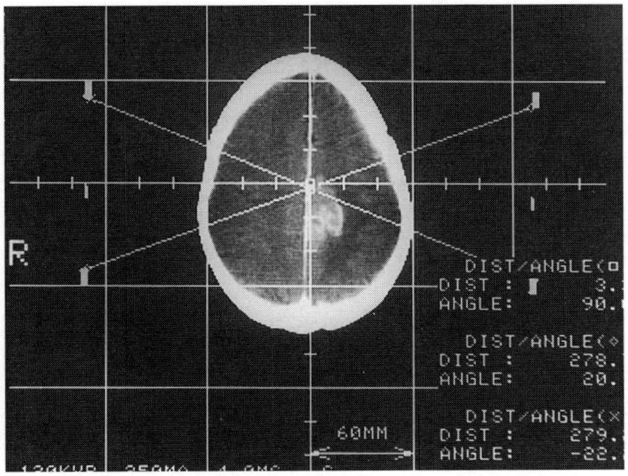

Fig. 3.2 Using the fiducials and the built-in scanner computer software the isocentre of the frame and CT scan are confirmed to coincide.

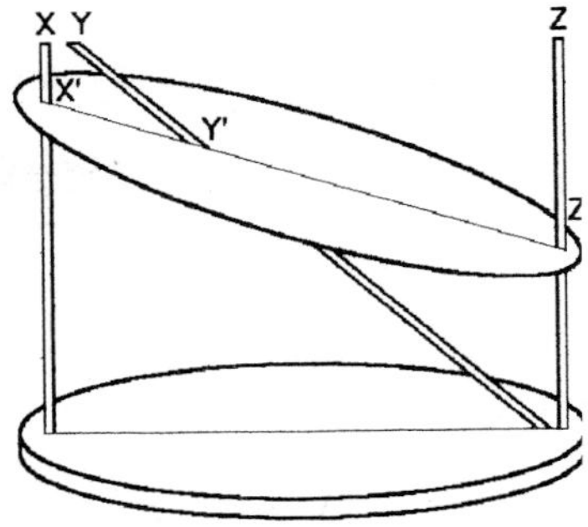

Fig. 3.4 The height above the reference plane (i.e. the stereotactic frame headring) of any point on the diagonal rod is determined by *y'z' /x' z'*(from Heilbrun 1984).

Brown–Roberts–Wells (BRW) system (Thomas et al 1984a). Over the next 15 years CT stereotaxy spread to such an extent that CT directed stereotactic biopsy using these various systems and others has become a routine neurosurgical procedure in many units, several of which have reported their experience in large retrospective series (Ostertag et al 1980, Apuzzo et al 1987, Thomas & Nouby 1989, Wild et al 1990, Lunsford 1990; Table 3.1).

The aim of all systems is to transform two dimensional coordinates from the CT image to a three dimensional point in stereotactic space and to provide a suitable choice of trajectories along which the biopsy needle may pass relative to the stereotactic frame and the patient's head and internal cerebral anatomy. For this, the antero-posterior, lateral and vertical stereotactic coordinates relative to the centre of the frame are required. In some systems (e.g. the Hitchcock frame) this is achieved by attaching the headring itself to the scanner table using a gantry system so that CT images lie exactly parallel to it (Fig. 3.1). In this way, using standard scanner computer software, the isocentre of the frame can be applied to any CT image a known distance away from the frame and Cartesian coordinates of the intended biopsy site obtained (Figs. 3.2 and 3.3). In other systems (exemplified by the BRW frame) the frame is independent of any particular CT scanner for coordinate calculations. Instead, a localizing frame is used which is attached to the headring. Most commonly this involves three sets of three rods (fiducials) arranged in 'N' shapes as a so called 'picket fence' (Fig. 3.4). The height above the reference plain of the headring of the diagonal rod of each 'N' on the desired CT image is determined by the ratio of the fixed distance between the two vertical rods and the variable distance between the diagonal rod and either of the accompanying vertical rods as revealed on the side of the CT image. The plane of the image relative to the headring is thus defined by these three points and therefore the target coordinates in stereotactic space can be obtained. These calculations require

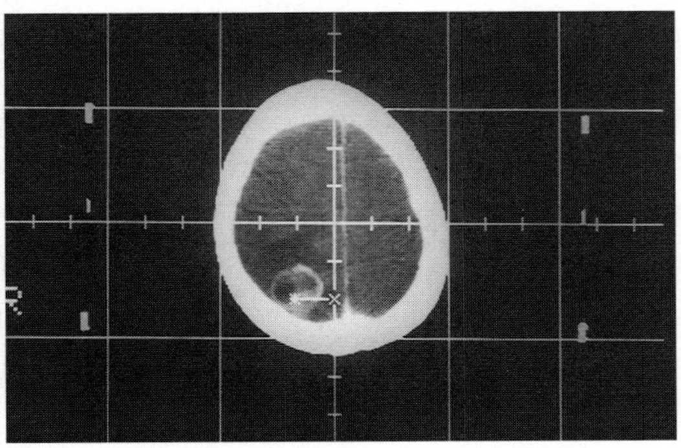

Fig. 3.3 The *x* coordinate is calculated at 20.9 mm (bottom right). The OM value of +38 mm (top left) gives the *z* coordinate.

independent computer software (e.g. the Epson HX-20 portable system used with the BRW frame). With this system the headring position and angle relative to the CT image is therefore not critical as long as it lies below the level of the intended target on the skull (to allow the localizing frame to be applied).

Having obtained target coordinates relative to the headring most modern systems utilize a system of arcs by which the biopsy needle apparatus itself is mounted on to the headring. This allows variable trajectory angles and skull entry points to be chosen. Variations of the arc system, originally expounded by Leksell in 1949, are used to achieve this end in the majority of the systems widely used today and allow great versatility in the choice available to the neurosurgeon. The authors have extensive experience with both the Hitchcock frame (Kitchen & Bradford 1991), the only British designed and manufactured system commercially available (D. P. Medical Systems, Surrey, UK), the BRW instrumentation and a recent modification of the latter, the Cosman–Roberts–Wells frame (Pell & Thomas 1991).

There are many variations on the exact procedural details used. For instance, it is quite possible to perform the entire operation including application and fixation of the headring and the biopsy itself under local anaesthesia. In this situation it is common to use a simple twist drill to make the skull opening. Both these practices are common on the Continent and in the USA (Heilbrun 1984). However, the majority of biopsies performed in the UK are under general anaesthesia and via a formal burr hole. The latter allows inspection of cortex and the ability to avoid or diathermy troublesome vessels. In addition, the slightly larger hole allows some flexibility in biopsying multiple targets with differing trajectory angles through the same skull opening.

Various biopsy needles are available. Most commonly used is the Sedan type side cutting needle with which a core of tissue is removed of approximately 5×2 mm (normal size needle). Our standard practice is to take four quadrant biopsies from each target, one of which is sent for immediate smear or frozen section examination, the rest being used for definitive histology. Tissue culture from these specimens is also possible (Thomas et al 1984b) as well as immunohistochemical studies, which are useful in the diagnosis of central nervous system (CNS) lymphoma (Feiden et al 1990; though in this series a 1×10 mm spiral needle was used). In addition, tumour cyst fluid may be aspirated through the Sedan needle and sent for cytological examination. Microrongeurs are an alternative used in some centres with the theoretical advantage of warning the surgeon when there is a likelihood of a vessel being caught up in the biopsy, indicated by an increased resistance on withdrawing the needle. In practice, however, the side cutting needle has not been shown to be any less safe and is generally preferred because of the quality of histological specimens it provides.

Once the neuropathologist has become accustomed to the small size of the tissue sent for examination, histological diagnosis is not a problem, and this is reflected in the high diagnostic yields reported, due principally to the high quality of the multiple tissue samples which can be accurately taken from various specific sites of interest within the target area (this ability to choose multiple targets at multiple locations is a great advantage in the accurate grading of gliomata in which histological variation within a tumour may occur). In addition, CT directed stereotactic biopsy procedures have provided much information regarding the histological basis of CT scan appearances. Several studies have compared samples taken from the hypodense centre, enhancing margin, and surrounding hypodensity of malignant gliomas (e.g. Hitchon et al 1985, Thomas et al 1984b, Kelly et al 1987, Greene et al 1989). Although figures vary, it is clear that there are frequently significant histological differences between the centre and edge of the lesion as defined by CT. Unidentifiable necrosis is more often found within the centre and a positive tissue diagnosis is more frequently obtained from the enhancing periphery, the exact percentages depending on the definition of a positive tissue diagnosis (in one series this included the presence of any tumour cells (97% yield, Kelly et al 1987) whilst in another, malignant glioma had to be specifically diagnosed (64% yield, Greene et al 1989)). What is clear is that a substantial proportion of biopsies taken from the enhancing edge of malignant gliomas are tumour free (46% quoted in Thomas et al (1985)) and it is common practice to take biopsies from both the centre and the edge for this reason. Furthermore, biopsies taken from hypodense areas surrounding the tumour proper often contain tumour cells. In one series this was 29% of biopsies taken up to 10 mm outside the enhancing edge. This fact is consistent with the more widespread abnormality revealed by MRI, although the enhancing rim as seen on CT almost certainly represents the extent of blood–brain barrier breakdown due to tumour growth (evidence from whole brain section studies (Burger et al 1983) have been corroborated by clinical work correlating CT and MRI appearances with histology and intraoperative impedance monitoring (Gorecki et al 1990).

It is hoped that the detailed analysis of multiple targets taken in and around malignant gliomas including histology and tissue culture, should provide the necessary information regarding tumour extent and intratumoural variability to allow the neurosurgeon, in the future, to plan appropriate treatment which may include aggressive local therapy where, for instance, tumour viability is less extensive than indicated by neuroimaging.

MRI DIRECTED STEREOTACTIC BIOPSY

Since the first report of the clinical application of MRI in 1980 by Hawkes et al, its use has become widespread in the neurosciences and its indications refined. Indeed, in many clinical situations it has become the imaging technique of choice. At present, clinicians are still evaluating its full potential, especially in imaging of the neuroaxis, where it has proved most useful.

Production of magnetic resonance images is considerably more complex than with CT, the final image depending on a number of variables, including the strength of the external magnetic field, the magnetic resonance signal of specific nuclei, and the T_1 and T_2 relaxation times of the tissues. Enhancement is possible using gadolinium though this phenomenon is not comparable to CT enhancement. MRI has, however, a number of advantages over CT, particularly in the field of neuroradiology. The patient is not exposed to any ionizing radiation. The high level of contrast between grey and white matter produces a greatly improved anatomical display (Doyle et al 1981) and computational artefacts due to compact bone seen with CT, especially in the posterior fossa, are absent in MRI (Young et al 1981). Coronal and sagittal slices can be produced directly without recourse to computer generated reconstructions from axial slices. Unfortunately, the inherent spatial accuracy of MRI is less than CT due to non-linearity in the field of the magnet as well as distortions induced by varying tissue susceptibility.

As might be expected with two fundamentally different techniques, images of the same cerebral lesion may have quite different characteristics on MRI as compared with CT. Indeed, it quickly became apparent that MRI could reveal lesions not visible on CT at all (Bydder et al 1982). MRI is certainly more sensitive than CT in detecting the presence and extent of neoplasms though the features are less specific and at the present time MRI is less accurate in histopathologically typing lesions than CT. In addition, MRI is poor at differentiating solid from cystic lesions and at delineating calcification. However, MRI is proving highly useful in the detection and differentiation of the focal CNS mass lesions found in the acquired immune deficiency syndrome (AIDS), and in this situation is superceding CT, as well as affecting surgical management with respect to the usefulness of biopsy with or without stereotaxy (Ciricillo & Rosenblum 1990).

The above findings and others have provided a strong stimulus for the development of MRI directed stereotactic techniques, in part to exploit the new diagnostic information and in part to achieved a better understanding of the image, as well as to address the distortion in the image caused by non-linearity of the field.

As with CT, the imaging technology awaited modifications of existing stereotactic hardware in order that tissue from targets visualized using

MRI could be obtained in this manner. A major constraint imposed on any frame by MRI was that it had to be completely free of ferromagnetic compounds to allow use within the strong magnetic field. In addition, closed conduction loops needed to be eliminated to avoid eddy current artefacts, and the instrument itself had to be compact enough to fit within the head coil of the MRI machine. A number of stereotactic frames have now been made MRI compatible and are generally constructed out of anodized aluminium, some with interposing insulated sections to prevent conduction loop formation. Non-conducting plastic is an alternative used in some systems.

By way of example the two most commonly used MRI compatible stereotactic frames will be described, namely the Leksell and BRW frames.

Leksell et al (1985) were among the first to describe modifications to an existing CT compatible frame. Manufactured by Elekta Instruments AB, Stockholm, Sweden, the Leksell frame was a target centred arc system constructed using an aluminium alloy for CT use. Tests confirmed that this standard frame caused minimal distortional artefacts from eddy currents and was highly suited to MRI. Skull fixation pins were made from glass fibre, and these attached to the frame with aluminium and plastic check holders. The coordinate scales were revised to correspond to the *x*, *y*, *z* system, which had been in general use in both CT and MRI stereotaxy. The CT localizers were replaced with similar plastic discs filled with vegetable oil, which was found to be the most suitable material (Leksell et al 1985) — with a T_1 value of 300 ms and a T_2 value of 200 ms at 6 MHz and 20°C (Wyper et al 1986). Fixation of the coordinate frame to the MRI scanner was by means of a glass fibre adaptor, instead of aluminium as used with CT. MRI is then performed in two planes, one parallel to the base plate the other coronally, although accuracy is said to be enhanced if sagittal scans are also performed. The target coordinates are then determined using the same principles as with CT (Leksell & Jernberg 1980).

The first cases of MRI directed stereotactic biopsies were reported in 1986 (Thomas et al 1986, Lunsford et al 1986) using, respectively, modified BRW (Trent Wells, Southgate, California, USA) and Leksell instrumentation. MRI compatibility was achieved by replacing the aluminium alloy base ring with one constructed of non-metallic paxolin and carbon fibre, and the stainless steel skull fixation pins with titanium ones. The localizing frame (Fig. 3.5) consisted of 12 rather than nine fiducials made from carbon fibre tubes filled with gadopentetic acid (Gd-DTPA), which gave a T_1 value of 200 ms, enabling them to be seen on appropriate magnetic resonance windows (Thomas et al 1986). The use of 12 fiducials necessitated a separate computer program to calculate the *x*, *y*, *z* target coordinates. These could then be fed into the standard BRW CT software in order to obtain the arc system frame settings. Current modifications of the BRW localizing frame (Fig. 3.6) allow target determination direct from sagittal and coronal, as well as axial, MRI planes.

There are a number of adverse factors affecting the accuracy of MRI directed stereotaxy. Inhomogeneities of the main magnetic fields and non-linearity of the orthogonal field gradients produce geometric image distortions which are due primarily to eddy current formation and are maximal in coronal and sagittal image sequencing (Wyper et al 1986). In addition, the

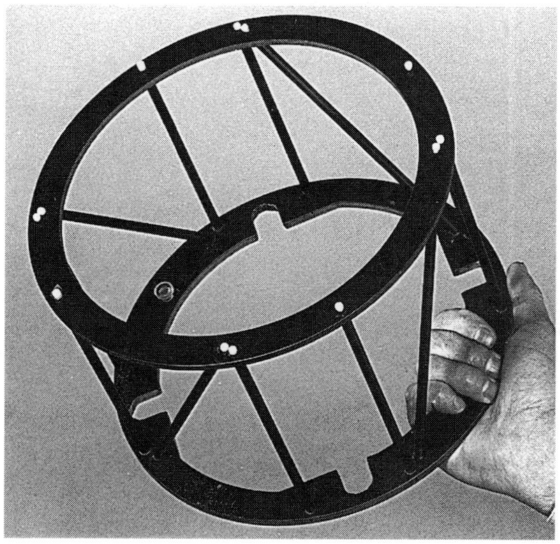

Fig. 3.5 The BRW localizing frame for MRI use. The 12 carbon fibre tubes (fiducials) are filled with Gd-DTPA or a dilute copper sulphate solution.

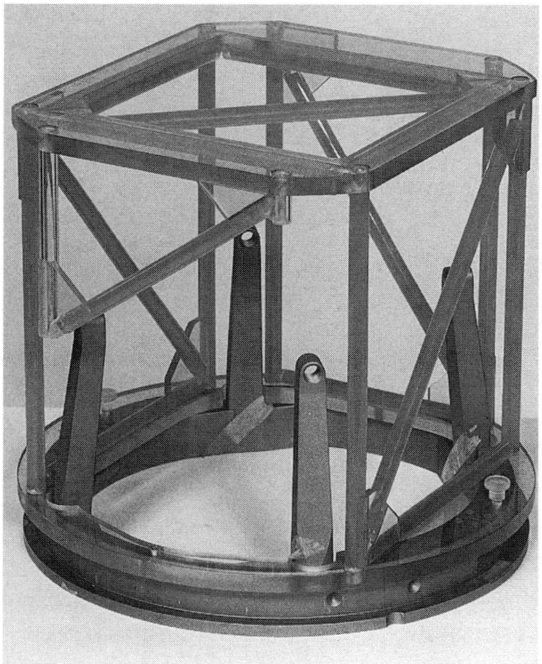

Fig. 3.6 Modified BRW base ring and localizer for MRI directed biopsy. This localizing frame allows biopsy of targets direct from coronal, sagittal as well as standard axial images.

voxel sizes are considerably larger than with CT, thus limiting resolution.

Lunsford et al (1986) performed intraoperative CT to confirm target location immediately following his three original cases of MRI directed biopsy using the Leksell frame, claiming an accuracy within 1 mm. This high degree of accuracy was largely confirmed by an experimental study by Wyper et al (1987), who found that MRI produced an accuracy better than 2 mm using an agar filled phantom and aluminium pellets as target points. Similarly, the BRW system has proved highly accurate. Bradford et al (1978a), using a perspex phantom and six target points, compared MRI localization with that obtainable via CT. The differences were 1 mm in the x axis, 3.75 mm in the y axis and 5 mm in the z axis. The z axis inaccuracy in this study was thought to be due to the 8 mm slice width used. Using 5 mm MRI scan slices in the axial plane, Heilbrun et al (1987) demonstrated an average error in the z axis of less than 2 mm. However, using information from axial, coronal and sagittal slices, targets could be localized to within one voxel in all three planes. The accuracy of target determination can potentially be further improved by correcting for field inhomogeneities as described by Schad et al (1987).

At present the accuracy of MRI is quite adequate for the stereotactic biopsy of mass lesions. Further studies are required, especially on non-linearity, to ascertain how suited it is to functional neurosurgery.

What is the current role of MRI directed stereotactic biopsy? It is now well established that this procedure is not only technically feasible but also accurate and reliable. In the USA, in particular, MRI has tended to be combined with other imaging techniques such as CT, digital subtraction angiography and even positron emission tomography to provide 'multimodality imaging', giving the neurosurgeon as much information as possible in each case undergoing stereotactic biopsy (Zhang et al 1990). However, in the UK it remains a useful adjunct to CT in the management of difficult cases, i.e. in those patients who require stereotactic biopsy of lesions which are not clearly delineated or seen at all on CT (Thomas et al 1987). In this context MRI has a particular niche in aiding stereotactic biopsies of brain stem lesions within the posterior fossa where MRI has a significant advantage over CT (because of diminished artefacts and because the lesions present early and are therefore small — see Fig. 3.7). In the largest series in the UK (Bradford et al 1987b, Thomas et al 1988) a transfrontal route is described using an ipsilateral, postcoronal, parasagittal burr hole and an entirely transparenchymal trajectory which avoids the posterior clinoid processes and the free edge of the tentorium. Preoperatively, MRI and CT scanning are performed and the most suitable image modality chosen for stereotaxy. This method of image directed stereotactic biopsy of brain stem lesions has been shown to be both safe and reliable (Coffey & Lunsford 1985, Hood et al 1986) and compares favourably with the several open methods previously described (Pool 1968, Lassiter et al

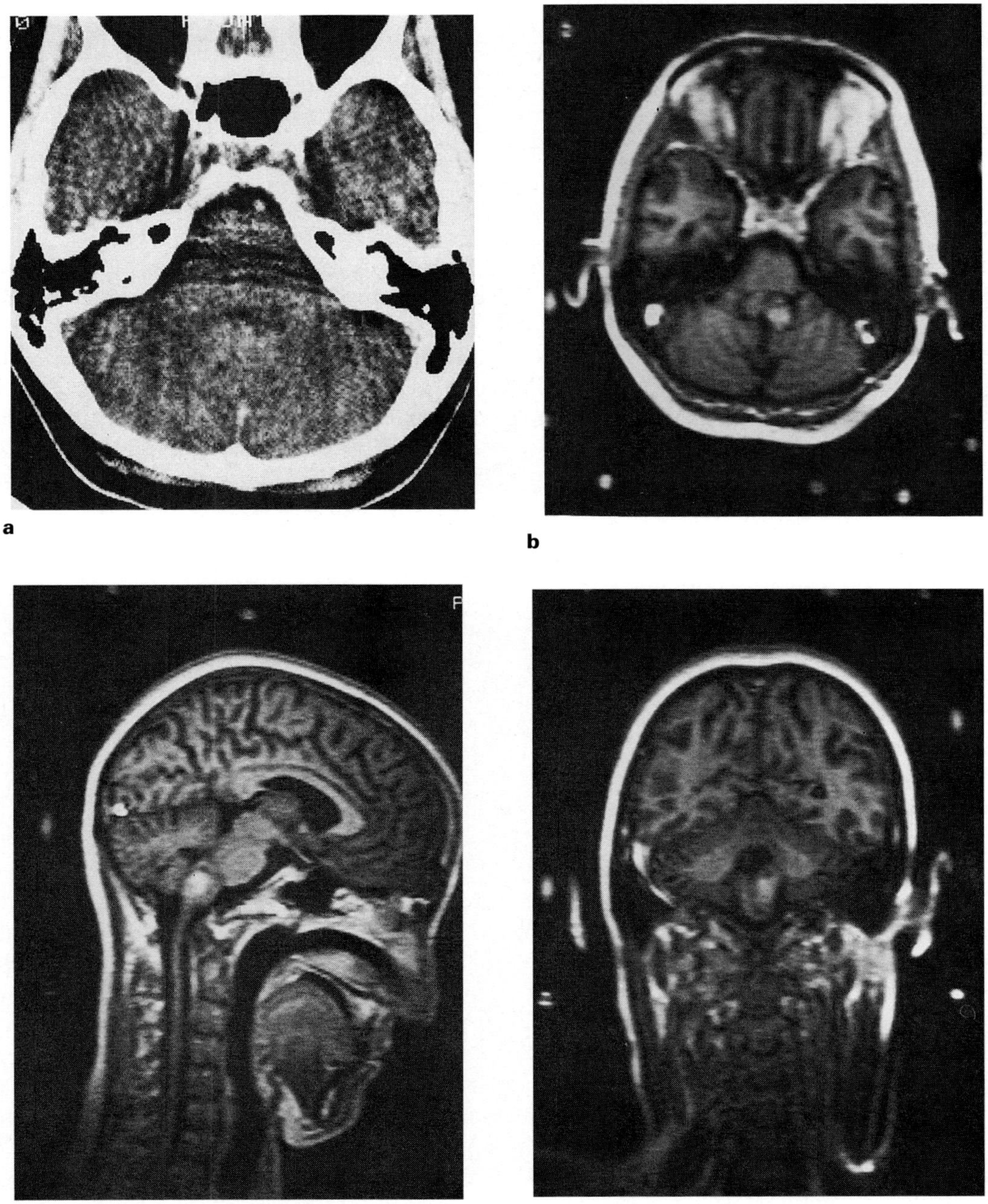

Fig. 3.7 **a** CT and **b–d** MRI scans of a 42-year-old woman who presented with an acute brain stem syndrome, including respiratory failure. The CT scan was reported as being normal, and considerable posterior fossa artefacts are evident. On MRI the lesion is clearly seen in all three planes. Subsequent MRI directed biopsy confirmed the lesion to be focal inflammatory demyelination. The patient partially recovered following a prolonged period of assisted ventilation to be independent and self-caring at home.

1971), though because of the small numbers of patients involved these complex cases should be referred to units concentrating such expertise.

Since its introduction at the National Hospital for Neurology and Neurosurgery, MRI directed stereotactic biopsies using the MRI compatible BRW frame have accounted for only 5% of image directed stereotactic tumour biopsies. This pattern partially reflects the relatively non-specific features displayed by many lesions on MRI with increased T_1 and T_2 signals. Targets are generally chosen within the T_1 weighted image as it less easy on the T_2 weighted image to distinguish tumour from surrounding oedema. Indeed, MRI seems no better than CT in this regard, and gadolinium appears not to improve the image any more than contrast enhanced CT does (Graif et al 1985). Clearly though, stereotactic biopsy represents an extension of the scope of MRI and promises to have valuable clinical and research applications, particularly in the definition of tumour boundaries and the study of tumour biology.

CONCLUSION

Advances in neuroradiology have not altered the fundamental principal of obtaining a tissue diagnosis of cerebral mass lesions. Instead, by combining with modern stereotactic techniques, CT and MRI directed biopsies have become safe and reliable procedures. In this way they have reinforced the importance of pathological definition not only for the individual patient but also in the meaningful evaluation of new treatments within controlled trials. In addition, our knowledge regarding the radiological image continues to accumulate. Clinically, CT directed stereotactic biopsy has become the principal and safest method by which to obtain tissue from within the brain.

REFERENCES

Apuzzo M L J, Chandrasoma T, Cohen D et al 1987 Computed imaging stereotaxy: experience and perspective related to 500 procedures applied to brain masses. Neurosurgery 20: 930–937

Bradford R, Bydder G M, Thomas D G T 1987a MRI-directed stereotactic biopsy of cerebral lesions. Acta Neurochirurgica (Suppl) 13: 25–27

Bradford R, Davis C H, Thomas D G T 1987b Stereotactic biopsy of intrinsic brain stem lesions. Journal of Neurology, Neurosurgery and Psychiatry 50: 1097

Burger P L, Dubois P J, Schold S C et al 1983 Computerized tomographic and pathologic studies of the untreated, quiescent, and recurrent glioblastoma multiforme. Journal of Neurosurgery 58: 159–169

Bydder G M, Steiner R E, Young I R et al 1982 Clinical NMR imaging of the brain: 140 cases. American Journal of Radiology 139: 215–236

Choksey M S, Valentine A, Shawdon H et al 1989 CT in the diagnosis of malignant brain tumours: do all patients require biopsy? Journal of Neurology, Neurosurgery and Psychiatry 52: 821–825

Ciricillo S F, Rosenblum M L 1990 Use of CT and MR imaging to distinguish intracranial lesions and to define the need for biopsy in AIDS patients. Journal of Neurosurgery 21: 720–724

Coffey R J, Lunsford L D 1985 Stereotactic surgery for mass lesions of the mid-brain ana pons. Neurosurgery 17: 12–18

Doyle F H, Gore J C, Pennock J M et al 1981 Imaging of the brain by NMR. Lancet ii: 53–57

Feiden W, Bise K, Steude U 1990 Diagnosis of primary cerebral lymphoma with particular reference to CT-guided stereotactic biopsy. Virchow's Archive (A) 417: 21–28

Frankel S A, German W J 1958 Glioblastoma multiforme. Review of 219 cases with regard to natural history, pathology, diagnostic methods, and treatment. Journal of Neurosurgery 15: 489–503

Gorecki J, Dolan E J, Tasker R R et al 1990 Correlation of CT and MR with impedance monitoring and histopathology in stereotactic biopsies. Canadian Journal of Neurological Sciences 17: 184–189

Graif M, Bydder G M, Steiner R E et al 1985 Contrast-enhanced MR imaging of malignant brain tumours. American Journal of Neurological Research 6: 855–863

Greene G M, Hitchon P W, Schelper R L, Yuh W, Dyste G N 1989 Diagnostic yield in CT-guided stereotactic biopsy of gliomas, Journal of Neurosurgery 71: 494–497

Hawkes R C, Holland G N, Moore W S et al 1980 Nuclear magnetic resonance (NMR) tomography of the brain: a preliminary clinical assessment with demonstration of pathology. Journal of Computer Assisted Tomography 4: 577–586

Heilbrun M P 1984 Computer tomography-guided stereotactic systems. Clinical Neurosurgery 31: 564–581

Heilbrun M P, Sunderland P M, McDonald P R et al 1987 Brown–Wells stereotactic frame modifications to accomplish magnetic resonance imaging guidance in three planes. Applied Neurophysiology 50: 143–152

Hitchcock E, Sato F 1964 Treatment of malignant gliomata. Journal of Neurosurgery 21: 497–505

Hitchon P W, Schelper R L, Barloom T 1985 Accuracy of CT scans in identifying tumor tissue. Applied Neurophysiology 48: 463–466

Hood T W, Gebarski S S, McKeever P E et al 1986 Stereotaxic biopsy of intrinsic lesions of the brain stem. Journal of Neurosurgery 65: 172–176

Kelly P J, Daumas-Duport C, Kispert D B, Kall B A,

Scheithaner B W, Illig J J 1987 Imaging-based stereotaxic serial biopsies in untreated intracranial glial neoplasms. Journal of Neurosurgery 66: 865–874

Kendall B E, Jakubowski J, Pullicino P et al 1979 Difficulties in the diagnosis of supratentorial gliomas by CAT scan. Journal of Neurology, Neurosurgery and Psychiatry 47: 485–492

Kitchen N D, Bradford R 1991 Experience with the Hitchcock Stereotactic Frame in a regional neurosurgical unit. Journal of Neurology, Neurosurgery and Psychiatry 55: 80

Lassiter K R L, Alexander E, Davis C H et al 1971 Surgical treatment of brain stem gliomas. Journal of Neurosurgery 34: 719–725

Leksell L 1949 A stereotactic apparatus for intracerebral surgery. Acta Chirurgica Scandinavica 99: 229–233

Leksell L, Jernberg B 1980 Stereotaxis and tomography. A technical note. Acta Neurochirurgica 15: 308–312

Leksell L, Leksell D, Schwebel J 1985 Stereotaxis and nuclear magnetic resonance. Journal of Neurology, Neurosurgery and Psychiatry 48: 14–18

Lunsford L D, Martinez J, Latchaw R E 1986 Stereotaxic surgery with a magnetic resonance and computerized tomography-compatible system. Journal of Neurosurgery 64: 872–878

Lunsford L D, Coffey R J, Cojocaru T et al 1990 Image-guided stereotactic surgery: a 10 year evolutionary experience. Stereotactic and Functional Neurosurgery 54/55: 375–387

Marshall L F, Jennett B, Langfitt T 1974 Needle biopsy for the diagnosis of malignant glioma. Journal of the American Medical Association 228: 1417–1418

Ostertag C B, Mennel H D, Kiessling M 1980 Stereotactic biopsy of brain tumours. Surgical Neurology 14: 275–283

Pell M, Thomas D G T 1991 The initial experience with the Cosman–Roberts–Wells stereotactic system. British Journal of Neurosurgery 5: 111–116

Pool J L 1968 Gliomas in the region of the brain stem. Journal of Neurosurgery 29: 164–169

Roth J G, Elvidge A R 1960 Glioblastoma multiforme: a clinical study. Journal of Neurosurgery 17: 736–750

Sandeman D R, Sandeman A P, Buxton P et al 1990 The management of patients with a supratentorial brain tumour. British Journal of Neurosurgery 4: 299–312

Schad L, Lott S, Schmitt F et al 1987 Correction of spatial distortion in MR imaging: a prerequisite for accurate stereotaxy. Journal of Computer Assisted Tomography 3: 499–505

Spiegel E A, Wycis H T 1952 Stereoencephalotomy. Grune and Stratton, New York

Tans J T J, de Jongh I E 1978 CT of supratentorial astrocytoma. Clinical Neurology and Neurosurgery 80–83: 156–168

Thomas D G T, Nouby R M 1989 Experience in 300 cases of CT-directed stereotactic surgery for lesion biopsy and aspiration of haematoma. British Journal of Neurosurgery 3: 321–326

Thomas D G T, Anderson R E, du Boulay G H 1984a CT-guided stereotactic neurosurgery: experience in 24 cases with a new stereotactic system. Journal of Neurology, Neurosurgery and Psychiatry 47: 9–16

Thomas D G T, Darling T L, Watkins B A et al 1984b A simple method for the growth of cell cultures from small biopsies of brain tumours taken during CT-directed stereotactic procedures. Acta Neurochirurgica (suppl) 33: 243–5

Thomas D G T, Davis C H, Ingram S et al 1986 Stereotaxic biopsy of the brain under MR imaging control. American Journal of Neurological Research 7: 161–163

Thomas D G T, Bradford R, Bydder G 1987 Magnetic resonance directed stereotactic brain biopsy. Journal of Neurology, Neurosurgery and Psychiatry 50: 645

Thomas D G T, Bradford R, Gill S et al 1988 Computer directed stereotactic biopsy of intrinsic brain stem lesions. British Journal of Neurosurgery 2: 235–240

Whittle I R, Gregor A 1991 The treatment of primary malignant brain tumours. Journal of Neurology, Neurosurgery and Psychiatry 54: 101–103

Wild A M, Xuereb J H, Marks P V et al 1990 Computerized tomographic stereotaxy in the management of 200 consecutive intracranial mass lesions. Analysis of indicators, benefits and outcome. British Journal of Neurosurgery 4: 407–415

Wyper D J, Turner J W, Patterson J et al 1986 Accuracy of stereotaxic localisation using MRI and CT. Journal of Neurology, Neurosurgery and Psychiatry 49: 1445–1448

Young I R, Burl M, Clark G J et al 1981 Posterior fossa: MR properties. American Journal of Roentgenology 137: 895–901

Zhang J, Levesque MF, Wilson CL et al 1990 Multimodality imaging of brain structures for stereotactic surgery. Radiology 175: 435–441

4. Principles and pitfalls of image directed stereotactic biopsy of brain lesions

L. S. Chin M. L. Levy C. H. Rabb P. T. Chandrasoma C. S. Zee M. J. Apuzzo

INTRODUCTION

The past decade has witnessed a dramatic increase in the amount, variety and detail of medical imaging available to clinicians. Those privileged to work in the neurological specialties have been at the forefront of this expansion. Through the use of computerized tomography (CT), magnetic resonance imaging (MRI), digital subtraction angiography (DSA) and positron emission tomography (PET) we are able to locate, identify and characterize lesions which were inaccessible to surgeons of a previous generation. These images, though sophisticated, do not replace the need for histological and microbiological assay in making accurate diagnoses. With this premise, the past decade has also witnessed a rebirth within the field of neurosurgery of the use of image directed stereotaxy. It couples the sophistication of medical imaging with modern computer and engineering principles, thus providing an accurate and reproducible means of obtaining tissue for further analysis. Specific applications include: (1) precise biopsy technique (Ostertag et al 1980, Fulling & Nelson 1984); (2) cyst or abscess aspiration (Rivas & Lobato 1985); (3) placement of temporary or permanent drains (Apuzzo & Sabshin 1983, Apuzzo et al 1984); (4) installation of single or multiple catheter arrays for volume or colloid based brachytherapy (Apuzzo & Sabshin 1983; Gutin et al 1984); (5) precise guidance of cerebroscopic instrumentation with concurrent biopsy, aspiration or excision (Iizuka 1975); (6) intraoperative point localization or guidance (Kelly et al 1984). At our institution (University of Southern California (USC)), we have had the privilege of using prototypes of the Brown–Roberts–Wells (BRW) and Cosman–Roberts–Wells (CRW) (Radionics, Burlington, Massachusetts, USA) systems while accumulating our experience (Apuzzo et al 1977, 1984a, 1987, Apuzzo & Sabshin 1983, Heilbrun 1983, Heilbrun et al 1983, Couldwell & Apuzzo 1990). This chapter outlines the insight and knowledge we have gained from our use of these two systems in over 3500 biopsy procedures.

CLINICAL SERIES OF IMAGE DIRECTED STEREOTACTIC BIOPSIES

Methodology

General principles

1. Rapid translation of accurate data from the imaging console to the operating room.
2. Efficient use of time during the procedure.
3. Performance of the procedure under local anaesthesia with the neuroanaesthesiologist standing by. This allows full cooperation of the patient and enhanced recognition of complications.
4. Minimization of tissue trauma and handling.
5. Close interaction with the neuroradiologist, neurosurgeon and neuropathologist during the procedure.

Stereotactic instrumentation

1. A nickel plated aluminium headring which is fixed to the scalp by four plastic and steel set pins. This ring acts as a platform for the localizer ring and arc system.
2. A localizing unit composed of six vertical and three diagonal carbon fibre rods that provide

fiducial points for establishing the target point in stereotactic space.

3. An arc centred guidance system (CRW) which allows for a limitless variety of settings, entry points and transits within the intracranial stereotactic space.

4. A phantom base consisting of a base ring (headring equivalent) and a movable pointed tip (phantom target) which allows confirmation of the accuracy in the target point settings and the arc ring system.

5. An Epson HX-20 programmable calculator.

Steps in point access

1. Application of the base ring (10 minutes). Following shaving and preparation of the scalp, selection of appropriate pin positions is made with the patient in the sitting position. This is most easily achieved in the operating room. In most case, the base ring is positioned in a plane defined by the tip of the nose and the inion. Observers at the foot of the operating table and lateral to the patient ensure that the ring is even while the planned pin penetration sites are marked on the scalp. These points are then infiltrated with 1% Lidocaine (lignocaine) with adrenaline. The two posterior pins are advanced first and then the ring is pushed forward until the skin contacts the pins. The anterior pins are then advanced and affixed to the skull until the pins are 'finger tight'. The posterior pins are secured in similar fashion. During this time, intravenous contrast medium is being administered. The patient is transported to the scanner with the anaesthesiologist in attendance.

2. Scan target (15 minutes). The localizer is attached to the base ring and a limited CT scan defining the proposed entry point and targets is performed. After the scan slice is selected for the target, pixel coordinates for the nine localizer rods and the target are recorded.

3. Entry point selection (5 minutes). The CRW system renders this step superfluous because the arc centred design allows an infinite number of entry points for any particular target setting. When the BRW system is used, the arc system is placed on the base ring and the settings adjusted to bring the probe tip to the planned entry site on the scalp. The arc-ring is then removed and the anteroposterior, lateral and vertical coordinates recorded.

Determination of the entry point must take into account: (a) lesion location, size and consistency, (b) intervening neural and vascular structures. In general, the entry point should minimize the length of transit through the brain and avoid eloquent areas. Maintaining an orthogonal relationship to the skull will ensure ease of entry through the skull and avoid stripping of the dura away from the inner table.

4. Data processing (10 minutes). The nine fiducial coordinates, target values and entry points (if applicable) are entered into the Epson HX-20 computer. Anteroposterior, lateral, and vertical values are derived and printed by the computer.

5. Arc system and phantom settings (10 minutes). The movable target on the phantom base is set at the previously calculated anteroposterior, lateral and vertical values. The arc system is brought into play and the corresponding axes are also fixed. By simulating the proposed transit with a probe, the accuracy of the settings can be verified. In addition, the actual biopsy cannula and forceps can be precisely calibrated to the phantom target point.

6. Completion of the surgical procedure (10–20 minutes). The arc-ring system is brought back to the patient and attached to the base ring. The actual biopsy technique will be described subsequently. After tissue is obtained, it is sent to the pathologist who then determines if the tissue is adequate for a definitive diagnosis. At this time the incision is closed with a single monofilament suture and the patient is sent for an immediate postoperative scan.

Biopsy instrumentation

A variety of instruments are available and provide satisfactory specimens. These include: (1) cup forceps, (2) a spiral needle, (3) a side cutting aspirator and (4) a needle core device. The needle core device is a No. 14 gauge cannula with a stylet for entry. A core is aspirated at the target site but is greatly dependent on lesion texture and proved to be unreliable in our hands. The side cutting aspirator is a modification of the needle coring device. It provides a 1.5 × 10 mm cylindrical specimen but is also dependent on lesion consistency for a good sample. We prefer to use a flexible cup forceps which provides consistent 1.5 mm^3 sized specimens and is less dependent on lesion characteristics. It also provides some assessment of tissue firmness as judged by resistance to palpation of the lesion with the probe tip.

Biopsy technique

The scalp entry point is infiltrated with 1% Lidocaine (lignocaine) with adrenaline and a 1 cm incision made. The arc system is attached to the base ring on the patient. A long 4.5 mm twist drill bit is used to make the craniostomy. The twist drill guide tube in the arc slide bushing is exchanged for a 2.7 mm guide tube. A sharp probe is used to penetrate the dura. The No. 13 gauge cannula is then advanced to the target site. The blunt stylet is removed and the biopsy forceps advanced to the predetermined set point and biopsies obtained. Different samples can be taken by advancing the probe slightly and also by rotating the direction of cup opening and closure. Aspiration for drainage and fluid analysis may be undertaken at this time.

Endoscopy technique

A 6.2 mm diameter endoscope with a barrel 20 cm in length has been employed for both cerebroscopy and ventriculoscopy. This instrument, produced by Karl Storz Endoscopy (Tuttlingen, Germany), provides visualization, irrigation and a port for aspiration or biopsy instrumentation. Submersible quartz fibres for transmission of laser energy may be introduced for haemostasis and lesion coagulation (Iizuka 1975, Sugita et al 1975, Apuzzo et al 1984, 1987b)

For a lesion at the foramen of Munro, a scan slice at the foramen is obtained and the appropriate target selected. A burr hole is made 1 cm anterior to the coronal suture in the midpupillary line. The dura is opened and a small corticopial window is fashioned with the biopolar forceps. The endoscopy sheath with a blunt stylet in place is then introduced through the rigid bushing to the target point. Irrigating fluid (Ringer's lactate) at body temperature is then introduced intermittently through adjustable side ports. Cyst puncture and aspiration is accomplished by using a sharp tipped stylet to puncture the wall; the cannula is then advanced into the cyst and aspiration performed (Rivas & Lobato 1985)

Neuroimaging

The CT and MRI scans are indispensible elements of the preoperative planning for a stereotactic procedure. The CT scan with contrast is the foundation upon which the accuracy of the procedure rests since most biopsies are CT guided. Proper setting of soft tissue windows and intravenous contrast allow separation of lesion from normal brain. Some lesions such as low grade neoplasms may enhance poorly. These patients may require a double dose of IV contrast medium and delayed scanning; in our experience, this procedure is very effective in clarifying otherwise poorly enhancing lesions. If CT is unable to resolve the lesion, another imaging modality may be needed to guide the stereotactic biopsy. Areas of contrast enhancement are generally the best areas to biopsy and obviously cystic or necrotic areas are less likely to yield a diagnostic specimen. The CT scan is also good at defining regions of calcification. For obvious reasons, these areas should not be targeted for biopsy. In patients with a previous craniotomy, the bone flap presents a challenge in deciding base ring pin fixation sites and entry point placement. Bone window settings are helpful in this aspect of surgical planning.

MRI represents a major advance in the diagnostic imaging of neurological diseases. Compared to CT, MRI provides: (1) increased soft tissue contrast between normal and abnormal tissue; (2) elimination of bone artefacts in the middle and posterior fossa; (3) direct coronal and sagittal imaging; (4) better characterization of vascular structures and lesions; (5) superior anatomical definition. For these reasons, MRI is more sensitive in the detection of primary and metastatic neoplasms, infarcts and infectious processes (Brandt-Zawadzki et al 1983, Bradley et al 1984). Furthermore, anatomical detail and pathological changes can be better defined by manipulating a variety of imaging parameters.

Despite the exquisite detail of plain MRI, the

University of Ulster LIBRARY

use of a contrast medium is as important in MRI as it is in CT. The contrast agent gadopentetate dimeglumine (Gd-DTPA) acts similarly to iodinated contrast medium by accumulating in areas of blood–brain barrier breakdown and slow flowing vascular structures (Brandt-Zawadzki et al 1986). Contrast enhanced MRI has been shown to be more sensitive than routine MRI for detecting metastatic foci (Healy et al 1987) (Fig. 4.1) It also better defines the margins of the lesion and areas of necrosis, thus providing valuable information on target selection (Zee et al 1991).

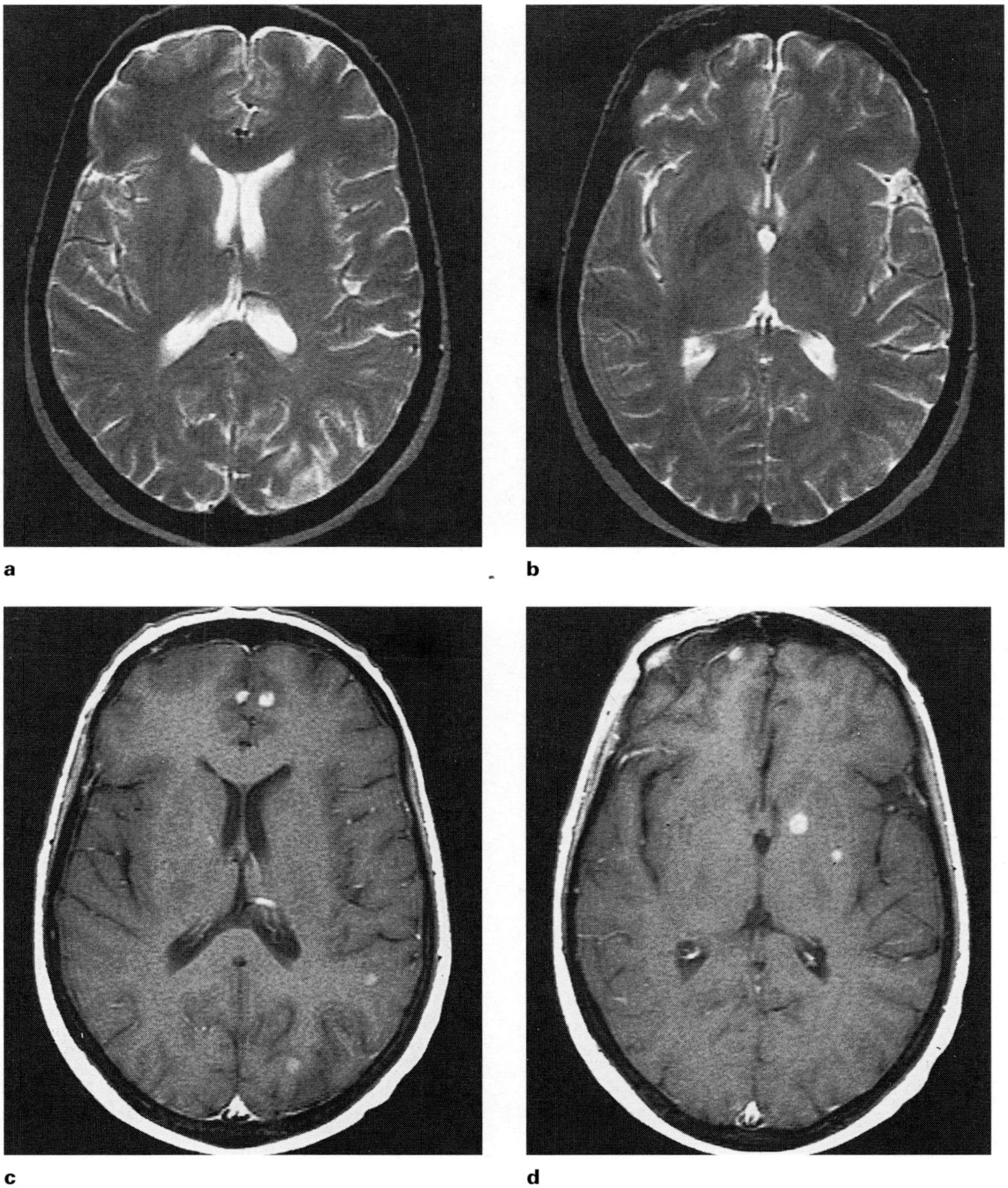

Fig. 4.1 **a,b** T_2 weighted MRI scan shows a single, small lesion in left putamen. **c**, **d**-T_1 scan with gadolinium enhancement reveals multiple small lesions in cortical and subcortical areas consistent with metastases.

The ability of MRI to characterize blood in different settings makes it crucial in the pre-operative planning of a biopsy. The presence of haemorrhage and the age of the haemorrhage is readily defined with T_1 and T_2 images (Mattle et al 1990). This provides insight into the nature of the lesion, its recent evolution, and possibly its response to an invasive procedure. A prime example is the cavernous angioma. This lesion is characterized by variable density in T_1 and T_2 images, consistent with haemorrhages of different ages and a haemosiderin ring (Fig. 4.2) (Gomon et al 1986, Tung et al 1990). Biopsy of this lesion is potentially fatal and its recognition must occur before surgery. Normal intracranial arteries and veins can also be distinguished using various imaging techniques (Von Schulthess & Higgins 1985, Bradley et al 1987, Kucharcyzk et al 1989). This allows for judicious planning of probe entry and brain transits in order to avoid a subdural or intracerebral haemorrhage.

State-of-the-art MRI is now able to provide three dimensional reformatting, which offers several advantages over conventional MRI. Extremely thin slices are possible and no gap exists between the slices. The result is a variety of reconstructed images, including multiplanar, oblique and curved (Menick et al 1990). The planned transit through the brain can be rehearsed and evaluated in the radiology suite prior to biopsy.

Pathological evaluation of the stereotactic biopsy

General principles and methods

The sample submitted for pathological evaluation varies in different centres from a 1 mm^3 fragment of tissue obtained with a biopsy forceps to several cores that may be up to 2 cm each in length obtained with the side cutting needle (Heilbrun 1983, Kelly et al 1984, Apuzzo et al 1987, Lunsford 1988, Ostertag 1988, Chandrasoma & Apuzzo 1989) At USC the typical sample consists of 1–3 pieces of tissue, each 1–3 mm^3 in volume. This is the smallest possible sample that can be obtained, and our success with stereotactic biopsy indicates that the sample size is not a factor that limits diagnostic accuracy.

In all cases, the stereotactic biopsy represents a

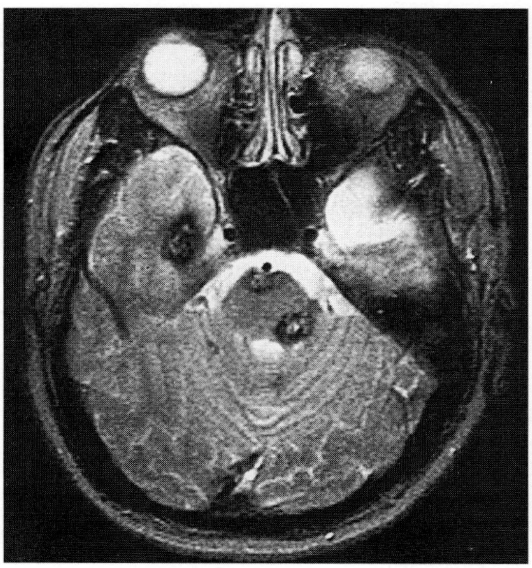

a

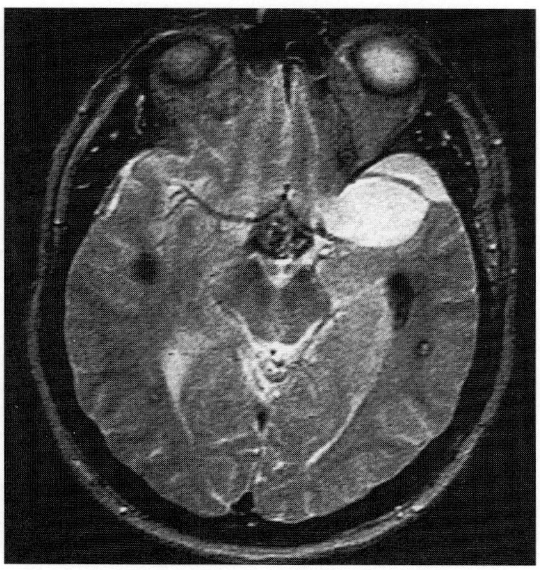

b

Fig. 4.2 Multiple cavernous angiomas are seen on T_2 weighted MRI in the pons, temporal lobe and suprasellar cistern. Note the characteristic speckled pattern indicating small haemorrhages of different ages and the dark haemosiderin ring marking the capsule formed from chronic haematoma. An arachnoid cyst of the left middle fossa is incidentally seen.

sample from within a larger lesion that has been visualized by radiological imaging. It is of critical importance in the evaluation of the biopsy that the pathologist be aware of how the sample relates to the radiological lesion. At USC, the neurosurgeon performing the biopsy discusses the clinical history and imaging studies with the pathologist, either in the operating room or the frozen section area before the specimen is handled. In this way, the stereotactic biopsy is converted into a clinicopathological problem rather than a blind evaluation of a pathological specimen. To attempt to do otherwise increases the likelihood of diagnostic error.

After removal from the brain, the specimen is immediately placed on a Telfa pad and taken in a Petri dish by the neurosurgeon to the frozen section area of the pathology department. The specimen is examined grossly by the pathologist, and a portion of the specimen is cut out with a sharp scalpel blade for preparation of the smear. We take approximately 25% of each biopsy fragment for the smear. The sample taken for the smear is random. We have attempted to use a dissecting microscope to direct the sampling, but this has not improved diagnostic accuracy over direct selection.

The small pieces from each fragment are placed in a horizontal row on a clean glass slide. A second slide is used to make the smear (Chandrasoma & Apuzzo 1989). The amount of pressure needed varies with the specimen, and can be gauged by the ease with which the tissue crushes when compressed between the two slides. With tissues that do not flatten out with pressure, it may be necessary to use multiple back and forth movements with the two slides to effect separation of the tissue. Such harsh handling of the tissue creates considerable artefacts, but provides a smear that is usually adequate for cytological examination, and is preferable to an unseparated crushed tissue fragment that is impossible to evaluate. The ease with which a tissue smears also helps determine the degree of cellularity in the tumour. Cellularity may be underestimated on the smear with tissues that spread out evenly, and overestimated with tissues that do not smear out well. With some experience, the pathologist develops the ability to assess cellularity on the smear so that it correlates well with the cellularity on permanent sections.

At the USC, the smear represents the primary technique for evaluating the biopsy in almost all cases. The only exception to this rule is in those very rare cases where the neurosurgeon reports that the specimen felt extremely hard during removal. In such cases, we proceed directly to frozen section, but this represents only 1% of biopsies. In the vast majority of stereotactic biopsies, we do not perform a frozen section as part of the evaluation.

In most cases, the sample provided by the stereotactic biopsy is adequate for diagnosis (Liwnicz et al 1982, Heilbrun 1983, Kelly et al 1984, Willems & Alva-Willems 1984, Apuzzo et al 1987a, Moriquand et al 1987, Lunsford 1988, Ostertag 1988, Chandrasoma & Apuzzo 1989). An inadequate specimen requires further biopsy attempts, either from the same target point with minor adjustment of the needle, or after a second target determination.

The further handling of the tissue depends on what is seen on the smear. Each case is treated as an individual problem, to optimize the information that is provided by the biopsy. This is predicated by the fact that the quantity of tissue is not sufficient to perform all tests on every case, thus, triage is mandatory. As examples, let us take the case of a smear showing an anaplastic astrocytoma (Fig. 4.3) and another showing brain with lymphocytic infiltration (Fig. 4.4). In the case of the astrocytoma, we freeze the tissue to permit immunoperoxidase evaluation of Ki-67, a proliferative antigen that is predictive of prognosis (Ostertag et al 1987, Sasaki et al 1988). In the case of an inflammatory lesion, we take a small sample for electron microscopy, because, in our experience, this has had the highest yield in identifying a viral aetiology. The tissue is then place in paraffin for serial sections, which permit immunoperoxidase stains for detecting various viral antigens, and then perform lymphocytic marker studies. Viral cultures, which have a low diagnostic yield, are done only if tissue remains.

Diagnosis of neoplasms

When the mass lesion is a neoplasm, a specific and accurate tissue diagnosis can be made in over

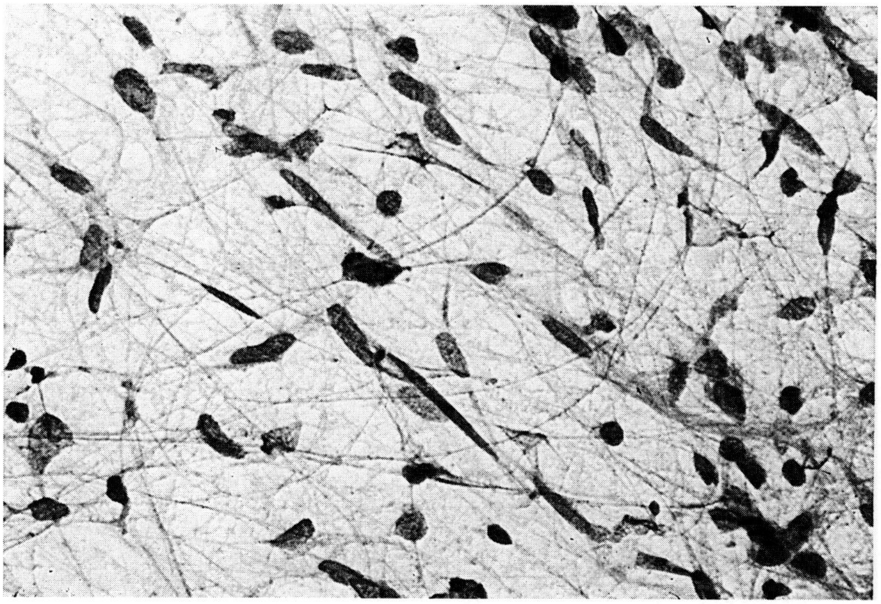

Fig. 4.3 Smear of an anaplastic astrocytoma showing hypercellularity and fibrillary, pleomorphic astrocytes which have enlarged, spindle shaped nuclei, and cytoplasmic fibrils. × 110.

95% of cases (Liwnicz et al 1982, Heilbrun 1983, Kelly et al 1984, Willems & Alva-Willems 1984, Apuzzo et al 1987a, Moriquand et al 1987, Lunsford 1988, Ostertag 1988, Chandrasoma & Apuzzo 1989). When the mass lesion is non-neoplastic, the expectation for a specific diagnosis is less. In these cases, the main value of the biopsy is to exclude a neoplasm.

Most intraparenchymal neoplasms have infiltrating edges, and the first distinction to be made

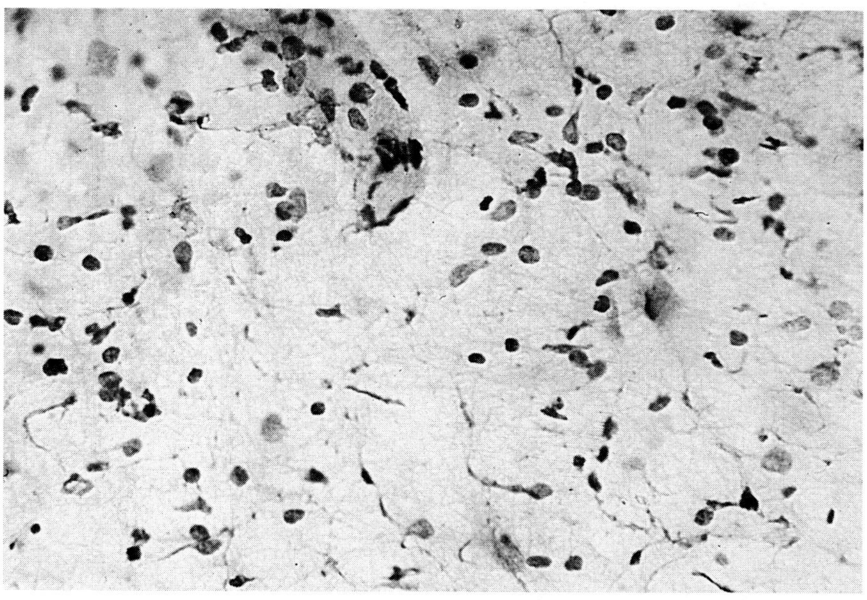

Fig. 4.4 Smear showing reactive gliosis and inflammation. Note the polymorphous cell population which includes many small rounded lymphocytes. × 70.

in a biopsy is whether the specimen is taken from the infiltrating edge of tumour into brain or from a region of pure tumour. The infiltrating edge of a neoplasm consists of normal brain or reactive glial tissue, oedema and neovascularity in addition to neoplastic cells. The diagnosis in biopsies from this area is extremely difficult and depends on the identification of single neoplastic cells in a background of normal or reactive glial tissue. This can be easy in a non-glial neoplasm such as metastatic carcinoma (Fig. 4.5), very difficult in an anaplastic glial neoplasm, and virtually impossible in a well differentiated glial neoplasm. When the biopsy is from an area where the neoplasm has completely replaced brain, the diagnosis is much easier. In these cases, the smear consists of only neoplastic cells without any normal brain in the background and the diagnosis only depends upon identifying the constituent cell type. In most well targeted stereotactic biopsies, the tissue is from the area that consists only of neoplasm.

Another consideration in the understanding of neoplasms of the brain is that they are not homogeneous, which can lead to sampling error. Such sampling error exists in all biopsies unless a total resection of the tumour is performed. The possibility of sampling error is highest in a stereotactic biopsy.

Homogeneous neoplasms include metastatic carcinoma, melanoma, malignant lymphoma, oligodendroglioma, ependymoma, craniopharyngioma and meningioma. Recognition of the abnormal cell population leads to a diagnosis which rarely requires further qualification. For example, the presence of neoplastic epithelial cells in a specimen is diagnostic of carcinoma, and there is a high level of confidence that this diagnosis will not change even if the entire lesion is studied.

Considerations in the diagnosis of the heterogeneous neoplasms will be addressed in the following sections on astrocytomas and pineal region tumours.

Astrocytic neoplasms

Astrocytomas are extremely complex neoplasms that have presented problems of classification and grading that have been contentious over several generations and have not been successfully resolved (Burger 1990). For the usual cerebral hemispheric astrocytomas, we use the three-tier classification originally put forth by Ringertz: astro-

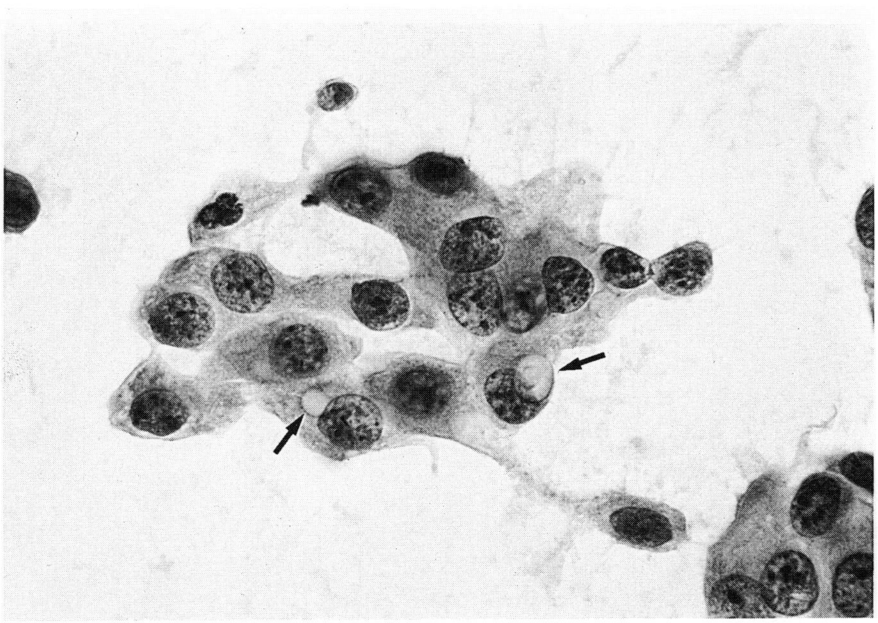

Fig. 4.5 Smear showing metastatic adenocarcinoma with cohesive groups of malignant epithelial cells. Note the presence of cytoplasmic vacuolation representing intracytoplasmic mucin (arrows). × 110.

cytoma (grade II astrocytoma in the World Health Organization system), anaplastic astrocytoma and glioblastoma multiforme (Ringertz 1950). A glioblastoma is an anaplastic astrocytoma with necrosis, thus recognizing that necrosis is the histological feature that predicts the worst biological behaviour among astrocytomas. Lesions that fall into the anaplastic astrocytoma and astrocytoma groups show a wide range of biological behaviour which is difficult to predict on the basis of histological features alone. We are currently using Ki-67 and flow cytometry to help predict prognosis.

The hallmark of smears of an astrocytic neoplasm is the presence of abnormal astrocytes which are larger and more angulated than normal astrocytes and contain prominent cytoplasmic fibres. The result is a fibrillary background as opposed to the granular, eosinophilic background seen in normal brain. In addition, endothelial proliferation can be accurately assessed on the smear. Target selection during stereotactic biopsy usually results in the avoidance of necrotic areas; therefore, there is a bias which underestimates the incidence of glioblastoma. Well differentiated astrocytomas show neoplastic astrocytes of low to moderate cellularity, little to moderate cytological atypia, and the absence of gemistocytes, endothelial proliferation, and necrosis. Correlation with the CT scan is important in this setting, because the identical biopsy would be considered inadequate if it were obtained from the periphery of a lesion, the possibility being that the biopsy in fact represents reactive gliosis.

Pineal germ cell neoplasms

Pineal germ cell neoplasms are heterogeneous lesions with areas of germinoma, teratoma, embryonal cell carcinoma, yolk sac carcinoma, and choriocarcinoma (Scheithauer 1984). In addition, there may be large areas of granulomatous inflammation in a pure germinoma (Fig. 4.6) (Scheithauer 1984, Krachoke et al 1988). We have had four germinomas where the initial biopsy showed granulomas and subsequent samples showed germinoma. A biopsy may show material that is diagnostic, yet may not be representative of the entire neoplasm. For this reason, the stereotactic biopsy results need to be combined with imaging characteristics and serum and cerebrospinal fluid tumour markers, i.e. α-fetoprotein and human chorionic gonadotrophin.

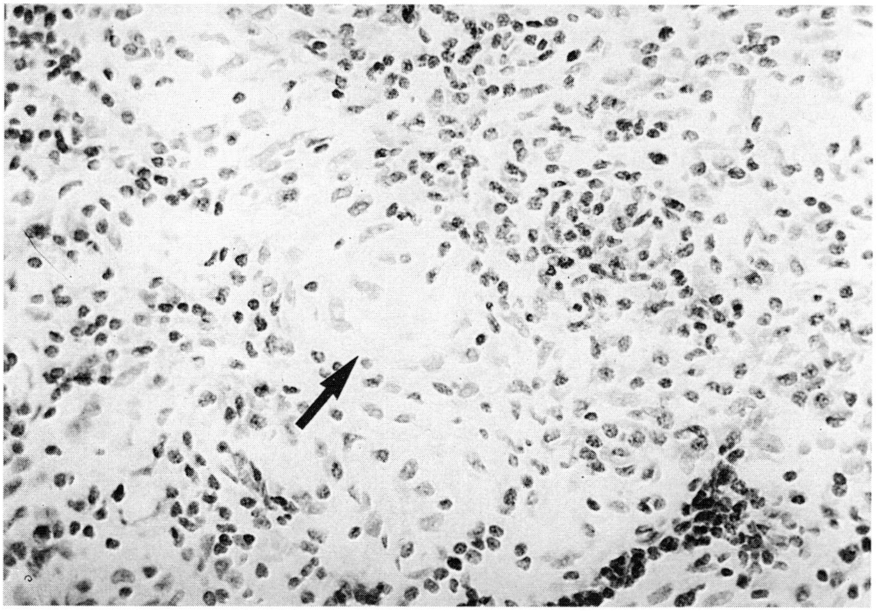

Fig. 4.6 Granulomatous inflammation in a germinoma obtained at stereotactic biopsy. The central epithelioid cell granuloma (arrow) is surrounded by numerous lymphocytes. No germinoma cells are present in this area. × 35.

Diagnosis of non-neoplastic lesions

The expectations of stereotactic biopsy are less for non-neoplastic lesions than for neoplasms. In most cases, the smear and sections show reactive gliosis and inflammatory cells, usually lymphocytes and plasma cells (see Fig. 4.4).

In a minority (approximately 20%) of cases with reactive gliosis and inflammation, a specific diagnosis can be made. These include cases where there are numerous foamy macrophages in the clinical setting consistent with cerebral infarction, and cases where a specific infectious agent is identified in the biopsy. Infections we have encountered include tuberculosis, coccidioidomycosis, mucormycosis, cryptococcosis, cysticercosis, herpes simplex and cytomegalovirus encephalitis, progressive multifocal leukoencephalopathy (Fig. 4.7), and toxoplasmosis (Fig. 4.8). We have also had cases where electron microscopy has demonstrated unspecified viral particles, providing evidence for viral encephalitis. In a biopsy that shows gliosis and inflammation on the smear, it is important to process the specimen in a manner that maximizes the probability of specific diagnosis. We take a piece for permanent sections from which multiple slides are cut for immunoperoxidase studies for viruses and toxoplasma. The next priority for tissue is for electron microscopy. If tissue remains, we take a sample for mycobacterial, fungal and viral culture before submitting the rest for routine sections.

In those cases where a specific diagnosis has not been made, the main concern is that a neoplasm has been missed by the biopsy. Those patients with a stereotactic biopsy diagnosis of reactive gliosis and inflammation are therefore followed carefully and a repeat biopsy done when clinically indicated. In our experience, it is uncommon for these cases to be neoplastic, but we have had a second biopsy reveal malignant lymphoma, Hodgkin's disease, anaplastic astrocytoma and pineal germinoma after an initial non-diagnostic biopsy.

The use of stereotactic biopsy in the acquired immune deficiency syndrome (AIDS) is controversial. In our experience, the occurrence of any mass lesion in the brain is associated with short survival in human immunodeficiency virus (HIV) positive patients. We utilize stereotactic biopsy in our institution only for mass lesions where a strong

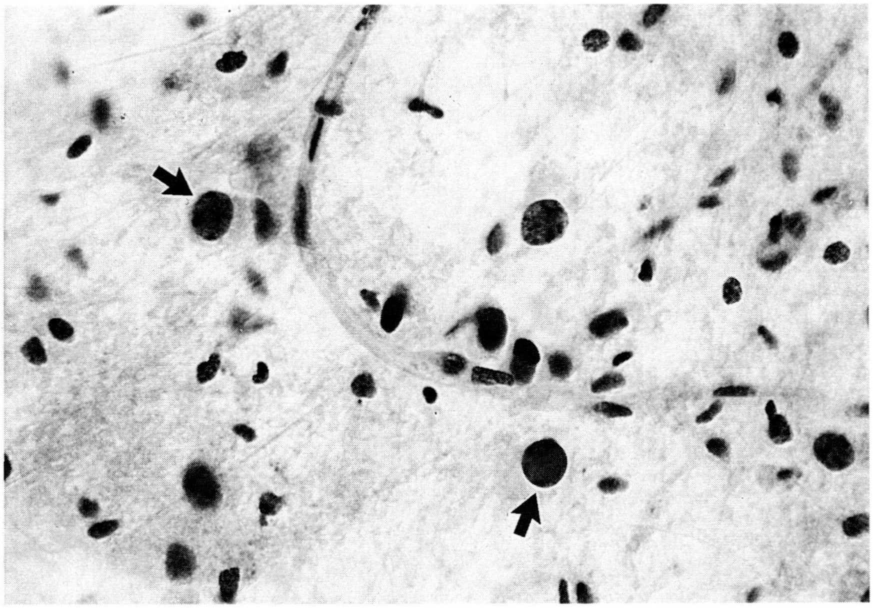

Fig. 4.7 Smear showing features diagnostic of progressive multifocal leukoencephalopathy (PML). Several nuclei show enlargement with the presence of smudgy ground glass appearance and chromatin clumping that is characteristic of PML (arrows). × 110.

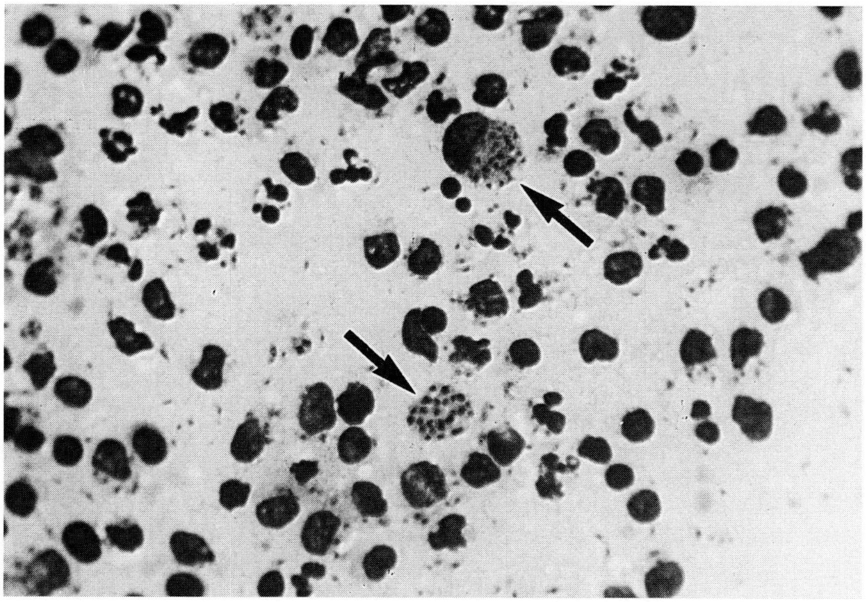

Fig. 4.8 Smear of cerebral toxoplasmosis showing numerous organisms, both intracellular (arrows) and extracellular, as cysts and individual trophozoites. × 110.

suspicion of malignant lymphoma exists after a trial of antitoxoplasma drugs.

Results and complications

Sites of biopsy are listed in Table 4.1 (Apuzzo et al 1987a). Of these biopsies, 69% were performed in the supratentorial space, 25.8% in the thalamus or midbrain, 4.2% in the cerebellum and 1% at the pontomedullary junction.

The variety of pathological diagnoses obtained during stereotactic biopsy is shown in Table 4.2 (Apuzzo et al 1987a). As expected, the largest group was neoplastic (70%), followed by infectious processes (17.8%), vascular (6.2%), nondiagnostic (4.4%) and miscellaneous (1.6%).

A failed diagnosis was given in 4.4% of our cases, the most common finding being necrosis or a chronic inflammatory process. This is similar to results obtained in other reports (Pecker et al 1979, Bosch 1980, Ostertag et al 1980, Lunsford 1988, Kelly 1991). Quite often a missed diagnosis occurs because the selected target was in the necrotic centre of a tumor or the enhancing area was missed. Careful preoperative study of the images and double dose contrast medium administration with delayed scan can obviate these difficulties. Multiple targets may need to be selected, and the procedure should continue until the pathologist has received an adequate specimen. A potentially difficult diagnosis must be discussed with the pathologist so that special tissue handling procedures may be used for further studies.

In our experience at USC (Table 4.3), only one death as a result of biopsy has occurred. This resulted from the diagnosis of a cavernous angioma which was not noted preoperatively. Seven haemorrhages had occurred which required surgical evacuation. Three haematomas occurred at the target site (two melanomas, one

Table 4.1 Target mass location

Location	Percentage
Centrum, basal ganglia	56.8
Para-third ventricle	27.8
Temporal lobe	6.8
Third ventricle	5.0
Pineal region	4.4
Lateral ventricle	2.8
Thalamus, midbrain	25.8
Cerebellar	4.2
Pontomedullary	1.0

Table 4.2 Pathological entities obtained at biopsy

Type	Percentage
Neoplastic	70.0
Anaplastic astrocytoma	
Astrocytoma	
Glioblastoma multiforme	
Metastatic carcinoma	
Ependymoma	
Oligodendroglioma	
Meningioma	
Lymphoma	
Germinoma	
Primitive neuroectodermal tumour	
Pituitary adenoma	
Craniopharyngioma	
Dermoid	
Teratoma	
Pineocytoma	
Ganglioglioma	
Pineoblastoma	
Infectious	17.8
Bacterial abscess	
Cysticercosis	
Toxoplasma abscess	
Herpes encephalitis	
Tuberculous abscess	
Tuberculous granuloma	
Coccidioidomycosis abscess	
Vascular	6.2
Haematoma	
Infarction	
Cavernous angioma	
Thrombosed arterioventricular malformation	
Nondiagnostic	4.4
Inflammation	
Gliosis	
Necrosis	
Granuloma	
Miscellaneous	1.6
Colloid cyst	
radionecrosis	

glioma); three were acute subdural haematomas; one was an epidural haematoma which occurred because the drill stop was not employed. No permanent neurological sequelae have resulted. There have been three transient focal seizures observed during transit of the probe and two generalized seizures. In all cases, rapid control was achieved by intravenous medication. Two infections have been observed. One was a superficial scalp infection following a burr hole biopsy, and the other was a subgaleal abscess after multiple catheters were inserted.

Specific considerations for complication avoidance

Application of the base ring

The presence of pin artefact on the CT scan is potentially disastrous as accurate targeting is precluded. Shaving the entire head allows the surgeon to examine the contours of the skull in relation to the projection of the lesion on coronal and sagittal MRI. This can direct pin placement so as to avoid artefacts. In addition, the pins must not be placed too close to the vertex as this may result in rostral ring migration.

Entry point, transit and target determination

In general, the anterior two-thirds of the cerebrum, centrum semiovale, basal ganglia, thalamus and brain stem may be acquired through the pericoronal entry. The posterior third of the cerebrum, the pineal region and temporal targets are approached via a superior parieto-occipital entry.

Targets from cortical and subcortical regions carry increased risk because of vascularity and should be avoided if possible. Biopsy from cyst or ventricular walls also increases the risk of haemorrhage because of the absence of a tamponade effect from surrounding brain and anticoagulant effects of cerebrospinal or cyst fluid on blood. Lesions at the frontal and temporal poles carry risk because tethering draining veins may tear if there is torsion of the pole during the biopsy. Finally, Sylvian and peri-Sylvian areas are dangerous because of vascularity (Fig. 4.9).

Of equal importance to selection of entry point and target is the technique used for cranial

Table 4.3 Complications associated with biopsy (USC experience)

Type		Total number
Death		1
Haemorrhage (symptomatic)		7
Acute subdural	3	
Melanoma	2	
Glioma	1	
Epidural	1	
Seizure		5
Focal	3	
Generalized	2	
Scalp infection		2

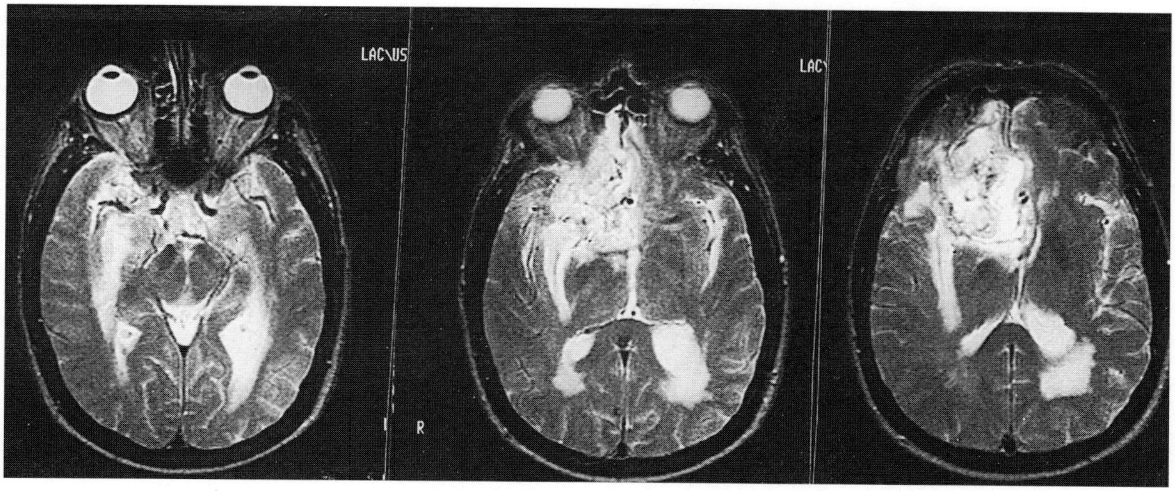

Fig. 4.9 A large, infiltrating mass in the right inferior frontal and Sylvian region is seen on T_2 weighted MRI. A right control entry point is preferred with specimens taken from the posterior aspect of the frontal portion away from the insula.

perforation. A perpendicular entry is performed as drilling on an angulated surface carries the risk of drill migration and stripping of underlying dura. Use of the twist drill requires that the underlying subarachnoid space be minimal to avoid injury to cortical draining veins (Fig. 4.10). When there is cortical atrophy and a generous subarachnoid space a burr hole is safer because the site of cortical entry is performed under direct vision (Fig. 4.11).

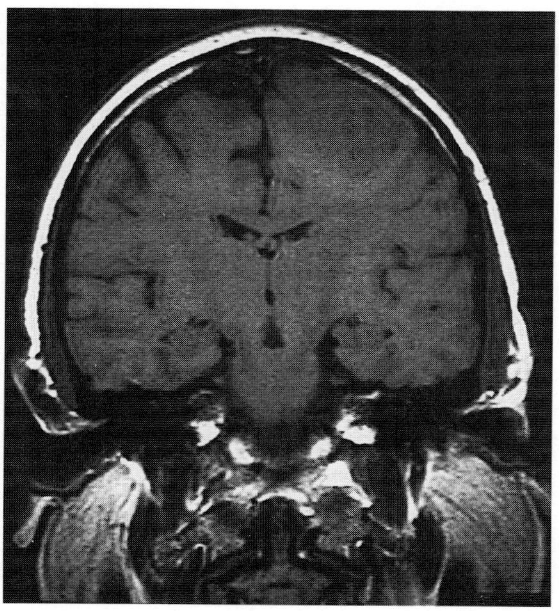

Fig. 4.10 A large, hypodense mass on T_1 MRI is shown infiltrating the left parasagittal cortical and subcortical area. Mass effect from the lesion has obliterated the overlying subarachnoid space. A twist drill entry directly over the mass is performed with biopsies taken from the centre.

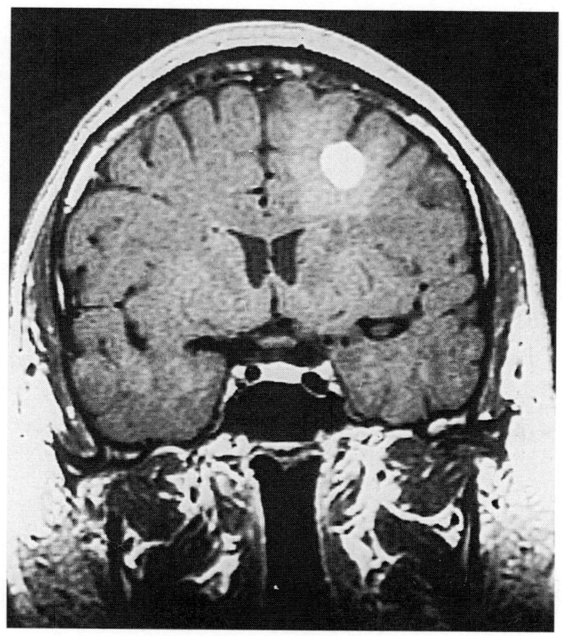

Fig. 4.11 A round enhancing lesion on T_1 MRI is present at the cortical–subcortical interface in the depths of a sulcus. A burr hole entry should be made over the lesion and the cortical entry performed under direct vision.

CONCLUSION

Image directed stereotactic biopsy of brain lesions is an effective and minimally invasive diagnostic method. Strategies have been evolved which maximize the precision of histological diagnosis and minimize the surgical complication rate. The principal target sites for which the method is indicated are those which are deep and otherwise inaccessible; however, any intracranial region is technically approachable in this way.

REFERENCES

Apuzzo M L J, Sabshin J K 1983 Computed tomographic guidance stereotaxis in the management of intracranial mass lesions. Neurosurgery 12: 277–285

Apuzzo MLJ, Heifetz MD, Weiss MH, Kurze T 1977 Neurosurgical endoscopy using the side viewing telescope: Technical note. Neurosurgery 46: 398–400

Apuzzo M L J, Chandrasoma P T, Zelman V et al 1984a Computed tomographic guidance stereotaxis in the management of lesions of the third ventricular region. Neurosurgery 15: 502–508

Apuzzo M L J, Chandrasoma P T, Cohen D et al 1987a Computed imaging stereotaxy: experience and perspective related to 500 procedures applied to brain masses. Neurosurgery 20: 930–937

Apuzzo M L J, Chandrasoma P T, Zelman V, et al 1987b Applications of stereotaxis. In: Apuzzo M L J (ed) Surgery of the third ventricle. Williams and Wilkins, Baltimore pp 751–792.

Backlund E O, Granberg P O, Hamberger B 1985 Transplantation of adrenal medullary tissue to striatum in parkinsonism. Journal of Neurosugery 62: 169–173

Bosch D A 1980 Indications for stereotactic biopsy in brain tumors. Acta Neurochirurgica (Wien) 54: 167–179

Bradley W G, Waluch V, Yadley R et al 1984 Comparison of CT and MR in 400 patients with suspected disease of the brain and cervical spinal cord. Radiology 152: 69–72

Bradley W G, Waluch V, Lai K et al 1987 Appearance of rapidly flowing blood on magnetic resonance imaging. American Journal of Roentgenology 143: 167–174

Brandt-Zawadzki M, Davis P L, Crooks L E et al 1983 NMR demonstration of cerebral abnormalities: comparison with CT. American Journal of Roentgenology 140: 847–854

Brandt-Zawadzki M, Berry I, Osaki L et al 1986 Gd-DTPA in clinical MR of the brain: 1. Intra-axial lesions. American Journal of Neuroradiology 7: 1–78

Burger P C 1990 Classification, grading and patterns of spread of malignant gliomas. In: Apuzzo M L J (ed) Malignant cerebral glioma. American Association of Neurological Surgeons, Illinois, pp. 3–18.

Chandrasoma P T, Apuzzo M L J 1989 Stereotactic brain biopsy. Igakushoin, New York, pp. 65–185.

Couldwell W T, Apuzzo M L J 1990 Initial experiences related to the use of the Cosman–Roberts–Wells stereotactic instrument. Journal of Neurosurgery 72: 145–148

Daumas-Duport C, Scheithauer B W, O'Fallon J et al 1988 Grading of astrocytomas: a simple and reproducible method. Cancer 62: 2152–2165

Fulling K H, Nelson J S 1984 Cerebral astrocytic neoplasms in the adult: contribution of histological examination to the assessment of prognosis. Seminars in Diagnostic Pathology 1: 152–163

Gomon J M, Grossman R L, Goldberg H L et al 1986 Occult cerebral vascular malformations: high field MR imaging. Radiology 158: 707–717

Gutin P H, Phillips T L, Wara W M et al 1984 Brachytherapy of malignant brain tumors with removable high activity iodine-125 sources. Journal of Neurosurgery 60: 61–68

Healy M E, Hesselink J R, Press G A et al 1987 Increased detection of intracranial metastases using intravenous gadolinium-DTPA. Radiology 165: 619–624

Heilbrun M P 1983 Computed tomography-guided stereotactic systems. Clinical Neurosurgery 31: 564–580

Heilbrun M P, Roberts T S, Apuzzo M L J et al 1983 Preliminary experience with Brown–Roberts–Wells computerized tomographic stereotaxic guidance system. Journal of Neurosurgery 59: 217–222

Iizuka J 1975 Development of stereotaxic endoscopy of the ventricular system. Confinia Neurologica 37: 141–149

Kelly P 1991 Stereotactic biopsy procedures. In: Kelly P (ed) Tumor stereotaxis. W B Saunders, Philadelphia, pp. 183–223.

Kelly P J, Kall B A, Goerss S G 1984 Computer-assisted stereotactic biopsies utilizing CT and digitized arteriographic control. Acta Neurochirurgica (Wien) 33S: 233–235

Krachoke S, Cosgrove M, Chandrasoma P T 1988 Granulomatous inflammation in pineal germinoma: a cause of diagnostic failure at stereotaxic brain biopsy. American Journal of Surgical Pathology 12: 655–660

Kucharcyzk W, Lemme-Pleghos L, Uske A et al 1989 Intracranial vascular malformations: MR and CT imaging. Radiology 156: 383–386

Liwnicz B H., Henderson K S, Masukawa T et al 1982 Needle aspiration cytology of intracranial lesions. Acta Cytologica 26: 779–786

Lunsford L D 1988 Diagnosis and treatment of mass lesions using the Leksell stereotactic system. In: Lunsford L D (ed) Modern stereotactic neurosurgery. Martinus Nijhoff, Boston, pp 145–168

Mattle H P, O'Reilly G V, Edelman R R et al 1990 Brain: spontaneous hemorrhage. In: Edelman R R, Hesselink J R (eds) Clinical magnetic resonance imaging. W B Saunders, Philadelphia, 483–515

Menick B, Atlas S W, Bobman S A 1990 High resolution DFr steady state MR imaging of the brain: clinical assessment. Presented at the Annual Meeting and Scientific Assembly of the Radiological Society of North America, Chicago

Moriquand C, Benabid A L, Breyton M 1987 Stereotaxic cytology of brain tumors: review of an eight year experience. Acta Cytologica 31: 756–764

Ostertag C B 1988 Reliability of stereotactic brain tumor biopsy. In: Lunsford L D (ed) Modern stereotactic neurosurgery. Martinus Nijhoff, Boston, pp 129–136

Ostertag C B, Mennel H D, Kiessling M 1980 Stereotactic biopsy of brain tumors. Surgical Neurology 14: 275–283

Ostertag C B, Volk B, Shibata T et al 1987 The monoclonal antibody Ki-67 as a marker for proliferating cells in stereotactic biopsies of brain tumors. Acta Neurochirurgica 89: 117–121

Pecker J, Scarabin J M, Vallee B et al 1979 Treatment of tumours of the pineal region: value of stereotactic biopsy. Surgical Neurology 12: 341–348

Ringertz N 1950 Grading of gliomas. Acta Pathologica, Microbiologica et Imunologica Scandinavica 27: 51–64

Rivas J J, Lobato R D 1985 CT-assisted stereotaxic aspiration of colloid cysts of the third ventricle. Journal of Neurosurgery 62: 238–242

Sasaki K, Matsumura K, Tsuji T et al 1988 Relationship between labeling indices of Ki-67 and BrdUrd in human malignant tumors. Cancer 62: 989–993

Scheithauer B W 1984 Neuropathology of pineal region tumors. Clinical Neurosurgery 32: 351–383

Sugita K, Matsuga N, Takoaka Y et al 1975 Stereotaxic exploration of para-third ventricle tumors. Confinia Neurologica 37: 156–162

Tung H, Giannotta S L, Chandrasoma P T et al 1990 Recurrent parenchymal hemorrhages from angiographically occult vascular malformations. Journal of Neurosurgery 73: 174–180

Von Schulthess G K, Higgins C B 1985 Blood flow imaging with MR: Spin-phase phenomena. Radiology 157: 687–695

Willems J G M S, Alva-Willems J M 1984 Accuracy of cytologic diagnosis of central nervous system neoplasms in stereotactic biopsies. Acta Cytologica 28: 243–248

Zee C S, Segall H D, Apuzzo M L J et al 1991 MR imaging of pineal region neoplasms. Journal of Computer Assisted Tomography 15: 56–61

5. Prognostic value of histopathology in stereotactic biopsy

T. Revesz F. Scaravilli

INTRODUCTION

Management of brain tumours depends crucially on histological diagnosis. It is now technically possible, with low morbidity, to obtain biopsy material by image directed surgery from any brain region. This is a recent development and formerly the hazards of surgical biopsy were thought to justify management purely on the basis of clinical and neuroradiological diagnoses. Thus, in 1966 Cheek & Taveras came to the conclusion in their study on thalamic tumours that successful treatment of these neoplasms could be achieved by radiotherapy, after a 'presumptive' diagnosis had been established exclusively by radiological means. A similar approach, which avoided cerebral biopsy, had previously been advocated by Posner & Horrax (1946) and Ward & Spurling (1948). One flaw of this method of treatment is that radiological investigations sometimes fail to establish the correct diagnosis, thus making it difficult to apply the most appropriate treatment. Neurosurgeons generally treat malignant cerebral gliomas by extensive removal of the tumour with histological examination followed by radiotherapy (Taveras et al 1962, Hitchcock & Sato 1964, Pool & Kamrin 1966, Jelsma & Bucy 1967, Wilson & Hoshino 1969, Marshall et al 1974, Posner & Shapiro 1975, Winger et al 1989, Nazzaro & Neuwelt 1990). However, in a number of cases this technique cannot be used either because the poor general condition of the patients or the localization of the neoplasm would entail unacceptable operative risk (Hallac & Bakay 1963, Hitchcock & Sato 1964, Marshall et al 1974). Under these circumstances different methods were obviously required, which would be accompanied by low morbidity and mortality. These new techniques included the free hand and stereotactic needle biopsies (Shetter et al 1977). With the former, a biopsy needle is manually directed towards a preselected target, sometimes under radiographic or fluoroscopic control through a standard trephination or a drill hole.

Stereotactic, non-computerized tomography directed, biopsies usually required the use of intraventricular contrast media. Superimposing the images on plain X-ray films a convenient target-to-film distance (usually 3 m) was used in order to avoid significant magnification (Conway 1973). Comparison of free hand and stereotactic biopsies (Shetter et al 1977) showed that the latter technique had undeniable advantages over the former. These included the rigid fixation of the skull, stable probe guidance and more accurate location of the tip of the needle, with consequent reduction of the average number of specimens required to achieve diagnosis. In addition, this technique reduced the risk of both temporary and permanent neurological complications, especially haemorrhage and brain swelling.

In the last two decades significant progress has been made in the field of radiological imaging techniques, including computerized tomography (CT) and magnetic resonance imaging (MRI). The combination of these methods and neurosurgical techniques applying new and more advanced stereotactic devices form the basis of image guided stereotactic cerebral biopsies (Apuzzo & Sabshin 1983, Heilbrun et al 1983, Kelly et al 1984, 1985, Apuzzo et al 1987). This new method of brain biopsy allows the neurosurgeon to sample virtually any intracerebral lesion, regardless of its size and location (Lunsford & Martinez 1984).

CT directed stereotactic procedures may be performed for one or more reasons: for diagnosis, treatment (e.g. implantation of a radioactive or chemotherapeutic agent), or decompression of a cyst.

The reliability and validity of the image directed biopsy is emphasized by reports from several institutions (Lobato et al 1982, Apuzzo & Sabshin 1983, De Divitiis et al 1983, Heilbrun et al 1983, Scerrati & Rossi 1984, Kelly et al 1985, 1987a, b, Ostertag 1988, Colbassani et al 1988, Chandrasoma et al 1989, Nakamine et al 1989). A successful diagnosis in 90–97% of cases with low mortality (0–3%) was reported. More recent investigations (Lunsford & Martinez 1984, Greene et al 1989) further confirmed the high diagnostic yield of the method. A further advantage is that CT directed stereotactic biopsy allows the pathologist to investigate several specimens from different regions of the same lesion. Indeed, it is quite common for a pathologist to receive from five to eight or even more specimens from a single biopsy. On the other hand, the limited size of the samples (up to 12 mm in length and 1 mm in diameter before fixation) often poses problems. The question arises, too, of how well the tissue samples represent the disease process investigated. Even a difference of a few millimetres between the calculated and the actual targets can result in major differences in the histological appearances of the tissue samples.

HISTOLOGICAL FINDINGS IN A CLINICAL SERIES OF IMAGE DIRECTED STEREOTACTIC BIOPSIES

Patients and neuropathological methods

Data from 419 image guided stereotactic brain biopsies at The National Hospitals for Neurology and Neurosurgery, Queen Square and Maida Vale, London, between 1981 and 1989 inclusive, were reviewed. Of these, 290 cases, carried out between 1981 and 1988, were included in the present study. The neurosurgical procedure applied has been described elsewhere (Bradford & Thomas 1990, Pell & Thomas 1991). In all cases one or more lesions had been demonstrated neuroradiologically before operation and the leading differential diagnosis was of brain tumour.

At operation several tissue samples from different targets (from 2 to 14) were taken for histological examination; in our institution the average size of a specimen was 10 x 1.0 mm. Each sample was laid on a histological slide and put in a separate Petri dish, quickly covered by the lid to avoid evaporation. The Petri dishes, labelled with the necessary information about the target biopsied, were quickly transferred to the neuropathological department for rapid examination. For the intraoperative diagnosis, smears were prepared from small selected fragments and stained with 1% toluidine blue and/or haematoxylin and eosin (McMenemey 1960, Marshall et al 1973, Barnard 1974, Adams et al 1981). The number of smears made varied from case to case. The general rule was that as soon as an intraoperative diagnosis had been made, all remaining samples were immersed in 10% buffered formalin and processed for embedding in paraffin wax.

On rare occasions small fragments of one or more specimens were placed in 3% glutaraldehyde and processed for electron microscopy.

Paraffin sections 4 μm in thickness were stained with routine and, where necessary, immunohistochemical methods. The histological slides were carefully labelled to provide information about the stereotactic source.

Whenever possible, the histological diagnosis of glial tumours also included numerical grading. The guideline of the World Health Organization's latest histological classification of tumours of the central nervous system (Zülch 1979, Barnard 1982) were generally followed, but some modifications were also taken into consideration (Russell & Rubinstein 1989). A standard four tier grading system, based on Kernohan's classification (Kernohan et al 1949), was implemented. This takes into account the main morphological features of gliomas, principally cellular density, pleomorphism, mitotic activity, the presence of necrosis and vascular proliferation.

The clinical history, including postoperative treatment, relapses and final outcome, was reviewed from the hospital notes. In some of the cases no follow-up information was found, and letters were sent to the referring hospitals and/or the general practitioners. In some cases where the patients died several years before the present study, and information could not be obtained from either the hospital files or the general practitioners, an attempt was made to get the follow-up data from the Family Practitioners' Committee, where the clinical records are usually stored for a few years after a patient's death.

In this study a group of 31 gliomas of varying malignancy, often posing diagnostic difficulties, was selected for study with the monoclonal antibody (PC10) that was raised against the 'proliferating cell nuclear antigen' (PCNA) (Bravo & McDonald-Bravo 1987, Waseem & Lane 1990). This antibody differs from Ki-67 in its ability to react in formalin fixed, paraffin embedded sections. The aim of this study, in part, was to assess the value of this immunohistochemical method in the small samples provided by the stereotactic biopsy technique. In each case five fields with the highest labelling indices were selected. Using x400 magnification and applying an ocular grid, both labelled and unlabelled tumour cell nuclei were counted; the index finally obtained represented the ratio between the two populations of cells. The results obtained with the antibody were subsequently correlated with the histological diagnosis and follow-up information.

Data from the different groups of patients with gliomas were studied with statistical methods. Frequency distribution of age, follow-up, survival times and duration of preoperative symptoms were calculated in all subgroups of patients with glial tumours. The probability of survival in each subgroup was also assessed, and survival curves according to Kaplan & Meier (1958) were drawn. The data were analysed by the log rank test (Peto et al 1977), the two-sample t test, Student's t test and the Wilcoxon rank sum test.

Results

Sex and age

Between 1981 and 1988 290 consecutive patients with a radiologically apparent cerebral lesion had image guided stereotactic brain biopsy; 179 of them were male, 111 female. The mean age was 45.1 years; 49.9% of the patients were younger than 45 years and 14.1% were aged under 25 years. The age distribution is shown in Figure 5.1.

Localization

The lesions were localized in the following regions; supratentorial (251), brain stem (30), pineal gland (7) and cerebellum (2) (Tables 5.1 and 5.2). In the 150 cases with glial tumours where a sufficient amount of follow-up information was available (81% of all gliomas), the site of the tumour was studied in further detail, and is shown in Table 5.3. In 29 of these cases the tumour was deeply situated, affecting predominantly the thalamus, basal ganglia or hypothalamus. In another 11 cases of this group the lesion was located in the deep areas of one of the lobes, and in eight cases the glial tumour was in the brain stem.

Previous treatment

Most patients had not received any form of treatment before undergoing the CT directed stereotactic biopsy. In seven of them, however, there had been a previous neurosurgical, non-stereotactic operation with a diagnosis of low grade astrocytoma in six. In the seventh patient the earlier neurosurgical operation had been carried out to insert a shunt for normal pressure hydrocephalus. In this case the presumptive diagnosis before the second, stereotactic intervention was brain abscess.

Other data

In 10 patients the CT directed biopsy was later repeated, usually for a recurrent tumour, and in a further three cases the procedure was followed by another free hand biopsy.

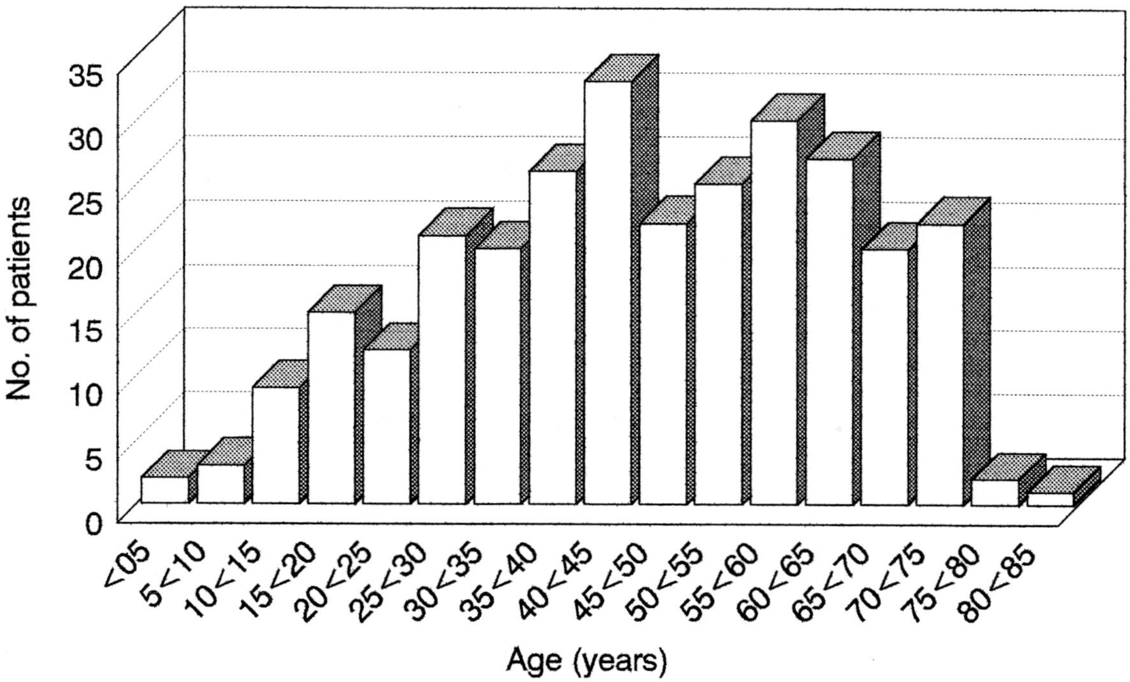

Fig. 5.1 Frequency distribution of age in 290 biopsies.

Morbidity and mortality

Three patients died within the first week, and 24 within the first month following the biopsy, most of the latter with very aggressive tumours.

Histological diagnosis

The histological diagnosis was established in 265 of the 290 cases (92%). In 78% a diagnosis of tumour was made. This group comprised 185 cases of glial tumour (63.7%), a few examples of which are illustrated in Figures 5.2–5.5. The glioma group also included 12 cases (4.1%) with the diagnosis of 'probable glioma', in which no attempt could be made to grade further the neolesions. Cerebral lymphoma (Fig. 5.6) was found in 11 cases (3.8%), while metastatic carcinoma and melanoma were diagnosed in 13 (4.5%) and one (0.3%) patients, respectively. In two cases (0.7%), owing to the limited size of the tissue sample, a malignant tumour was diagnosed, but we were unable to characterize it further. Tables 5.4 and 5.5 show the details of histological diagnosis in the 225 tumour cases. In the remaining cases either the presence of a tumour could not be confirmed histologically or a diagnosis was made of a non-neoplastic lesion (see also Table 5.6). 'No tumour' was the most frequent diagnosis in this group (25 cases, 8%). In 15 cases (5.2%) haemorrhage was present with or without evidence of a vascular malformation, eight of these were in the brain stem. 'Non-specific inflammatory changes' and 'encephalitis without specific features' were the diagnoses in nine cases (3.1%). In this series three patients suffering from the acquired immune deficiency syndrome (AIDS) underwent stereotactic biopsy. One of these patients had a cerebral lymphoma, another had progressive multifocal leukoencephalopathy (PML) and the biopsy of a third patient showed non-specific inflammatory changes only. PML was diagnosed in a further patient known to have been treated with immunosuppressive drugs. A few examples of non-neoplastic lesions are illustrated in Figures 5.7–5.9.

Histological diagnosis and follow-up information

The amount of information available was considered satisfactory in 222 cases (76.5% of all

Table 5.1 Localization of 225 tumours

	Hemisphere	Thalamus/ basal ganglia	Hypothalamus	Pineal gland	Brain stem	Cerebellum
Astrocytoma (low grade)	40	6	2	0	8	2
Astrocytoma (grade 3)	33	9	3	0	2	0
Glioblastoma	40	6	0	0	2	0
Oligodendroglioma	20	0	0	0	0	0
Probable glioma	8	2	2	0	0	0
Medulloblastoma	0	0	0	0	1	0
PNET	1	0	0	0	0	0
Pineoblastoma	0	0	0	2	0	0
Pineocytoma	0	0	0	1	0	0
Germinoma	0	0	2	2	0	0
Cerebral lymphoma	6	2	3	0	0	0
Meningioma	1	0	0	0	1	0
Epidermoid cyst	0	0	0	1	0	0
Craniopharyngioma	0	0	1	0	0	0
Metastatic carcinoma	10	1	0	0	2	0
Metastatic melanoma	1	0	0	0	0	0
Malignant tumour	1	0	0	1	0	0
Total	161	26	13	7	16	2

the biopsies). In 13 patients the results of a second brain biopsy, and in a further eight, autopsy findings were available. Of the 185 glioma cases, the proportion with adequate follow-up data was even higher (150 cases, 81% of all gliomas, Fig. 5.10). The descriptive statistical data of these 150 patients, including the mean age, the mean follow-up periods and the mean intervals between the first symptoms and the time of surgery are summarized in Table 5.7. In the low grade glioma group (51 patients) the mean age was 38.6 years; 17.6% of these patients were under the age of 20 years, 25% under the age of 30 years and 72.5% under the age of 45 years. In contrast, in the grade 3 astrocytoma (38 patients) and glioblastoma multiforme (36 patients) groups the mean age of the patients was 49.7 and 50.1 years, and the proportion of the patients under 45 years was 36.8 and 27.8% respectively. Data from two large groups consisting of grade 1 and 2 astrocytomas

Table 5.2 Localization of 65 non-neoplastic lesions

	Hemisphere	Thalamus/ basal ganglia	Hypothalamus	Pineal gland	Brain stem	Cerebellum
No tumour	21	1	1	0	2	0
Oedema	3	0	0	0	1	0
Non-specific inflammation	7	0	0	0	2	0
Tuberculosis	0	0	1	0	0	0
Sarcoidosis	0	0	1	0	1	0
PML	2	0	0	0	0	0
Demyelinating process	1	0	0	0	0	0
Radiation necrosis	1	0	0	0	0	0
Infarct	4	1	0	0	0	0
Haemorrhage, including malformations	5	2	0	0	8	0
Total	44	4	3	0	14	0

Table 5.3 Localization of 150 gliomas with follow-up information

	Astrocytoma (low grade)	Astrocytoma (grade 3)	Glioblastoma (grade 4)	Oligodendroglioma	Probable glioma
Frontal	21	5	6	10	3
Parietal	6	12	13	2	3
Temporal	6	8	7	2	0
Occipital	1	1	1	0	0
Corpus callosum	1	1	1	1	0
Thalamus/ basal ganglia	6	8	6	0	2
Hypothalamus	2	3	0	0	2
Brain stem	6	0	2	0	0
Cerebellum	2	0	0	0	0
Total	51	38	36	15	10

and grade 3 and 4 astrocytomas/glioblastomas, respectively, were analysed. With regard to age (Fig. 5.11), a statistically significant difference was found between the low grade and high grade glioma groups (p< 0.001, t test). Moreover, the length of preoperative symptoms and signs was considerably longer in the low grade astrocytoma group (21.2 and 5.9 months, respectively, p< 0.001, t test). In the low grade astrocytoma group, 62.7% of the patients with follow-up were alive at the time of the completion of our study (mean follow-up period 30 months). In this group there was only 5.5 years' difference in mean age between those who were dead (mean age 42.8 years) and those who were still alive (mean age 37.3 years, p< 0.1, t test). However, the mean follow-up period for patients who were dead at the time of the study was considerably shorter (12.3 months) than the mean follow-up time in the second group (40.3 months). In the grade 3 and 4 astrocytoma/glioblastoma groups none of the patients was alive at the time of our study (mean survival periods were 9.1 and 7.1 months, respectively). The mean duration of preoperative symptoms and signs was longer in the grade 3 astrocytoma group than in the grade 4 astrocytoma/glioblastoma group (8.4 v5 3.3 months, p< 0.05, t test). This difference appears to be accounted for by the inclusion in the former group of five patients whose symptoms lasted at least 1 year. Indeed, two of these patients had a previous, histologically confirmed low grade

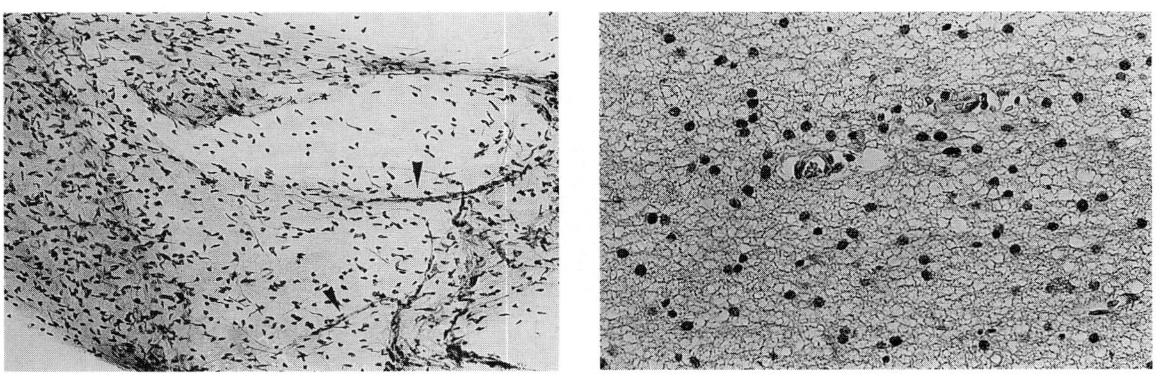

a **b**

Fig. 5.2 Photomicrographs of **a** smear preparation and **b** paraffin section of an occipital low grade astrocytoma. In **a** slender vessels are seen (arrowheads). In **b** tumour cells are loosely arranged in a fibrillary background. There is no significant pleomorphism and no mitotic figures are seen. **a**, toluidine blue (x 50); **b**, haematoxylin and eosin (x 210).

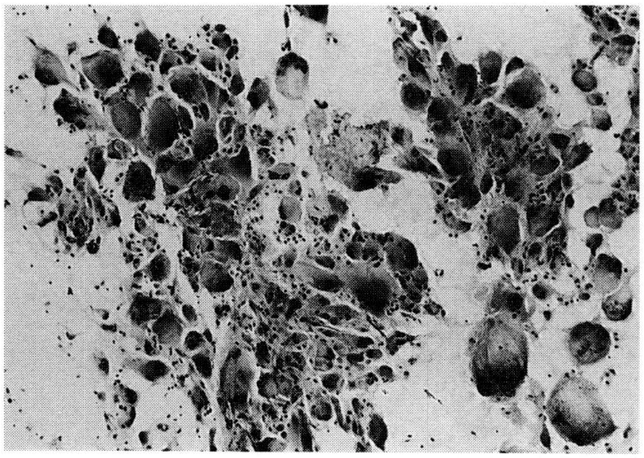

a

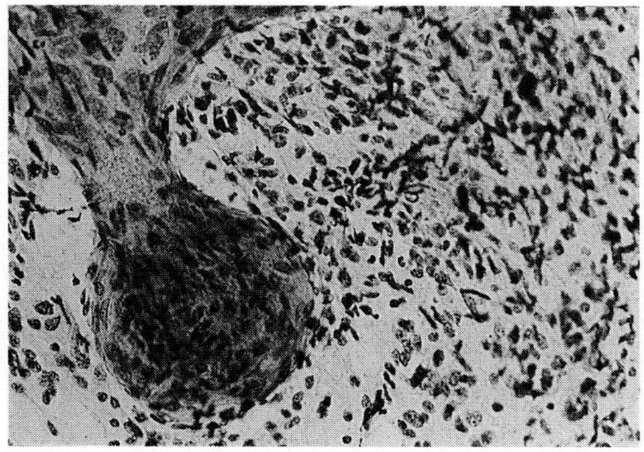

b

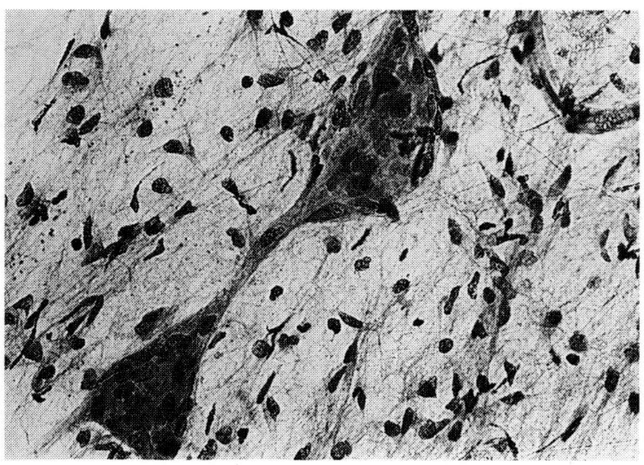

c

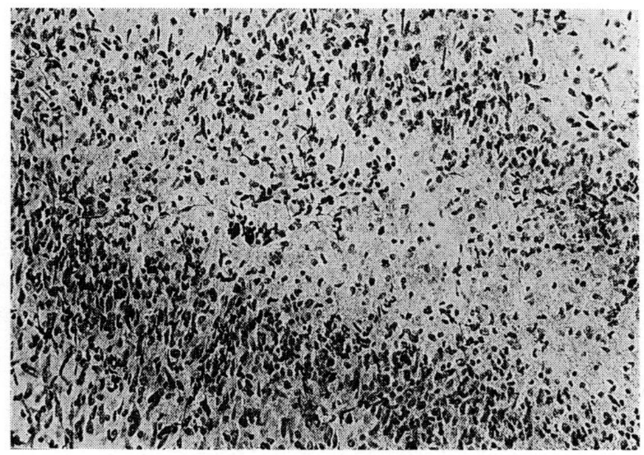

d

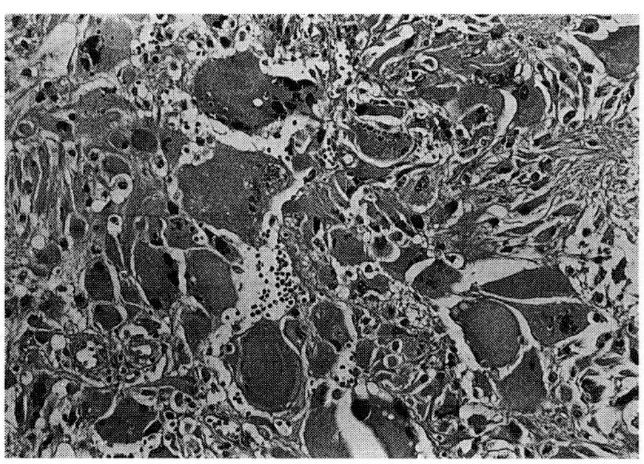

e

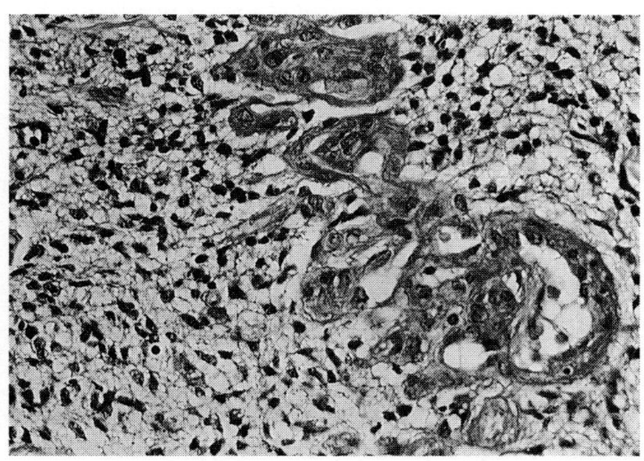

f

Fig. 5.3 **a–d** Smear preparations and **e, f** paraffin sections of gliomas showing various features suggestive of a high grade tumour. In **a** and **e** smear and paraffin section of the same tumour show considerable pleomorphism and large bizarre multinucleated tumour cells. In **d** the smear preparation shows a central area of necrosis surrounded by a palisade of viable tumour cells. Smear preparations (**b** and **c**) and paraffin section (**f**) show endothelial proliferation characteristic of high grade gliomas. **a,** toluidine blue (x 50); **b,** toluidine blue (x 260); **c,** toluidine blue (x 210); **d,** toluidine blue (x 105); **e,** haematoxylin and eosin (x 105); **f,** haematoxylin and eosin (x 210).

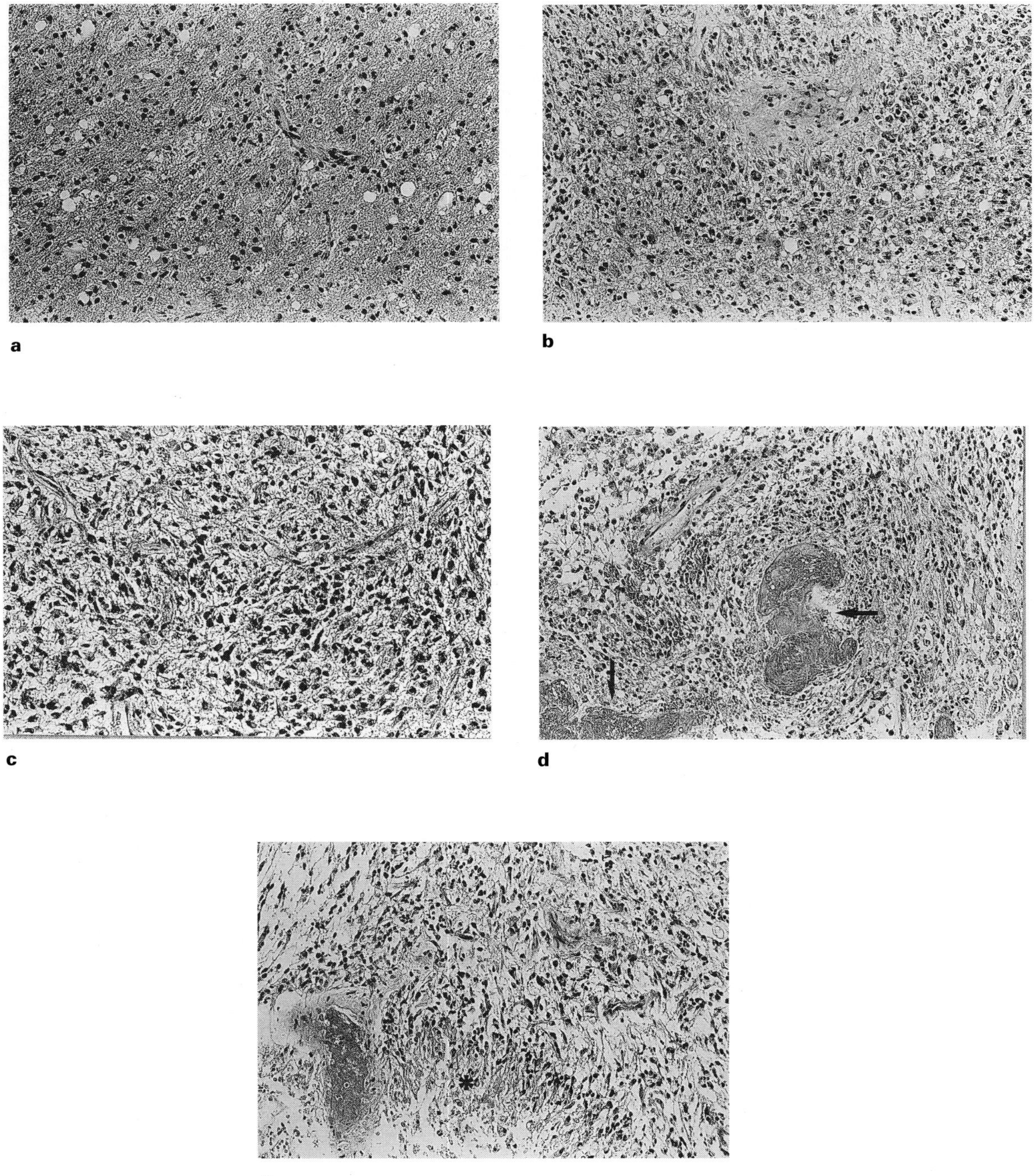

Fig. 5.4 **a–e** Photomicrographs of different targets removed from sequential regions at various distances from the centre of the tumour. The most peripheral sample (**a**) shows moderate cellularity and little pleomorphism. Nearer the centre there is increased cellularity (**b** and **c**), and other features of a glioblastoma, including large, thrombosed vessels (arrows, **d**) and necrosis are also seen (asterisk, **e**). **a–e**, haematoxylin and eosin (x 105).

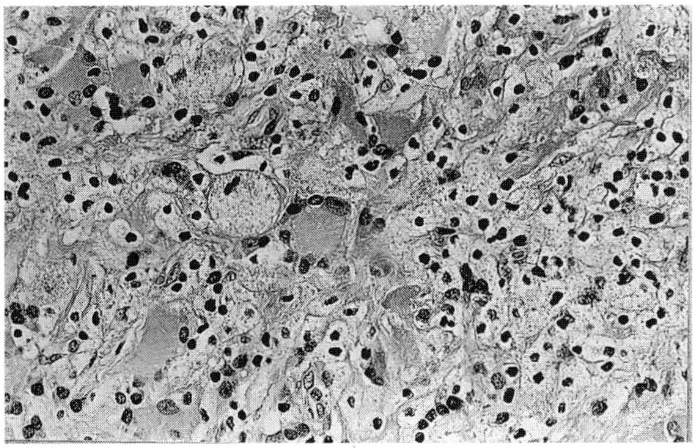

Fig. 5.5 Photomicrograph of a lipidized malignant glioma showing pleomorphic tumour cells, some of which are multinucleated and have foamy cytoplasm. Haematoxylin and eosin (x 210).

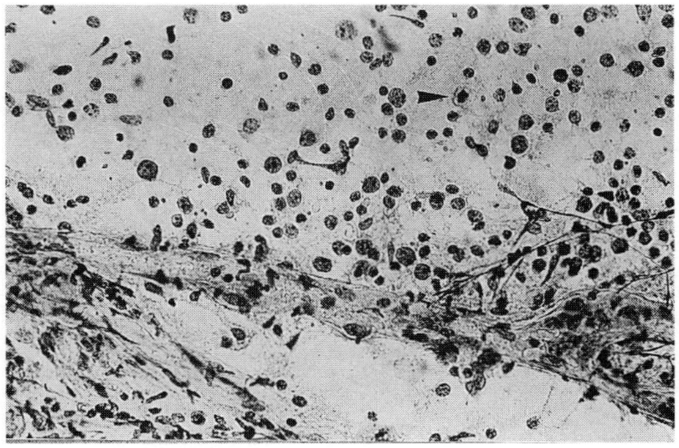

Fig. 5.6 Smear preparation showing a lymphoma consisting of a monolayer of round, moderately pleomorphic tumour cells. A mitosis is also seen (arrowhead). Toluidine blue (x 210).

astrocytoma and had presented with signs of relapse shortly before the stereotactic biopsy. In the oligodendroglioma and mixed oligoastrocytoma group (20 patients), 15 had adequate follow-up data. In these, both the duration of the preoperative symptoms and the postoperative follow-up periods were relatively long, the mean values being 30.3 and 43.4 months, respectively. The mean age of the patients in this group was 44.2 years; none of the patients was under 20 years of age, and more than 50% were aged between 35 and 45 years. In the heterogeneous group of 'probable gliomas' the mean age of the patients was 38.0 years, while the mean follow-up time and the length of the preoperative symptoms were 27.3 and 48.3 months, respectively.

Table 5.4 Histological diagnosis: Glial tumours[a]

	Number of cases	Percentage
Low grade astrocytoma	58	20.0
Grade 3 astrocytoma	47	16.2
Grade 4 astrocytoma/ Glioblast. m.	48	16.5
Oligodendroglioma	20	6.9
Probable glioma	12	4.1
Total	185	63.8

[a] For all biopsies n = 290 (100%); for all tumours n = 225 (77.6%).

Correlation between grading of gliomas and survival time

One of the main aims of our study was to test the value of the four tier grading system of gliomas in a situation where the diagnosis is based on limited amount of tissue. We therefore investigated how survival time, a general indicator of malignancy, correlated with the position given on our grading system. The analysis of survival probabilities showed no statistical difference between the grade 3 astrocytoma and the grade 4 astrocytoma/ glioblastoma multiforme groups on the Kernohan grading scale ($p < 0.5$, log rank test, Fig. 5.12). This analysis also showed that, on the basis of survival probabilities, a group comprising all cases of low grade astrocytomas (grades 1 and 2) could be convincingly separated from a single group of malignant gliomas consisting of all grade 3 and 4 cases. The difference between these two large groups with regard to survival probabilities was statistically significant ($p < 0.001$, log rank test). The survival curves of Kaplan & Meier (1958) in the low grade astrocytoma and the malignant glioma groups are demonstrated in Figure 5.13. The survival curve of the low grade astrocytomas strikingly demonstrates the presence of a group of patients with shorter survival times. Age strongly influenced outcome (Fig. 5.11). After survival analysis with stratifying for age had been carried out, the difference in survival time between the low grade and high grade groups

Table 5.5 Histological diagnosis: non-glial tumours[a]

	Number of cases	Percentage
Medulloblastoma	1	0.3
PNET	1	0.3
Pineoblastoma	2	0.7
Pineocytoma	1	0.3
Germinoma	4	1.4
Meningioma	2	0.7
Epidermoid cyst	1	0.3
Craniopharyngioma	1	0.3
Cerebral lymphoma	11	3.8
Metastatic carcinoma	13	4.5
Metastatic melanoma	1	0.3
Malignant tumour	2	0.7
Total	40	13.8

[a] For all biopsies n = 290 (100%); for all tumours n = 225 (77.6%).

Table 5.6 Histological diagnosis: non-neoplastic lesions or negative results[a]

	Number of cases	Percentage
No tumour	25	8.6
Infarct	5	1.7
Oedema	4	1.4
Non-specific inflammat. process	9	3.1
Tuberculosis	1	0.3
Haemorrhage, including malformations	15	5.2
Sarcoidosis	2	0.7
Radiation necrosis	1	0.3
PML	2	0.7
Demyelinating process	1	0.3
Total	65	22.4

[a] For all biopsies n = 290 (100%).

could still be detected ($p < 0.001$, log rank test), thus confirming that factors other than age influenced the final outcome. Localization of the tumour appeared to influence survival, but this was observed only in the low grade astrocytoma group. In cases in which the tumour was deep or was located in the brain stem the probability of survival was lower than in cases with a lobar neoplasm ($p < 0.03$, log rank test, Fig. 5.14). This trend could not be confirmed in the high grade glioma group ($p > 0.3$, log rank test, Fig. 5.15). Also, the presence or absence of necrosis did not have any influence on survival within the group of malignant gliomas ($p > 0.3$, log rank test, Fig. 5.1). More recent evaluation of the same cases with the Daumas-Duport grading scheme (Daumas-Duport et al 1988) shows that a different prognosis is found in grade 3 and 4 tumours.

Follow-up information in cases with a 'probable glioma' diagnosis

In this group, follow-up confirmed the presence of a glial tumour in 10 of the 12 (Table 5.9) cases. In three cases the image guided brain

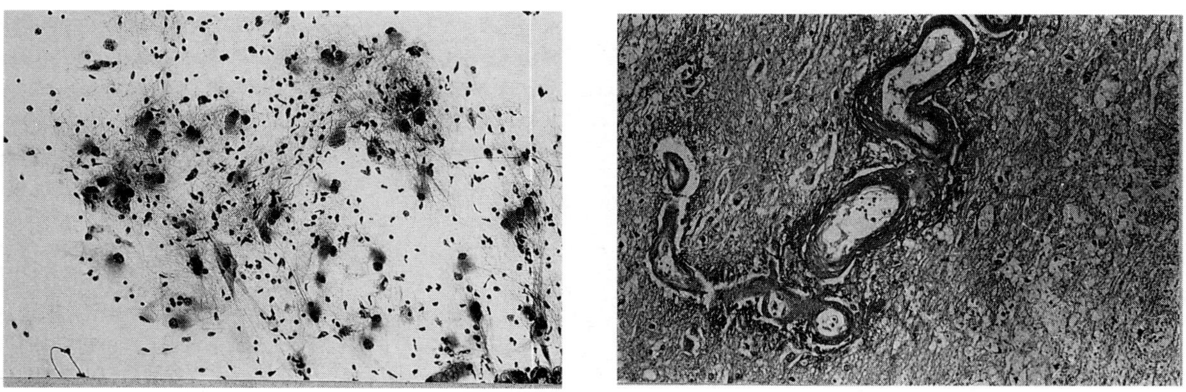

a **b**

Fig. 5.7 **a** Smear preparation and **b** paraffin section of an intracerebral mass. In **a** the presence of large astrocytes with abundant cytoplasm and numerous processes is suggestive of a reactive non-neoplastic process. **b** shows features of delayed effects of irradiation with fibrinoid degeneration of blood vessel walls, and sparse reactive astrocytes in the surrounding tissue. **a**, toluidine blue (x 210); **b**, haematoxylin and eosin (x 105).

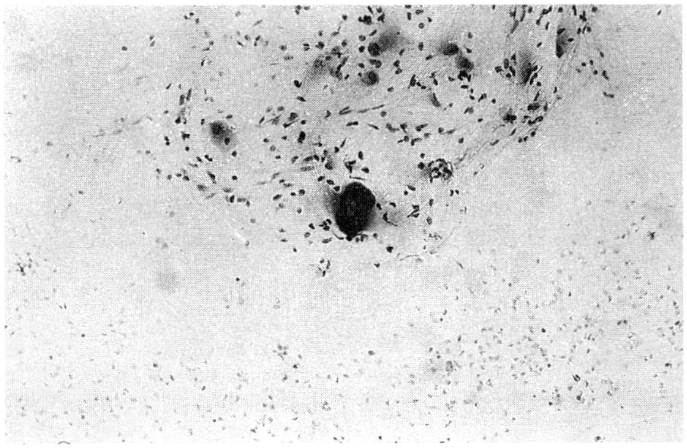

Fig. 5.8 Smear preparation showing a large bizarre astrocyte surrounded by others with the characteristics of 'reactive cells'. This appearance in smears is suggestive of PML. Toluidine blue (x 105).

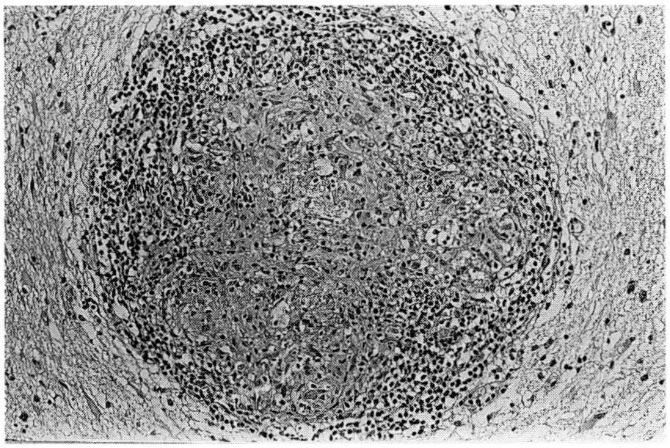

Fig. 5.9 Photomicrograph of a hypothalamic lesion showing a non-caseating (sarcoid) granuloma. Haematoxylin and eosin (x 105).

biopsy was followed by another neurosurgical intervention and the histological examination confirmed a low grade astrocytoma in two cases and a glioblastoma multiforme in one case. The postoperative clinical course was obviously that of a low grade astrocytoma in four cases, and that of a malignant glioma in two cases. No follow-up information was available for two patients.

Follow-up information in cases where a 'no tumour' diagnosis was established

The histological findings were non-contributory in a recurrent case in which a previous biopsy established the diagnosis of a glioma. A second image directed brain biopsy or a free hand biopsy showed a high grade glioma in three cases, and single cases of a low grade astrocytoma, a metastatic carcinoma and a metastatic carcinoid tumour. The subsequent clinical course confirmed a low grade astrocytoma in five cases, a malignant glioma in two patients (in one with post mortem confirmation), and a metastatic carcinoma with a known primary oat cell carcinoma in one case. In five cases the subsequent clinical course was not that of a brain tumour. No follow-up information was available in this group for five cases (Table 5.10).

Follow-up data in cases with a diagnosis of 'oedema'

This diagnosis was given in four cases, in all of which follow-up data were available. In two cases, the subsequent clinical course confirmed the presence of a brain tumour: low grade glioma in one and lymphoblastic lymphoma with cerebral deposits in another. The information in the third case suggested focal encephalitis; in the fourth, a demyelinating condition (Table 5.8).

Follow-up data in cases with a diagnosis of 'infarct'

In two of the cases the diagnosis of an infarct was mistakenly given. The lipid laden cells seen in the first biopsy were interpreted as foamy macrophages. In this case a second, non-stereotactic biopsy revealed that this process was in fact a lipidized glioma (see Fig. 5.5). In the second case the diagnosis of an infarct clearly resulted from surgical sampling error, being based on the presence of necrotic tissue, foamy macrophages and reactive astrocytes. Post mortem investigation disclosed a cerebral lymphoma.

Value of smear preparations

In the vast majority of the cases with a tumour (225 biopsies) the diagnosis was based on both the smear preparations and on paraffin wax embedded sections (some cases are illustrated in

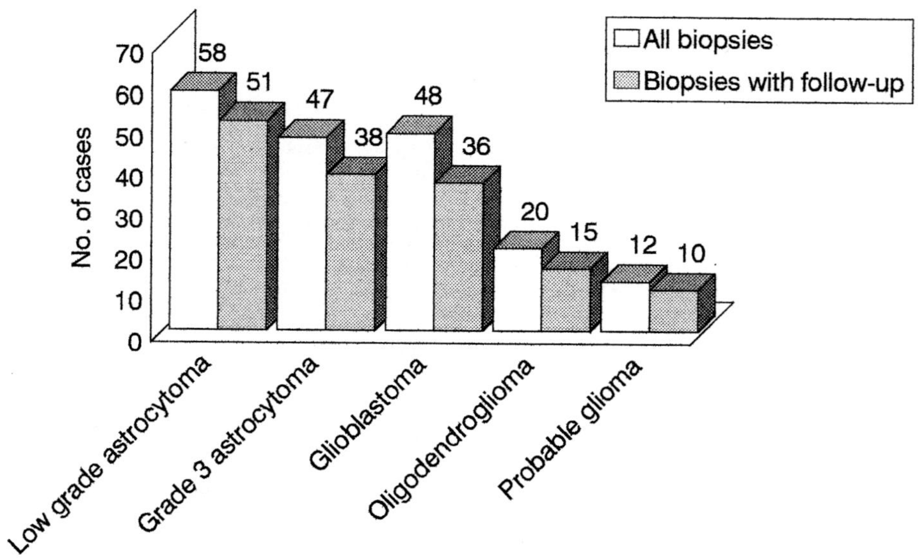

Fig. 5.10 Bar chart demonstrating the proportion of gliomas with adequate follow-up information.

Figures 5.2, 5.3 and 5.6–5.8. However, in a proportion of cases, the amount of tissue was sufficient only for smear preparations (12 cases) and, consequently, the diagnosis was based entirely on the appearances of the smears. In a small number of cases (three cases) the definitive sections did not confirm the diagnosis suggested by the smear preparation. In one of these the intraoperative diagnosis was of an oligodendroglioma, and the definitive sections showed an adenocarcinoma. In the second case the histological appearances of the definitive sections were consistent with a cerebral lymphoma, while the smear appearances (a large number of pleomorphic astrocytic cells were present) had been suggestive of a glioma. In the third case the intraoperative diagnosis was of glioblastoma multiforme, but the definitive sections disclosed an anaplastic carcinoma. In 18 cases the diagnosis at the time of surgery was uncertain. This involved the differential diagnosis between low grade glioma and reactive astrogliosis, or astrocytoma or oligodendroglioma, and also uncertainties regarding the grade of the tumour.

Table 5.7 Gliomas with follow-up information: statistical data of patients[a]

	Mean age (years)	Follow-up time (months)	Duration of preoperative signs (months)
Low grade glioma	38.6	30	21.2
Grade 3 astrocytoma	49.7	9.1	8.4
Grade 4 glioma	50.1	7.1	3.3
Oligodendroglioma	44.2	43.4	30.3
Probable glioma	38.0	27.3	48.3

[a] n = 150 (81% of all gliomas).

PCNA study

Of 31 cases investigated, 16 were originally diagnosed as low grade astrocytoma, four cases as grade 3 astrocytoma and 11 as grade 4 astrocytoma or glioblastoma multiforme. The labelling indices observed in the three groups ranged from 0 to 35.6% (mean 6.41%, standard deviation 9.49%) in the low grade, from 2.9 to 13% (mean 7.75%, standard deviation 4.46%) in the grade 3 astrocytoma, and from 8.7 to 69% (mean 26.46%, standard deviation 24.4%) in the grade 4 astrocytoma and glioblastoma multiforme groups (Fig. 5.1). It is important to note that three patients in the low grade astrocytoma group, whose tumours exhibited a high labelling index (up to 35.6%), died shortly

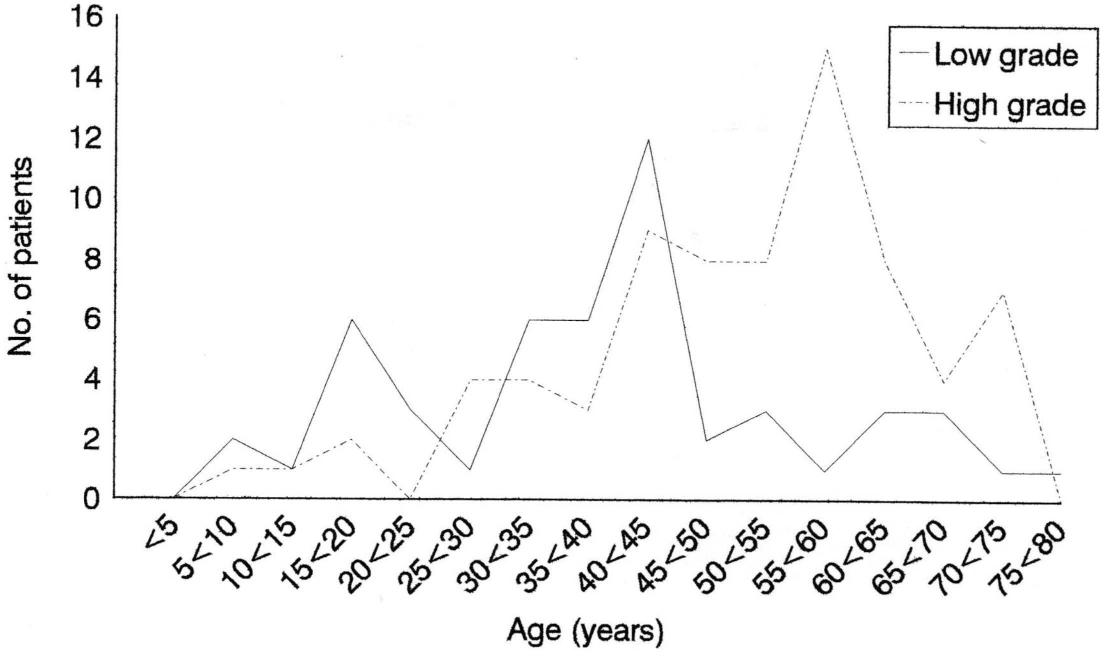

Fig. 5.11 Patients with low grade astrocytoma were significantly younger than those with high grade glioma (t test, $p < 0.001$).

after the biopsy (from 3.5 to 8 months). These three cases were responsible for the high standard deviation of the low grade group. Statistical analysis showed that the difference obtained between the values of labelling indices from the low grade astrocytoma group and a common group of grade 3 and 4 tumours was statistically significant ($p < 0.01$, Student's t test).

Summary

Image guided, stereotactic brain biopsies have become routine diagnostic procedures with high target accuracy, high diagnostic yield, and low morbidity and mortality (Ostertag et al 1980, Apuzzo et al 1984, Kelly et al 1984, Apuzzo et al 1987). In addition, they represent the method of choice for sampling deep lesions that hitherto had been inaccessible for conventional neurosurgical procedures (Apuzzo et al 1984, Kelly et al 1985, Coffey et al 1988, Frank et al 1988, Franzini et al 1988, Giunta et al 1988, Thomas et al 1988, Kelly 1989).

In our current series of 290 biopsies a definitive histological diagnosis was made in 265 cases (92%). In a small proportion of cases, however, the microscopical appearances were either non-specific or normal, and no certain diagnosis could be established. The proportion of this latter group is slightly higher in our material than in some of the other series in which non-diagnostic biopsies are mentioned (Ostertag et al 1980, Apuzzo et al 1987, Lunsford 1988).

In the current study the diagnosis was usually based on both smears and paraffin embedded sections. Smears are, in our opinion, superior to frozen sections, since they can be carried out using only a small portion of the specimen, allowing the remainder to be embedded in paraffin wax. Smears can be prepared easily and quickly, and their diagnostic accuracy, both in stereotactic and non-stereotactic biopsies, is estimated to be around 90% (Marshall et al 1973, Ostertag et al 1980, Kleihues et al 1984, Willems & Alva-Willems 1984). The value of the smear preparations is confirmed in our material, where diagnostic error was made in three cases (1.0%), and discrepancies between the smear and the definitive diagnosis, mainly related to tumour grading, or the type of the tumour, were found in

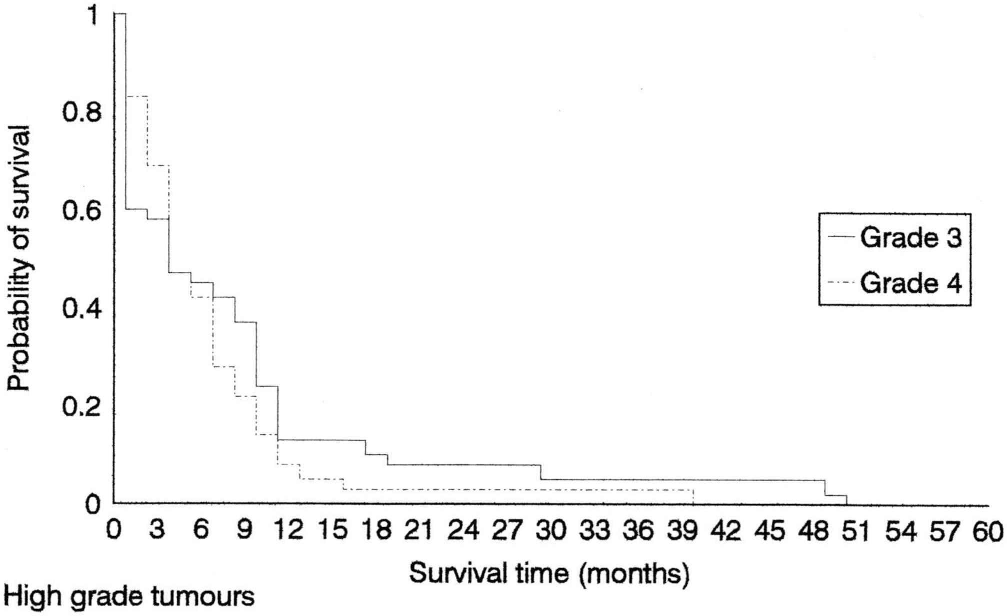

Fig. 5.12 Survival curves of patient groups with grade 3 and grade 4 astrocytic gliomas showed no difference in survival probabilities (log rank test, $p < 0.5$).

another 18 (6.2%). In the series of Kleihues et al (1984) a similar relatively small disparity between diagnosis on smears and paraffin sections is found. One of the difficulties in the interpretation of the smear preparations is to distinguish reactive astroglia from infiltrating glial tumour cells. Reactive gliosis can accompany a wide variety of brain lesions, including gliomas, metastases, lymphomas, haematomas and infarcts. The use of glutaraldehyde fixed and haemalum–phloxine stained paraffin sections, and haemalum–phloxine stained smears, has been recommended by Daumas-Duport et al (1987) as a useful means of differentiating reactive from neoplastic glia.

The diagnosis of tumour was made in the majority of biopsies in the current series (225 cases, 77.6% of all the biopsies).

Gliomas were found to form the single largest group not only of all the tumours (82.2%), but also of all the biopsies (63.8%). The proportion of neoplasms varies in different series according to the number of non-neoplastic lesions included (Ostertag et al 1980, Apuzzo et al 1987, Colbassani et al 1988, Friedman et al 1989). Among the tumours, low grade astrocytomas formed a significant proportion (20% of all biopsies and 31.3% of all gliomas). Low grade astrocytomas are known to be found in higher numbers in stereotactic series (Kleihues et al 1984, Ostertag 1980) than in non-stereotactic biopsies, autopsy or epidemiological series (Green et al 1976, Schoenberg et al 1976, McKeran and Thomas 1980, Poirier et al 1985). It is interesting that oligodendrogliomas and mixed oligoastrocytomas were also more frequently encountered in our series. Kelly et al (1987a) also reported a higher proportion of these tumours among a selected series of gliomas diagnosed by stereotactic biopsy, but this has not been reported by others (Ostertag et al 1980, Kleihues et al 1984, Apuzzo et al 1987, Friedman et al 1989). The explanation for the higher incidence of oligodendroglial tumours in some of the more recent series remains uncertain.

In our material the majority of the primary brain tumours of neuroectodermal origin were examples of the astrocytic series. There were no ependymomas, and some other rare tumours, such as pleomorphic xanthoastrocytoma, are also

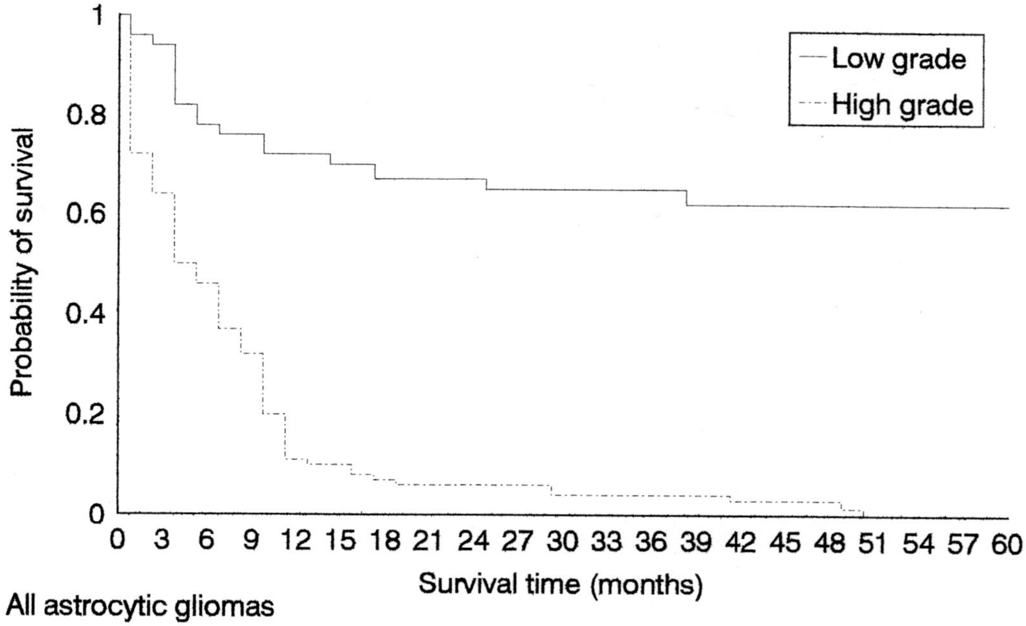

Fig. 5.13 Survival curves showing significant difference in probability of survival between the two large groups of patients with low or high grade gliomas (log rank test, $p < 0.001$).

not represented. The proportion of metastatic carcinomas was 4.5% (5.8% of all tumours) in the current material. Neurosurgical series are generally known to have a lower incidence of metastatic neoplasms, usually from 4 to 8% (Green et al 1976, Zülch 1986), than autopsy series, which give figures of 20–25% or even higher (Zimmerman 1969, Green et al 1976, Poirier et al 1985).

Cerebral lymphoma was found in 3.8% of all the biopsies (4.9% of all the tumours), all of them being of B cell origin and one case occurring in association with AIDS. In other stereotactic series, lymphomas constitute 0.5–15% of all the tumours (Bosch 1980, Kleihues et al 1984, Kelly et al 1985, Davis et al 1987, Lunsford 1988, Feiden et al 1990). It is important to note that cerebral lymphomas may show considerable reduction in size on the CT scan with regressive tissue changes histologically if the biopsies are taken during corticosteroid therapy (Feiden et al 1990, Geppert et al 1990).

Since the histological diagnosis of stereotactic biopsies is based only on a limited amount of tissue, and the numerical grading systems applied in the diagnosis of gliomas are based on, and have been mainly tested by, studies using non-stereotactic biopsies (Nelson et al 1983, Burger et al 1985), it is important for the pathologist to establish the validity of the histological diagnoses made. In our series, follow-up data were available in 150 of 185 gliomas, and their subsequent clinical course confirmed this. In addition, it is important to note that in this material a basic distinction between low grade and high grade astrocytic tumours could be made. These results also underline that a clear and convincing separation of grade 2 and grade 3 astrocytic tumours can be achieved by Kernohan grading. A more detailed grading by this system, however, could not be justified in this material. Cohadon et al (1985) came to a similar conclusion with regard to a two tier grading system in their large series of gliomas, where diagnosis was based in most of the cases on stereotactic biopsy material. However, reanalysis of the authors' material by the grading system of Daumas-Duport et al (1988) does show a significant difference in survival between grades 3 and 4 (unpublished data). This finding supports those who criticize the Kernohan approach as inadequate to describe tumour progression (Nelson et al 1983, Burger et al 1985). In fact,

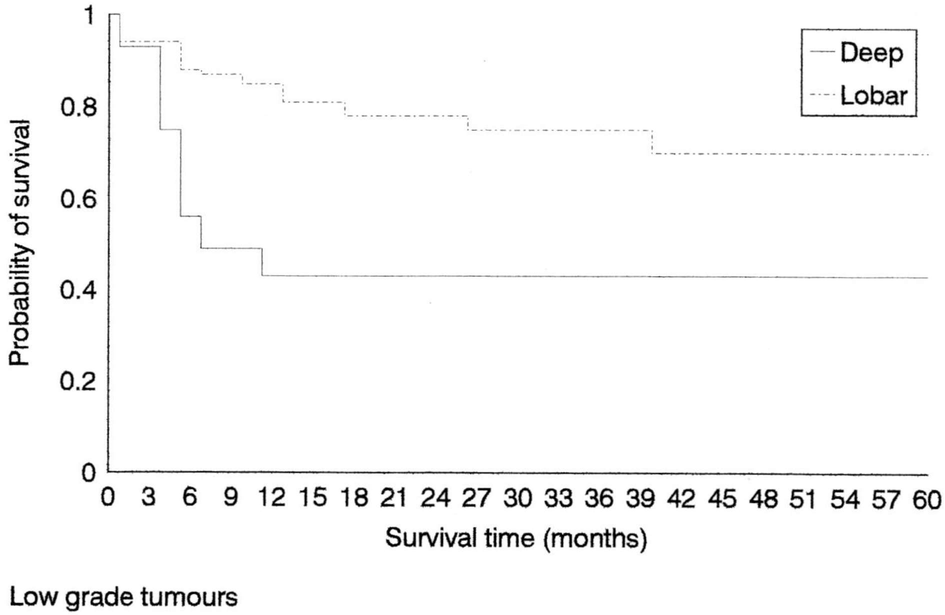

Fig. 5.14 Survial curves showing that patients with deeply seated low grade astrocytoma had lower survival probabilities than those with more superficial tumours (log rank test p> 0.02).

using the Kernohan grading system, two main groups emerge in which there are relatively minor differences between grades 1 and 2 on the one hand, and grades 3 and 4 on the other (Rubinstein personal communication). The probability of survival in our low grade glioma group (72% at 1 year and 61.9% at 5 years) is comparable to that described by others (Hoshino 1984, Cohadon et al 1985). However, the survival probabilities (64%, 46%, 11% and 5.5% at 3, 6, 12, and 24 months, respectively) observed in the high grade glioma group are lower than those given by other series in which the diagnoses were based on stereotactic biopsies (Cohadon et al 1985, Coffey et al 1988). However, the current series is rather selective, consisting of cases collected in a referral centre. We have confirmed that age is an important factor, but is not exclusive in influencing survival in patients with an astrocytic glioma (Nelson et al 1983, Burger et al 1985, 1987). When similar cases of stereotactic biopsy are analysed using the Daumas-Duport grading, the survival probabilities of grade 3 cases are 52, 37 and 2.3% at 12, 24 and 48 months, respectively, while at the same time intervals the probabilities for grade 4 cases are 10, 4 and 2%, respectively.

Our overall success rate of diagnosing gliomas and also grading them in most of the cases, was 92%. This relatively high diagnostic yield is likely to have resulted from the histological examination of multiple samples taken from different stereotactic targets (Daumas-Duport et al 1987, Greene et al 1989). This approach appears to be valuable as it provides tissue samples from the main areas of malignant gliomas, described as the hypodense centre, hyperdense margin and hypodense periphery on CT scans with contrast enhancement (Kelly et al 1987a, Greene et al 1989). Indeed, Greene et al (1989) showed that in cases of previously untreated malignant gliomas a correct diagnosis could be most consistently achieved if tissue samples were taken from areas seen as the hypodense centre and enhancing margin on the CT scan, while in the recurrent cases there was a tendency for the hypodense periphery to provide better material. The work of the latter authors also suggested that tumour could be identified up to 10 and 15 mm outside the enhancing margin in untreated and recurrent gliomas, respectively. Burger et al (1988) by comparing whole brain histological sections with radiological images of

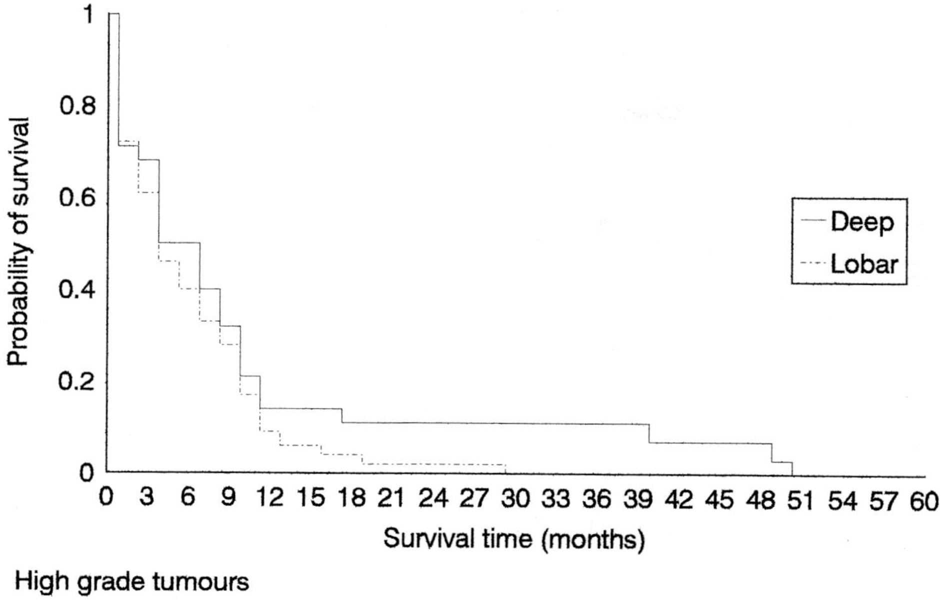

Fig. 5.15 In the high grade glioma group the localization of tumour did not influence survival (log rank test p> 0.3).

CT scans, demonstrated tumour distribution and spread in cases of untreated glioblastoma. This study showed that contrast enhancement on the CT scan, a feature considered to be directly related to the degree of neovascularization in high grade gliomas (Kelly et al 1987b), corresponded to the viable, densely cellular areas on histological sections. However, the extent of tumour spread, determined in vivo by the edges of the perifocal low density area on the CT scans, varied considerably on the histological sections. Indeed, malignant gliomas may extend far beyond the limits of the low density area seen on the CT scan, and isolated tumour cells may infiltrate even beyond the outer edge of the 'oedematous zone' defined by T_2 weighted MRI scans (Kelly et al 1987a, Lunsford 1988, Johnson et al 1989). For this reason, gliomas often appear to be more extensive on histological section than are widely believed (Barnard and Geddes 1987). These findings further emphasize the importance of looking at serial stereotactic biopsy specimens in order to be able to assess the extent of tumour cell infiltration, and to delineate the boundaries of gliomas (Thomas et al 1985, Daumas-Duport et al 1987, Parkins et al 1991).

It is important to note that follow-up information gave us the diagnosis of glial or non-glial tumour in 18 cases (6.2%) originally diagnosed as 'no tumour', 'oedema' or 'infarct'. In the 'probable glioma' group no attempt was originally made at grading (12 cases, 4.1% of all biopsies). Follow-up information, available in 10 cases, confirmed the presence of a low grade or malignant glioma in all of them. Kleihues et al (1984) found that in 4.5% of their biopsies a glioma was diagnosed but no grading could be attempted. These authors also investigated the accuracy and reliability of their diagnoses in 87 tumour cases (out of 600) by follow-up or autopsy. In their series, diagnostic discrepancies were encountered in 11 cases and, of these, five were obviously due to sampling error. In a

Table 5.8 Follow-up information in four cases with 'oedema' diagnosis[a]

Clinical course of glioma	1
Clinical course of lymphoma	1
Clinical course of encephalitis	1
Clinical course of demyelination	1

[a] Number of cases with 'oedema' diagnosis: 4.

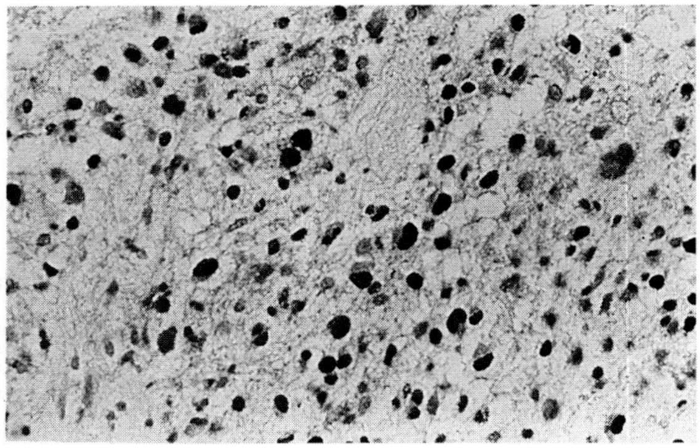

Fig. 5.16 Photomicrograph of a paraffin section immunostained with PC10 (PCNA antibody). A large proportion of the nuclei react with the antibody and appear homogeneously dark (x 210).

further three cases the follow-up revealed a higher grade of malignancy, but it was questionable whether this was the result of sampling error or tumour progression. In the remaining three cases the discrepancy was the result of a diagnostic error due to limited sample size. Chandrasoma et al (1989) reported 30 patients whose cerebral mass lesions were biopsied by a CT guided stereotactic technique, and who later underwent resection of the mass. In this study the histological diagnosis was appropriate for the direction of clinical management in 28 of the 30 cases. However, correlation between the stereotactic and resection diagnoses was exact in 19 cases only. In nine cases the correlation was imperfect, but this did not have significant clinical impact. Serious diagnostic error occurred in a case of pineal germinoma, in which large areas of granulomatous inflammation were biopsied. Of the 68 cases studied by Scerrati and Rossi (1984), out of 68 cases stereotactic surgery was followed by a craniotomy and removal of the tumour in 14 patients, and the tumour was studied after post mortem in a further five cases. The comparison of the follow-up data with the original histological diagnosis confirmed the value of the stereotactic biopsies in all but one case.

One of the main aims of histological numerical grading of gliomas is to assess malignancy and suggest the appropriate therapy. In addition to conventional histology, the implementation of newer, supplementary immunohistochemical and

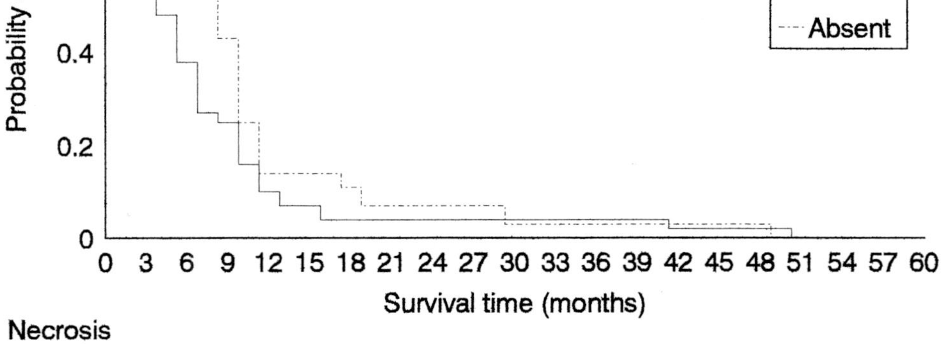

Fig. 5.17 Patients with high grade glioma without necrosis did not have better survival probabilities than those whose tumour showed necrosis (log rank test p> 0.3).

Table 5.9 Follow-up information in 10 cases with 'probable glioma' diagnosis[a]

Low grade astrocytoma on new biopsy	2
High grade glioma on new biopsy	1
Previously biopsied glioma	1
Clinical course of low grade astrocytoma	4
Clinical course of high grade glioma	2

[a] Number of cases with 'probable glioma' diagnosis: 12.

molecular biological techniques can help to characterize the proliferative capacity of gliomas (Libermann et al 1985, Bigner et al 1988, Humphrey et al 1988). Increased vimentin expression and decreased glial fibrillary acidic protein immunoreactivity have been found in high grade gliomas (Yoshimine et al 1987), but this tendency appears to be rather vague. Immunohistochemical detection of other antigens, such as the epidermal growth factor receptor (Bigner et al 1988, Reifenberger et al 1989), protein kinase C (Wechsler & Reifenberger 1989), somatostatin receptors (Reubi et al 1987), α-1-antitrypsin (Sawaya et al 1987) and plasminogen activator (Sawaya & Highsmith 1988) may have relevance in grading of gliomas. Immunohistochemical demonstration of tumour cell nuclei in the S phase of the cell cycle, by the bromodeoxyuridine (BUdR) method, is often used in cell kinetic studies (Hoshino et al 1985, 1989, Germano et al 1989, Morimura et al 1989). The BUdR index has been found to correlate with clinical survival as well as with histological features, such as necrosis and vascular proliferation (Germano et al 1989, Hoshino et al 1989). Immunostaining for antigens, supposed to be markers of proliferating cells, appear to be of considerable practical importance. The monoclonal antibody Ki-67 is raised against a nuclear antigen expressed in all phases of the cell cycle except G_0. It has been found in association with the DNA matrix and is expressed by proliferating human cells (Gerdes et al 1984). It is likely that a relationship exists between proliferation index (the fraction of labelled cells compared to all tumour cells) and histological diagnosis and numerical grade in human tumours, including gliomas (Burger et al 1986, Giangaspero et al 1987, Ostertag et al 1987, Deckert et al 1989, Böker et al 1990). Ki-67 immunoreactivity in glioblastoma multiforme has been shown to have striking intratumoural heterogeneity, and caution should be used in interpreting the results of this immunostain, especially when they are used as prognostic criteria (Deckert et al 1989, Parkins et al 1991). A further limiting factor in the application of the Ki-67 immunostain is that it can be used only on frozen sections. A recently introduced antibody (PC10) raised against the PCNA, may be of potential use in investigating cell proliferation in gliomas. PCNA staining has been shown to be localized at the intranuclear sites, where DNA synthesis is taking place (Bravo & McDonald-Bravo 1987, Waseem & Lane 1990). This method has the advantage over the Ki-67 immunostain that it can be used on formalin fixed and paraffin embedded material, thus allowing retrospective studies. Our own preliminary results suggest that this antibody may be useful in the assessment of the proliferative capacity of gliomas.

Although the number of inflammatory conditions in our series is relatively small (14 cases), our conclusion is that stereotactic biopsy is of limited value only in their diagnosis. This limitation is due to the fact that the small amount of tissue available may not contain specific elements, such as granulomas or fibrinoid necrosis of the vessel walls that may allow a certain diagnosis to be made. One of the exceptions to this rule appears to be the biopsies carried out in AIDS. Although this group of patients can suffer from a large variety of neurological conditions (Gray et al 1988),

Table 5.10 Follow-up information in 20 cases with 'no tumour' diagnosis[a]

High grade glioma on new biopsy	3
Low grade glioma on new biopsy	1
Carcinoma on new biopsy	1
Carcinoid on new biopsy	1
Previously biopsied glioma	1
Clinical course of low grade astrocytoma	5
Clinical course of high grade glioma	2
Clinical course of oat cell primary	1
Clinical data do not confirm tumour	5
Total	20

[a] Number of cases with 'no tumour' diagnosis: 25.

biopsies are usually required to establish the differential diagnosis between the two commonest types of space occupying lesions, toxoplasmosis and cerebral lymphoma. Both smear preparations and paraffin sections may provide valuable information, and can help to establish the diagnosis. In the case of toxoplasmosis, both smears and paraffin sections may show cysts containing the parasite, and lymphomas can be diagnosed by the presence of the characteristic lymphoid tumour cells. In addition to these two conditions, PML is also commonly diagnosed. PML can be recognized on smears by the presence of the large 'tumour-like' astrocytes. The diagnosis is further helped by the demonstration of the virus by electron microscopy and/or immunohistochemical and molecular biological techniques.

CONCLUSION

In a large series of stereotactic biopsies the histological investigation of specimens was found to provide valuable information about the nature of a variety of lesions. The predictive value of the small biopsies was found to be good in glial tumours, and the separation of low grade and high grade astrocytic neoplasms was possible. This finding is supported by the data provided by survival analysis.

REFERENCES

Adams J H, Graham D I, Doyle D 1981 Brain Biopsy. The smear technique for neurosurgical biopsies. Chapman and Hall, London.

Apuzzo M L J, Sabshin J K 1983 Computed tomographic guidance stereotaxis in the management of intracranial mass lesions. Neurosurgery 12: 277–285

Apuzzo M L J, Chandrasoma P T, Zelman V, Gianotta S L, Weiss M H 1984 Computed tomographic guidance stereotaxis in the management of lesions of the third ventricular region. Neurosurgery 15: 502–508

Apuzzo M L J, Chandrasoma P T, Cohen D, Zee C S, Zelman V 1987 Computed imaging stereotaxy: experience and perspective related to 500 procedures applied to brain masses. Neurosurgery 20: 930–937

Barnard R O 1974 Tumour biopsy in brain tumour. In: Vinken P J, Bruyn B W (eds) Handbook of clinical neurology, North-Holland, Amsterdam, pp 708–726

Barnard R O 1982 The classification of tumours of the central nervous system. Neuropathology and Applied Neurobiology 8: 1–10

Barnard R O, Geddes J F 1987 The incidence of multifocal cerebral gliomas. A histologic study of large hemisphere sections. Cancer 60: 1519–1531

Bigner S H, Burger P C, Wong A J, Werner M H, Hamilton S R, Muhlbaier L H 1988 Gene amplification in malignant human gliomas: clinical and histopathologic aspects. Journal of Neuropathology and Experimental Neurology 47: 191–205

Bosch D A 1980 Indications for stereotactic biopsy in brain tumours. Acta Neurochirurgica 54: 167–179

Böker D K, Stark H J, Gullotta F, Nadstawek J, Schultheiss R 1990 Immunohistochemical demonstration of the Ki-67 antigen in paraffin-embedded tumor biopsies. Clinical Neuropathology 9: 51–54

Bradford R, Thomas D G T 1990 Advances in surgery for malignant brain tumour. In: Thomas D G T (ed) Neuro-oncology, Edward Arnold, London, pp 148–163

Bravo R, MacDonald-Bravo H 1987 Existence of two populations of cyclin/proliferating cell nuclear antigen during the cell cycle: association with DNA replication sites. Journal of Cell Biology 105: 1549–1554

Burger P C Green S B 1987 Patient age, histologic features, and length of survival in patients with glioblastoma multiforme. Cancer 59: 1617–1625

Burger P C, Vogel F S, Green S B, Srike T A 1985 Glioblastoma multiforme and anaplastic astrocytoma. Pathologic criteria and prognostic implications. Cancer 56: 1106– 1111

Burger P C, Shibata T, Kleihues P 1986 The use of the monoclonal antibody Ki-67 in the identification of proliferating cells: application to surgical neuropathology. American Journal of Surgical Pathology 10: 611–617

Burger P C, Heinz E R, Shibata T, Kleihues P 1988 Topographic anatomy and CT correlations in the untreated glioblastoma multiforme. Journal of Neurosurgery 68: 698–704

Chandrasoma P T, Smith M M, Apuzzo M L J 1989 Stereotactic biopsy in the diagnosis of brain masses: comparison of results of biopsy and resected surgical specimen. Neurosurgery 24: 160–165

Cheek W R, Taveras J M 1966 Thalamic tumors. Journal of Neurosurgery 24: 505–513

Coffey R J, Lunsford L D, Taylor F H 1988 Survival after sterotactic biopsy of malignant gliomas. Neurosurgery 22: 465–473

Cohadon F, Aouad N, Rougier A, Vital C, Rivel J, Dartigues J F 1985 Histologic and non-histologic factors correlated with survival time in supratentorial astrocytic tumors. Journal of Neuro-oncology 3: 105–111

Colbassani H J, Nishio S, Sweeney K M, Bakay R A E, Takei Y 1988 CT-assisted stereotactic brain biopsy: value of intraoperative frozen section diagnosis. Journal of Neurology Neurosurgery and Psychiatry 51: 332–341

Conway L W 1973 Stereotaxic diagnosis and treatment of intracranial tumors including an initial experience with cryosurgery for pinealomas. Journal of Neurosurgery 38: 453–460

Daumas-Duport C, Sheithauer B W, Kelly P J 1987 A

histologic and cytologic method for the spatial definition of gliomas. Mayo Clinic Proceedings 62: 435–449
Daumas-Duport C, Sheithauer B, O'Fallon J, Kelly P 1988 Grading of astrocytomas; a simple and reproducible method. Cancer 62: 2152–2162
Davis D H, Kelly P J, Marsh W R, Kall B A, Goerss SJ 1987 Computer-assisted stereotactic biopsy of intracranial lesions Applied Neurophysiology 50: 172–177
De Divitiis E, Spaziante R, Cappabianca P, Caputi F, Pettinato G, Del Basso De Caro M 1983 Reliability of stereotactic biopsy. A model to test the value of diagnoses obtained from small fragments of nervous system tumours. Applied Neurophysiology 46: 295–303
Deckert M, Reifenberger G, Wechsler W 1989 Determination of the proliferative potential of human brain tumors using the monoclonal antibody Ki-67. Journal of Cancer Research and Clinical Oncology 115: 179–188
Feiden W, Bise K, Steude U 1990 Diagnosis of primary cerebral lymphoma with particular reference to CT-guided stereotactic biopsy. Virchows Archiv. A, Pathological Anatomy and Histopathology 417: 21–28
Frank F, Fabrizi A P, Frank-Ricci R, Gaist G, Sedan R, Peragut J C 1988 Stereotactic biopsy and treatment of brain stem lesions: combined study of 33 cases (Bologna-Marseille). Acta Neurochirurgica (suppl) 42: 177–181
Franzini A, Allegranza A, Melcarne A, Giorgi C, Ferraresi S, Broggi G 1988 Serial stereotactic biopsy of brain stem expanding lesions. Considerations of 45 consecutive cases. Acta Neurochirurgica (suppl) 42: 170–176
Friedman W A, Sceats D J, Nestok B R, Ballinger W E 1989 The incidence of unexpected pathological findings in an image-guided biopsy series: a review of 100 consecutive cases. Neurosurgery 25: 180–184
Geppert M, Ostertag C B, Seitz G, Kiessling M 1990 Glucocorticoid therapy obscures the diagnosis of cerebral lymphoma. Acta Neuropathologica 80: 629–634
Gerdes J, Lemke H, Baisch H, Wacker H H, Schwab U, Stein H 1984 Cell cycle analysis of a cell proliferation-associated human nuclear antigen defined by the monoclonal antibody Ki-67. Journal of Immunology 133: 1710–1715
Germano I M, Ito M, Cho K G, Hoshino T, Davis R L, Wilson C B 1989 Correlation of histopathological features and proliferative potential of gliomas. Journal of Neurosurgery 70: 701–706
Giangaspero F, Doglioni C, Rivano M T, Fileri S, Gerdes J, Stein H 1987 Growth fraction in human brain tumors defined by the monoclonal antibody Ki-67. Acta Neuropathologica 74: 179 –182
Giunta F, Marini G, Grasso G, Zorzi F 1988 Brain stem expansive lesions: stereotactic biopsy for a better therapeutic approach. Acta Neurochirurgica (suppl) 42: 182–186
Gray F, Gherardi R, Scaravilli F 1988 The neuropathology of the acquired immune deficiency syndrome (AIDS). Brain 111: 245–266
Green J R, Waggener J D, Kriegsfeld B A 1976 Classification and incidence of neoplasms of the central nervous system. Advances in Neurology 15: 51–55
Greene G M, Hitchon P W, Schelper R L, Yuh W, Dyste G N 1989 Diagnostic yield in CT-guided stereotactic biopsy of gliomas. Journal of Neurosurgery 71: 494–497
Hallac I, Bakay L 1963 New instrument for brain biopsy. Journal of Neurosurgery 20: 529–530
Heilbrun M P, Roberts T S, Apuzzo M L J, Wells T H, Sabshin J K 1983 Preliminary experience with Brown–Roberts–Wells (BRW) computerized tomography stereotaxic guidance system. Journal of Neurosurgery 59: 217–222
Hitchcock E, Sato F 1964 Treatment of malignant gliomata. Journal of Neurosurgery 21: 497–505
Hoshino T 1984 A commentary on the biology and growth kinetics of low-grade and high-grade gliomas. Journal of Neurosurgery 61: 895–900
Hoshino T, Nagashima T, Murovic J, Levin E M, Levin V A, Rupp S M 1985 Cell kinetic studies of in situ human brain tumors with bromodeoxyuridine. Cytometry 6: 627–632
Hoshino T, Prados M, Wilson C B, Cho K G, Lee K S, Davis R L 1989 Prognostic implications of the bromodeoxyuridine labeling index of human gliomas. Journal of Neurosurgery 71: 335–341
Humphrey P A, Wong A J, Vogelstein B, Friedman H S, Werner M H, Bigner D D, Bigner S H 1988 Amplification and expression of the epidermal growth factor receptor gene in human glioma xenografts. Cancer Research 48: 2231–2238
Jelsma R, Bucy P C 1967 The treatment of glioblastoma multiforme of the brain. Journal of Neurosurgery 27: 388–400
Johnson P C, Hunt S J, Drayer B P 1989 Human cerebral gliomas: correlation of postmortem MR imaging and neuropathologic findings. Radiology 170: 211–217
Kaplan E L, Meier P 1958 Non-parametric estimation from incomplete observations. Journal of American Statistical Association 53: 457–481
Kelly P J 1989 Stereotactic biopsy and resection of thalamic astrocytomas. Neurosurgery 25: 185–195
Kelly P J, Alker G J, Kall B A, Goerss S 1984 Method of computed tomography based stereotactic biopsy with arteriographic control. Neurosurgery 14: 172–177
Kelly P J, Earnest F, Kall B A, Goerss S J, Scheithauer B 1985 Surgical options for patients with deep-seated brain tumors: computer-assisted stereotactic biopsy. Mayo Clinic Proceedings 60: 223–229
Kelly P J, Daumas-Duport C, Kispert D B, Kall B A, Scheithauer B W, Illig J J 1987a Imaging-based stereotaxic serial biopsies in untreated intracranial glial neoplasms. Journal of Neurosurgery 66: 865–874
Kelly P J, Daumas-Duport C, Scheithauer B W, Kall B A, Kispert D B 1987b Stereotactic histologic correlations of computed tomography — and magnetic resonance imaging — defined abnormalities in patients with glial neoplasms. Mayo Clinic Proceedings 62: 450–459
Kernohan J W, Mabon R F, Svien H J, Adson A W 1949 Symposium on a new and simplified concept of gliomas. A simplified classification of gliomas. Proceedings of the Staff Meetings of the Mayo Clinic 24: 71–75
Kleihues P, Volk B, Anagnostopoulos J, Kiessling M 1984 Morphologic evaluation of stereotactic brain tumour biopsies. Acta Neurochirurgica (suppl) 33: 171–181
Libermann T A, Nusbaum H R, Razon N, Kris R, Lax I, Soreq H, Whittle N, Waterfield M D, Ullrich A, Schlessinger J D 1985 Amplification, enhanced expression, and possible rearrangement of EGF receptor gene in primary human brain tumours of glial origin. Nature 313: 144–147
Lobato R D, Rivas J J, Roger R 1982 Stereotactic biopsy of brain lesions visualised with computed tomography. Applied Neurophysiology 45: 426–430

Lunsford L D 1988 Diagnosis and treatment of mass lesions using the Leksell stereotactic system. In Lunsford L D (ed) Modern stereotactic neurosurgery, Martinus Nijhoff, Boston, pp 145–168

Lunsford L D, Martinez A J 1984 Stereotactic exploration of the brain in the era of computed tomography. Surgical Neurology 22: 222–230

McKeran R O, Thomas D G T 1980 The clinical study of gliomas. In: Thomas D G T, Graham D I (eds) Brain tumours, Butterworth, London, pp 194–230

McMenemey W H 1960 An appraisal of smear-diagnosis in neurosurgery. American Journal of Clinical Pathology 33: 471–479

Marshall L F, Adams H, Doyle D, Graham D I 1973 The histological accuracy of the smear technique for neurosurgical biopsies. Journal of Neurosurgery 39: 82–88

Marshall L F, Jennett B, Langfitt T W 1974 Needle biopsy for the diagnosis of malignant glioma. Journal of the American Medical Association 228: 1417–1418

Morimura T, Kitz K, Budka H 1989 In situ analysis of cell kinetics in human brain tumors. A comparative immunocytochemical study of S phase cells by a new in vitro bromodeoxyuridine-labeling technique, and of proliferating pool cells by monoclonal antibody Ki-67. Acta Neuropathologica 77: 276–282

Nakamine H, Yokote H, Itakura T et al 1989 Non-Hodgkin's lymphoma involving the brain. Diagnostic usefulness of stereotactic needle biopsy in combination with paraffin-section immunohistochemistry. Acta Neuropathologica 78: 462–471

Nazzaro J M, Neuwelt E A 1990 The role of surgery in the management of supratentorial intermediate and high-grade astrocytomas in adults. Journal of Neurosurgery 73: 331–344

Nelson J S, Tsukada Y, Schoenfeld D, Fulling K, Lamarche J, Peress N 1983 Necrosis as a prognostic criterion in malignant supratentorial, astrocytic gliomas. Cancer 52: 550–554

Ostertag C B 1988 Reliability of stereotactic brain tumor biopsy. In Lunsford L D (ed) Modern stereotactic neurosurgery. Martinus Nijhoff, Boston, pp 129–136

Ostertag C B, Mennel H D, Kiessling M 1980 Stereotactic biopsy of brain tumors. Surgical Neurology 14: 275–283

Ostertag C B, Volk B, Shibita T, Burger P, Kleihues P 1987 The monoclonal antibody Ki-67 as a marker for proliferating cells in stereotactic biopsies of brain tumours. Acta Neurochirurgica 89: 117–121

Parkins C S, Darling J L, Gill S S, Revesz T, Thomas D G T 1991 Cell proliferation in serial biopsies through human malignant brain tumours: measurement using Ki67 antibody labelling. British Journal of Neurosurgery 5: 289–298

Pell M F, Thomas D G T 1991 The initial experience with the Cosman–Roberts–Wells stereotactic system. British Journal of Neurosurgery 5: 111–116

Peto R, Pike M G, Armitage P et al 1977 Design and analysis of randomised clinical trials requiring prolonged observations of each patients: analysis and examples. British Journal of Cancer 35: 1–39

Poirier J, Gray F, Gherardi R, Favolini M 1985 Histopathologie des tumeurs du systeme nerveux. Masson, Paris, p 9

Pool J L, Kamrin R P 1966 The treatment of intracranial gliomas by surgery and radiation. Progress in Neurological Surgery 1: 258–299

Posner J B, Shapiro W R 1975 Brain tumor: current status of treatment and its complications. Archives of Neurology 32: 781–784

Posner M, Horrax G 1946 Eye signs in pineal tumors. Journal of Neurosurgery 3: 15–24

Reifenberger G, Prior R, Deckert M, Wechsler W 1989 Epidermal growth factor receptor expression and growth fraction in human tumours of the nervous system. Virchows Archiv. A, Pathological Anatomy and Histopathology 414: 147–155

Reubi J C, Lang W, Maurer R, Koper J W, Lambert S W J 1987 Distribution and biochemical characterisation of somatostatin receptors in tumors of the human central nervous system. Cancer Research 47: 5758–5764

Russel D S, Rubinstein L J 1989 Pathology of tumours of the nervous system. Edward Arnold, London, pp 84–86

Sawaya R, Highsmith R 1988 Plasminogen activator activity and molecular weight patterns in human brain tumours. Journal of Neurosurgery 68: 73–79

Sawaya R, Zuccarello M, Highsmith R 1987 Alpha-1-antitrypsin in human brain tumors. Journal of Neurosurgery 67: 258–262

Scerrati M, Rossi G F 1984 The reliability of stereotactic biopsy. Acta Neurochirurgica (suppl) 33: 201–205

Schoenberg B S, Schoenberg D G, Christine B W, Gomez M R 1976 The epidemiology of primary intracranial neoplasms of childhood. A population study. Mayo Clinic Proceedings 51: 51–56

Shetter A G, Bertuccini T V, Pittman H W 1977 Closed needle biopsy in the diagnosis of intracranial mass lesions. Surgical Neurology 8: 341–345

Taveras J M, Thompson H G, Pool J L 1962 Should we treat glioblastoma multiforme? A study of survival in 425 cases. American Journal of Roentgenology 87: 473–479

Thomas D G T, Powell M P, Bradford R. Darling J L, Olney J, Barnard R O 1985 Correlation of CT-directed target site with histology and cell culture in cerebral glioma. Applied Neurophysiology 48: 460–462

Thomas D G T, Bradford R, Gill S, Davis C H 1988 Computer-directed stereotactic biopsy of intrinsic brain stem lesions. British Journal of Neurosurgery 2: 235–240

Ward A, Spuling R G 1948 The conservative treatment of third ventricle tumors. Journal of Neurosurgery 5: 124–130

Waseem N H, Lane D P 1990 Monoclonal antibody analysis of the proliferating cell nuclear antigen (PCNA): structural conservation and detection of a nucleolar form. Journal of Cell Science 96: 121–129

Wechsler W, Reifenberger G 1989 Application of immunohistochemistry for tumor grading in human neuro-oncology. In: Fields W S (ed) Primary brain tumor, Springer-Verlag New York, pp 133–141

Willems J G M S, Alva-Willems J M 1984 Accuracy of cytologic diagnosis of central nervous system neoplasms in stereotactic biopsies. Acta Cytologica 28: 243–249

Wilson C B, Hoshino T 1969 Current trends in the chemotherapy of brain tumors with special reference to glioblastomas. Journal of Neurosurgery 31: 589–603

Winger M J, MacDonald D R, Cairncross J G 1989 Supratentorial anaplastic gliomas in adults. Journal of Neurosurgery 71: 487–493

Yoshimine T, Maruno M, Ushio Y, Hayakawa T, Nakajima Y, Mogami H 1987 Intermediate filaments and anaplastic change of ENU-induced gliomas: immunohistochemical study with vimentin and astroprotein (GFAP). Journal of Neuro-oncology 5: 377–385
Zimmerman H M 1969 Brain tumors: their incidence and classification in man and their experimental production. Annals of the New York Academy of Sciences 159: 337–359
Zülch K J 1979 Histological typing of tumours of the central nervous system. World Health Organization, Geneva
Zülch K J 1986 Brain tumors. Their biology and pathology, 3rd edn. Springer-Verlag, Berlin

6. Stereotactic excision of brain tumours

P. J. Kelly

INTRODUCTION

Intracranial tumours can be localized by imaging based stereotactic techniques. In the simplest sense, point-in-space stereotactic procedures can be used to centre a bone flap directly over superficial lesions and can be used to locate subcortical lesions (Kelly & Alker 1980, 1981, Moore et al 1989). However, the volumetric information inherent in computerized tomography (CT) and magnetic resonance imaging (MRI) data can guide more thorough tumour resections. This concept prompted development of early manual systems for the transposition of CT scanning information into stereotactic space (Kelly et al 1978, 1979, Kelly & Alker 1980). These manual systems for volumetric stereotaxis are well described in earlier reports. They were accurate and used available CT software and commercially available stereotactic frames. Unfortunately, these methods required many hours for surgical planning and were cumbersome to use intraoperatively. We soon found that without an operating room computer system, volumetric stereotactic procedures were neither practical nor time efficient. The computer system was added to the surgical instrumentation in 1980 and custom software developed for this application (Kelly et al 1982a,b, 1983).

In the stereotactic technique which is practised at the present time, computer interpolation of stereotactic CT and MRI defined tumour contours produces a three dimensional target volume in stereotactic space (Kelly et al 1984, Kelly 1987). This volume may then be interactively resected by computer assisted stereotactic craniotomy. Over the past 10 years, instrumentation and techniques have evolved which make it possible to resect tumours from deep seated and centrally located regions of the brain efficiently and safely (Kelly 1989, 1990).

We have found that imaging based volumetric stereotactic techniques provide the following advantages in tumour excision. First, tumours can be approached and located in deep seated regions of the brain in the safest possible manner. Second, bone flaps need be no larger than the largest cross-sectional diameter of the tumour. Finally, volumetric stereotactic techniques help the surgeon identify the plane between tumour and surrounding brain parenchyma since the computer presents to the surgeon a scaled image which shows the cross-sectional configuration and size of the tumour at any defined depth.

The following sections will describe the instrumentation and methods for volumetric stereotactic tumour excision.

INSTRUMENTATION

COMPASS stereotactic system

A new stereotactic system evolved from a Todd–Wells frame which had been modified for CT compatibility (Kelly et al 1988b).

The COMPASS stereotactic system (Stereotactic Medical Systems, New Hartford, New York, USA), specifically designed for volumetric tumour stereotaxis, consists of a fixed arc-quadrant, three dimensional slide and removable headholder. It can be fixed on to a semipermanent base unit or mounted on to the lateral support rails of a standard operating table (Fig. 6.1).

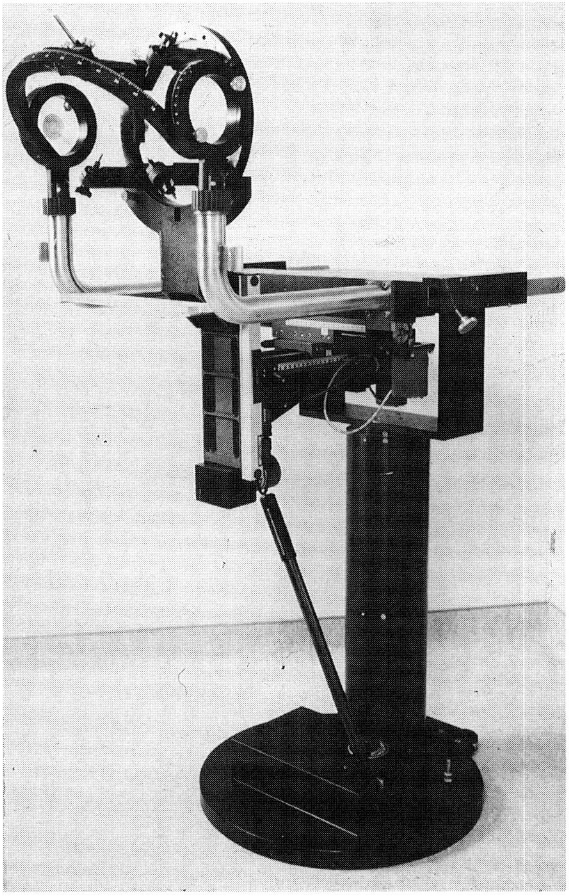

Fig. 6.1 The COMPASS stereotactic system consists of a three dimensional slide, a stereotactic headholder and a fixed arc-quadrant. With *x*, y, *z* degrees of freedom, the slide places a target within the focal point of the arc-quadrant. The frame can be operated manually, electronically or by means of computer controlled stepper motors. Stereotactic coordinates are read out on mechanical scales or optical encoders. In addition to its placement on a semipermanent base as shown here, the stereotactic instrument can be attached to the side rails of a standard operating table.

In an arc-quadrant stereotactic frame the patient's head, fixed in a rigid headholder, is moved with three orthogonal degrees of freedom (x, y and z) in order to position an intracranial target point on to the focal point of a fixed sphere which is defined by the arc-quadrant. A probe inserted perpendicular to the tangent of the arc-quadrant and to a depth equal to its radius will arrive at the focal point of the arc-quadrant. All approaches to the target point are therefore described by two angles: collar (the angle from the horizontal plane) and arc (the angle from the vertical plane). Thus, there are six simple mechanical adjustments: three axes (x, y and z), two angles (collar and arc) and a probe depth. In addition, the patient's head in the headholder can be rotated to any position which provides a comfortable working situation for the surgeon.

An 'N' shaped CT localization system was developed and eventually reported (Goerss et al 1982). This was based on the inclined plane concept described by Goodenough et al (1975) and also used by Brown (1979), Perry et al (1980) and Boethius et al (1980).

Computer support

At present, computer support for volumetric stereotaxis and the COMPASS system consists of a Sun 4 workstation with a Vicom VME image processor. Custom software for data acquisition, surgical planning and simulations and interactive surgery has been developed. The computer and image processing system hardware is housed in the computer facility located directly above two operating rooms equipped for stereotaxis (Fig. 6.2).

Stereotactic retractors

A stereotactic retractor system developed for the resection of deep tumours with the COMPASS system consists of cylindrical retractors, dilators and an arc-quadrant adaptor (Kelly et al 1988c). The retractor is a thin walled hollow cylinder 140 mm in length and 2 cm in diameter. Indexing marks on the retractor shaft are provided for measurement of insertional depth with respect to the stereotactic arc-quadrant. The retractor cylinder is directed perpendicular to the tangent and towards the focal point of the stereotactic arc-quadrant. Dilators which fit inside the retractor cylinder are 1 cm longer than the retractor. The distal end of the dilator is wedge shaped, which spreads and dilates an incision to the diameter of the retractor so that the retractor cylinder can be advanced.

The retractor maintains exposure and creates a shaft from the surface of the brain to the

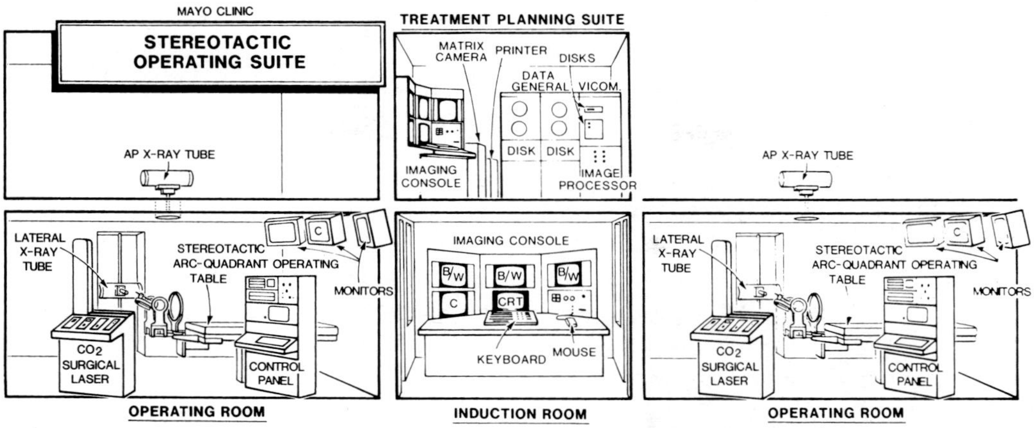

Fig. 6.2 Two operating rooms equipped for stereotactic surgery. Fixed tube anteroposterior and lateral laser collimated teleradiographic equipment are used for functional procedures, and for confirmation of probe placement. Video display monitors suspended from the ceiling present computer generated tumour volume reconstructions. A computer room with a planning console is located on the floor directly above the operating room. A second imaging console is located in the induction room between the operating rooms for interoperative stereotactic calculations and surgical planning.

superficial aspect of deep seated tumours. In addition, the retractor also has a known configuration (a cylinder). Since it is directed to a given depth by the stereotactic arc-quadrant, the distal end of the retractor also has a known location in stereotactic space. It therefore provides a fixed stereotactic reference structure in the stereotactic surgical field. Computer generated slice reconstructions of the CT/MRI defined tumour volume are related to the position of the distal end of the retractor (Kelly 1988, 1990, Kelly et al 1988c).

Accessory instruments

A variety of custom made extra long instruments are necessary in the stereotactic resection of deep tumours. Bipolar forceps with a working shaft length of 150 mm are required to control bleeding in the surgical field when working through the stereotactic retractors. In addition, 150–160 mm long suction tips, dissectors and alligator scissors are also used.

'Heads-up' display for the operating microscope

Computer generated slice images are transmitted to a small video monitor mounted on the operating microscope. This image is optically scaled to actual size and superimposed on the surgical field viewed through the microscope. Thus, the surgeon sees the actual surgical field and the superimposed computer generated CT and MRI based rendition of that field through the microscope. In addition, when the image of the cylindrical retractor reflected into the microscope by the heads-up display unit is superimposed over the distal end of the retractor in the surgical field, the microscope is optically indexed to the stereotactic surgical field.

Carbon dioxide laser system

The carbon dioxide laser is not essential for stereotactic tumour excision. It is, however, convenient for dissecting around and for the vaporization of deep seated tumours exposed through a narrow aperture stereotactic retractor. Furthermore, the laser is relatively haemostatic and the zone of thermal injury with laser incision is usually 300 mmg or less. This is an important feature when resecting tumours located in the thalamus or brain stem.

INTERACTIVE STEREOTACTIC RESECTION

In general, the operating room computer system monitors and displays the position of stereotactically placed cranial trephine defects and stereotactically directed instruments in relation to computer generated image reconstructions of the tumour volume. Computer assisted stereotactic laser microsurgical procedures are performed in three phases — database acquisition, surgical planning and the interactive procedure — as discussed below.

Data acquisition

The replaceable stereotactic headholder is secured to the patient's skull by a flanged carbon fibre pin fixation system inserted into drill holes in the outer table of the skull. Local anaesthesia is employed. Micrometer measurements of the exposed length of the carbon fibre pin extending beyond the fixed vertical support elements of the headholder are recorded and used when replacing the headholder for subsequent data acquisition or surgical procedures.

Following frame application, the patient undergoes stereotactic CT, MRI and digital angiographic examinations as described below.

A CT table adaptation plate receives the stereotactic headholder CT localization system, which consists of nine carbon fibre localization rods arranged in the shape of the letter 'N' located on either side of the head and anteriorly to create nine reference marks on each CT slice. Stereotactic CT scanning is done on a General Electric 9800 CT scanning unit gathering 5 mm slices through the lesion, utilizing a medium body format.

Stereotactic MRI examinations are performed on a General Electric 1.5 T Signa unit. The MRI localization system consists of capillary tubes filled with copper sulphate solution, which are arranged in basic 'N' shaped sets located bilaterally, anteriorly, posteriorly and superiorly. These create reference marks on each transverse, coronal or sagittal MRI scan, from which stereotactic coordinates may be calculated for any point on that image.

Stereotactic digital angiography is performed utilizing the standard femoral catheterization and radiographic techniques used in diagnostic angiography. A DF adaptation plate fixes to the table of the General Electric DF 3000 and 5000 digital angiographic units and receives the stereotactic headholder. A localization system which consists of four lucite plates which each contain nine radiopaque reference markers fixes to the base ring of the stereotactic headholder. The lucite plates are positioned on each side of the patient's head, anteriorly and posteriorly. The radiopaque markers create 18 reference marks on each anteroposterior and lateral digital angiography image. Calculation of magnification in any depth plane, and establishment of a distortion correction grid which corrects for non-uniformity of the images, is possible because of the known mathematical relationships between the fiducial marks and their projected locations on the digital angiography images. Furthermore, the distances between the reference marks on the lucite plates, the measured distances between those marks on the radiographs, the calculated magnification factors and the distortion grid permit calculation of stereotactic coordinates for any point or points on intracranial blood vessels and display of the correct position of CT and MRI derived stereotactic target points and volumes on angiographic images.

Orthogonal and 6° oblique arterial and venous phases are obtained in orthogonal and 6° rotated stereoscopic pairs. 6° indexing marks on the base ring of the stereotactic headholder base ring are aligned to ensure precise 6° rotation for the stereoscopic pair (Fig. 6.3).

Surgical planning

Following data acquisition, the archived magnetic data tapes from the CT, MRI and digital angiography examinations are transferred from respective host computers to the operating room computer system. The nine reference marks on each CT slice and MR image are detected automatically by an intensity detection algorithm. This suspends the position of each slice in a three dimensional computer image storage matrix. The 18 reference marks on the arterial and venous digital angiography images are digitized by box cursor manipulated by the mouse subsystem (Fig. 6.4).

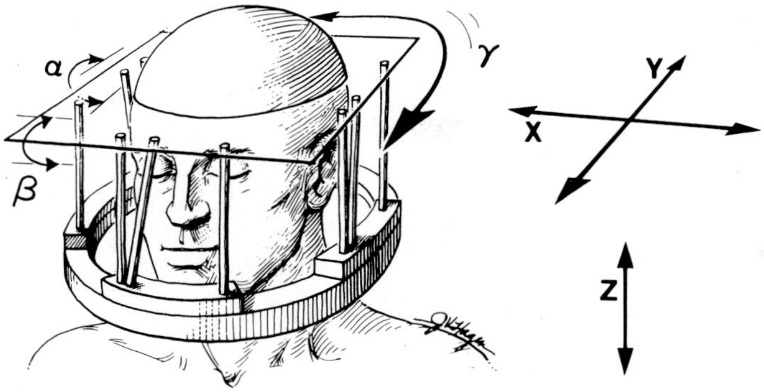

a

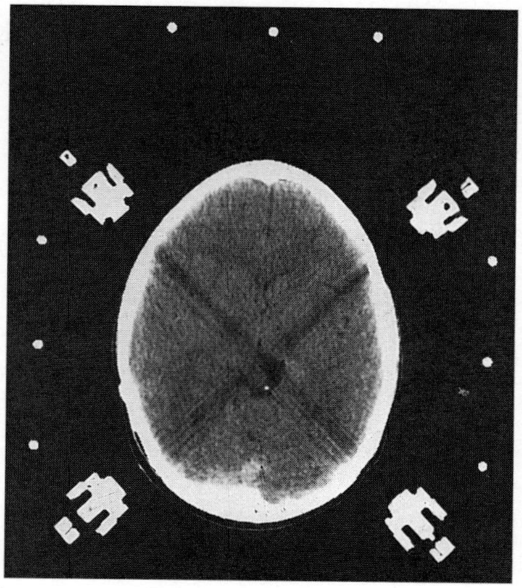

b

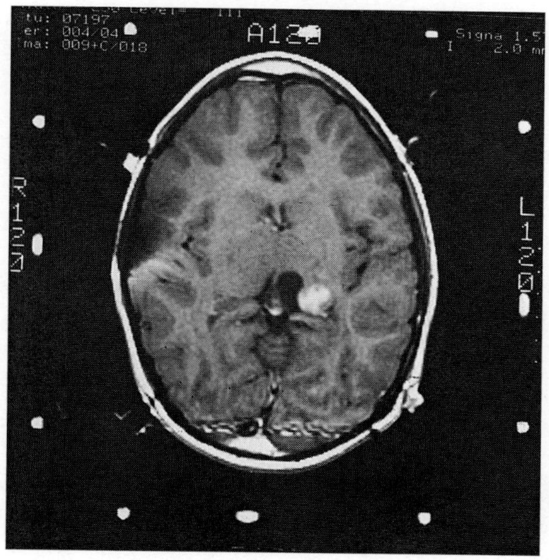

c

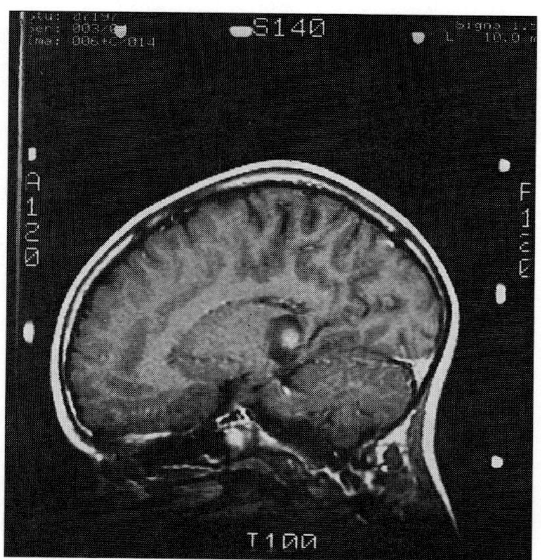

d

Fig. 6.3 **a** Stereotactic CT and MRI examinations are performed with 'N' shaped localization devices attached to the base ring of the stereotactic head frame, which results in a series of reference marks on each CT and MRI scan, from which image rotation (γ), anteroposterior and right–left slice tilts and stereotactic coordinates may be calculated.
b Stereotactic CT scan showing a left thalamic tumour. Note reference marks produced by the localization system. Same patient on gadolinium acid enhanced stereotactic axial (c) and sagittal MRI (d).

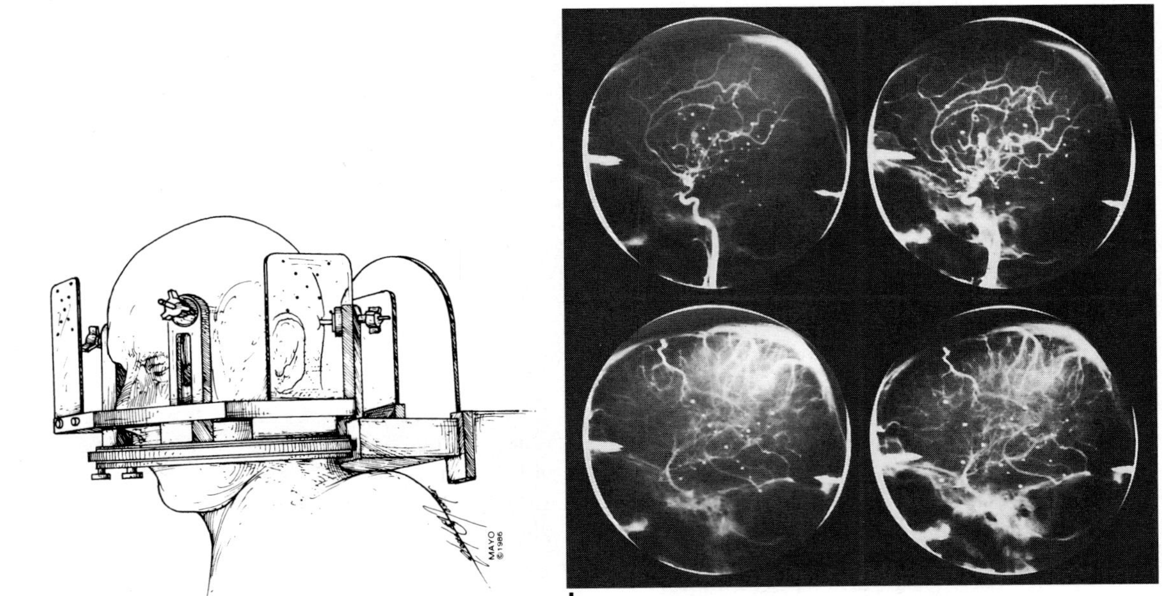

a b

Fig. 6.4 **a** The angiographic localization system consists of four lucite plates each with nine radiopaque markers situated bilaterally, anteriorly and posteriorly. **b** Stereotactic stereoscopic angiogram. Note the 18 reference marks produced by the localization system. Identification of deep segments of arteries and veins which are apparent in stereoscopic pairs indicate the position of the sulci and fissures.

Interpolation of tumour volume

The procedure used to create a tumour volume in stereotactic space is as follows. The surgeon first traces around the outline of the lesion defined by the various imaging modalities on all sequential slice images which show the lesion. Thus, a series of contours is established for the boundary defined by CT contrast enhancement, CT hypodensity, T_1 and T_2 weighted signal abnormalities of the MRI and the gadolinium enhanced boundaries. Each of these digitized contours is suspended in the computer image matrix. A computer program then interpolates intermediate slices at 1 mm intervals between the digitized contours (Kelly et al 1982, 1984). Volumes are now created in defined stereotactic space by filling in each of the digitized and interpolated slices with 1 mm cubic voxels. Finally, a central target point is digitized on a CT or MRI slice. Stereotactic coordinates for this point are calculated. These coordinates (x, y and z) are actually mechanical stereotactic frame settings which position that point onto the focal point of the stereotactic arc-quadrant. The interpolated tumour volume is constructed around that point and all subsequent image displays and frame translations relate to that point.

Volumes defined by CT and MRI are assigned identifying grey level. Slices through the volumetric image matrix are displayed individually or all together on a raster display monitor.

Determination of surgical trajectory

The surgical trajectory (viewline) is now determined. The viewline is the surgical approach to a specified central point within the tumour volume (which will be positioned at the focal point of the stereotactic arc-quadrant). This is defined mathematically and expressed as angles from the horizontal and vertical planes, which are, in fact, collar and arc angle settings on the stereotactic frame, respectively.

The three dimensional shape of the lesion, and the location of important overlying cortical regions, subcortical white matter pathways and vascular structures are considered in determining the optimum surgical approach. Ideally, tumours should be approached through non-essential brain tissue and in a direction parallel to major white matter fibre tracts. In addition, deep sulci, localized stereotactically from stereotactic MRI or stereoscopic digital angiography, provide a route for the approach to and exposure of deep seated lesions. In this case an entry point in the superficial aspect of the sulcus is selected and the trajectory or viewline is determined from target and entry points. The actual surgical approach can be simulated on the computer screen in order to view its relationships to the tumour volume and overlying and surrounding anatomical structures (Fig. 6.5).

Patient rotation

The base ring of the COMPASS stereotactic headholder is circular, and the patient's head can be rotated to any position which will provide a comfortable working position for the surgeon. Indexing marks on the base ring with 5° intervals align with a reference mark on the yoke of the three dimensional slide system. Thus, a patient with a right central laterally lying tumour is operated in the left side down lateral decubitus body position with the head and base ring of the headholder rotated to 270°. This rotation parameter is entered into the computer, which adjusts the x, y and z stereotactic frame settings and updates arc and collar angles to account for this rotation. Therefore, the final viewline parameters will depend on patient rotation and arc and collar angles.

Surgical procedures

The technical aspects of the surgical procedure will depend on whether the lesion is located superficially or deep. In both procedures, the patient is positioned and the base ring fixed in the receiving yoke of the three dimensional slide system at the proper rotation position after the x, y and z adjustments for the target have been inputted.

In superficial lesions, the stereotactic instrument is used to centre a circular trephine over the tumour. A computer representation of the circular trephine is superimposed by the heads-

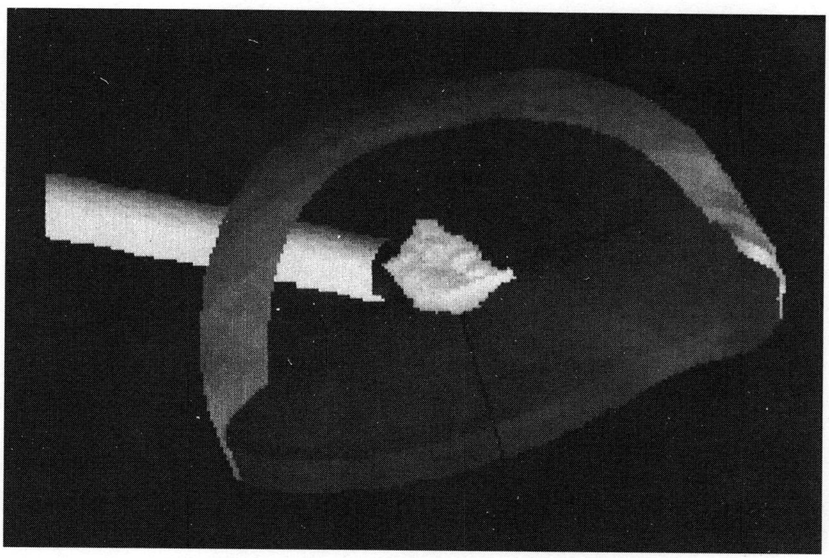

Fig. 6.5 The computer has calculated a tumour volume in stereotactic space. The surface of the skull detected by an automatic intensity detection program is also presented as surface display. Here, a posterior thalamic tumour is approached by means of a 2.0 cm stereotactically directed cylindrical retractor through the superior parietal lobule. The clipping plane on the lateral surface of the skull allows one to appreciate the relationship between the retractor and tumour.

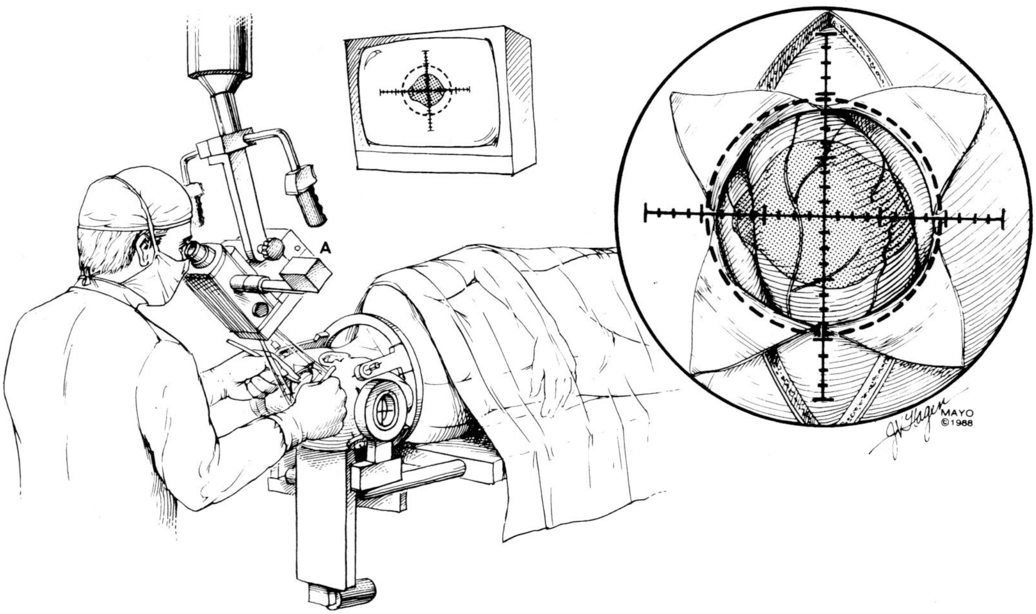

Fig. 6.6 Illustration of stereotactic craniotomy performed for resection of a superficial tumour. The computer generated image corresponds to the outline of the stereotactically placed trephine and the imaging defined limits of the lesion are scaled to size and superimposed upon the surgical field by the heads-up display unit of the operating microscope. This helps the surgeon identify and develop a plane around superficial lesions. (From Kelly (1998).)

up display in the operating microscope on to the actual trephine in the surgical field. Slices from the CT and/or MRI defined tumour volumes are then displayed in proper stereotactic relationship to the trephine. These orient the surgeon as to the location of the tumour boundaries during dissection around and removal of the lesion. Deep tumours are removed through a cylindrically shaped retractor utilizing a carbon dioxide laser. In these procedures the distal end of the retractor itself provides the reference structure to which the computer displayed tumour slices are related.

Superficial lesions

Procedural Aspects. The patient is placed under general endotracheal anaesthesia. The stereotactic head frame is replaced by inserting the flanged carbon fibre pins into the pin holes in the skull and duplicating the micrometer settings recorded during the data acquisition phase. The patient is then positioned in the stereotactic frame. The headholder rotation angle as determined in planning is set. After preparing and draping the head, the stereotactic arc-quadrant is positioned and arc and collar approach angles set. Through a stab wound in the scalp a pilot hole is drilled in the outer table of the skull by a stereotactically directed 1/8" (3 mm) drill. The scalp is opened by linear incision. A craniotomy is performed using a power trephine centred on the pilot hole. The size of the trephine selected is equal to or slightly larger than the diameter of the largest cross-sectional slice of the tumour reformatted along the surgical viewline.

The computer displays into the heads-up display unit of the operating microscope the configuration of the trephine in relationship to the reformatted tumour outlines (Fig. 6.6). The surgeon first scales the image and moves the microscope so that the graphics image of the trephine is superimposed over the actual trephine in the surgical field. A section of cortex having the same size and configuration as the most superficial computer generated tumour slice image is removed with bipolar forceps and scissors. Cortex is non-viable when tumours extend to within 1 cm of the surface. A plane is then developed around the tumour utilizing a carbon dioxide laser or bipolar forceps. The tumour slice images provide a template which aids in the identification of this plane.

The natural tendency for neurosurgeons is to enter the lesion and internally debulk it. This should not be done in stereotactic excisions, however, since the walls of the decompression cavity within the lesion will fall in on themselves and render subsequent slice images inaccurate. Therefore, in stereotactic excisions, it is best to first isolate the lesion from surrounding brain tissue and keep the specimen intact. The surgeon interacts with the computer by means of a sterile joystick, controller system mounted on the operating table and the menu system, which is displayed in the microscope by means of the heads-up display unit. Intermediate and high grade gliomas can be removed as intact specimens with negligible bleeding. In addition, infiltrated areas of brain parenchyma in low grade gliomas located in non-essential brain tissue can also be resected in a similar manner. For correlation to the appropriate image slice phase, the depth of the surgical working plane is determined as follows: first, the distance from the arc-quadrant to the outer table of the skull is measured (m) and this distance is subtracted from 135 mm (r is the radius of the arc-quadrant). The zero slice plane at the focus of the arc-quadrant is therefore this remaining distance (r-m) below the outer table of the skull. Marks are made on the bipolar forceps for convenient reference.

Deep tumours

The open stereotactic approach to periventricular, basal ganglia or thalamic tumours requires stereotactic retractors, extra long bipolar forceps and dissecting instruments.

The stereotactic retractors are mounted on an internal stereotactic arc-quadrant. The position of these retractors is also indicated on the computer display terminal in the operating room and in the heads-up display unit of the operating microscope (Fig. 6.7). The position of the cylindrical retractor is shown as a circle in the computer display in relationship to the tumour slice. During surgery, the computer generated image of the retractor is superimposed on the actual view of the retractor in the operating microscope.

A variety of surgical approaches have been developed for various deep tumour locations. These include transcortical, transsulcal, trans-Sylvian and interhemispheric exposure. The actual approach selected depends on the proximity of the tumour to deep sulci which can be split microsurgically and spread wide enough to provide adequate exposure. The approach to thalamic tumours depends on whether they are located anteriorly (and thus approached anterior superiorly), posterior dorsally (and exposed through the lateral ventricle by way of the superior parietal lobule) or posterior ventrally (and approached posterior laterally). The issue here is the preservation of normal thalamic tissue. Multiplanar MRI is invaluable in defining the anatomical relationships between tumour and normal structures in order to select the best surgical approach trajectory for stereotactic craniotomy.

The stereotactic resection of deep tumours is performed under general anaesthesia and the patient is replaced in the stereotactic head holder and positioned in the stereotactic frame. The selected target point within the tumour volume is positioned on to the focal point of the stereotactic arc-quadrant. In cystic tumours, intraventricular tumours or those near the ventricular system, the following step may be necessary in order to monitor possible movements of the tumour during the procedure. A series of 0.5 mm stainless steel reference balls are deposited at 5 mm intervals along the surgical viewline in the tumour by a stereotactically directed biopsy cannula inserted through a ⅛" (3 mm) drill hole in the skull. Anteroposterior and lateral radiographs are obtained (Fig. 6.8). The position of these steel balls on subsequent radiographs following exposure of the lesion may indicate shifts in the position of the tumour which can be adjusted in the computer software for updated accurate tumour slice images.

The scalp is opened with a linear incision. A

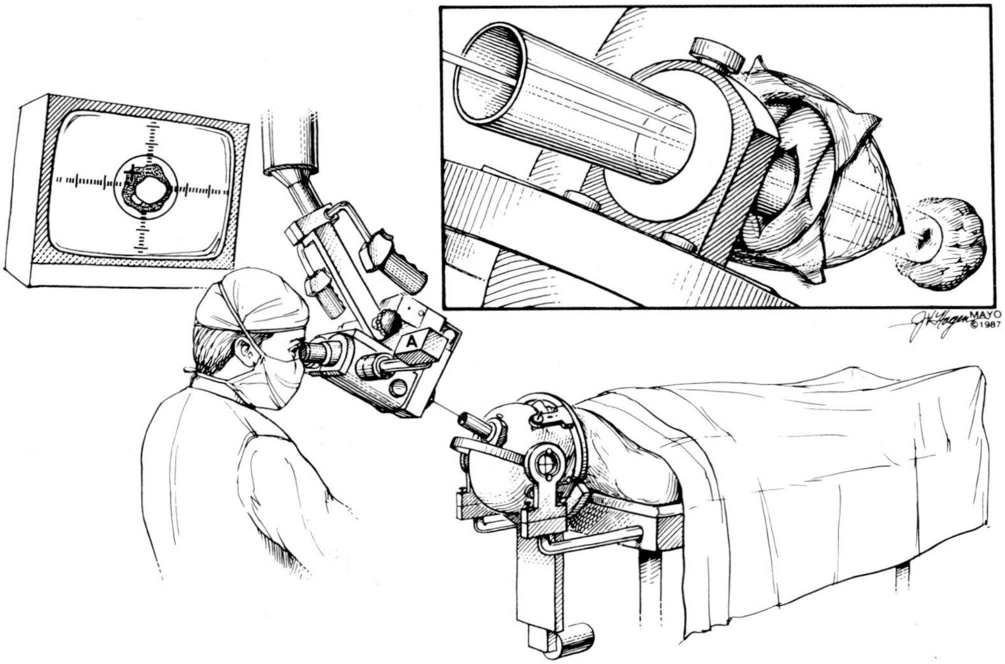

Fig. 6.7 Deep tumours are resected through a stereotactically directed cylindrical retractor mounted on the arc-quadrant. The computer monitor displays the position of the distal end of the retractor with respect to slices through the imaging defined tumour volume cut perpendicular to the surgical viewline. (From Kelly (1988).)

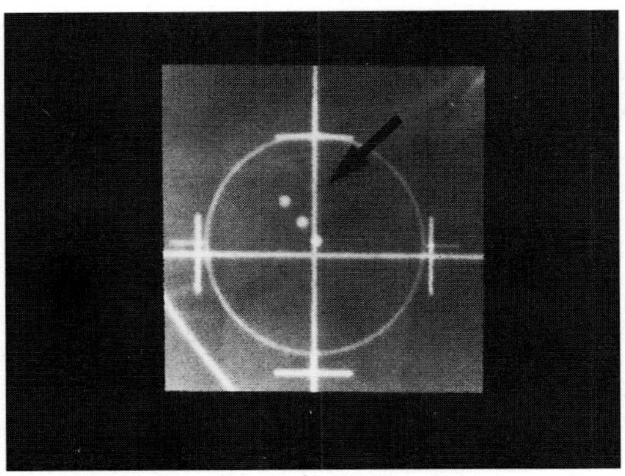

Fig. 6.8 Coned down lateral radiograph demonstrating stereotactically placed steel balls within a small partially cystic thalamic astrocytoma. Subsequent stereotactic radiographs as the surgery progresses may demonstrate possible shifts of the neoplasm. Shifts measured off these radiographs will allow adjustment of the tumour volume within the three dimensionally constructed computer image matrix for subsequent updated image displays, which account for possible tumour movements during surgery.

$1\frac{1}{2}$" (40 mm) trephine craniotomy is performed and a cruciate opening of the dura accomplished. A linear incision is made in the cortex and then the subcortical white matter incision is progressively deepened with the stereotactically directed carbon dioxide laser. Alternatively, a convenient sulcus can be split microsurgically and the cortical incision made in the depths of this sulcus.

The direction of the subcortical incision should be through non-essential brain tissue and in a direction parallel to major white matter fibres. As the incision is deepened, the stereotactic retractor is advanced to maintain the developing exposure.

The computer has calculated the range of the tumour along the surgical viewline. At the outer border of the tumour, the laser beam is deflected laterally and a dilator placed through the retractor and the retractor is advanced. This creates a shaft from the surface to the outer border of the tumour. Using the computer display as a guide, the surgeon creates a plane of dissection around the lesion with the laser, advances the retractor and deepens the incision circumscribing the tumour. Tumour tissue within the retractor is then removed with 65–85 W of defocused laser power. The tumour is removed slice by slice, extending from the most superficial slices to the deepest. Haemostasis is secured utilizing the extra long bipolar forceps. Anteroposterior and lateral teleradiographs are obtained to document the progress of the procedure and record possible movements of the reference balls (which are removed as they are encountered during the procedure).

Tumours larger than the retractor opening can be removed as follows. First, one side of the tumour is positioned under the retractor and with the laser the surgeon creates a plane between this side of the tumour and brain tissue. The display image is then translated on the computer display terminal to position the other side of the lesion under the retractor. The computer calculates new stereotactic frame adjustments which are duplicated on the stepper motor driven slide mechanism of the frame by means of a remote control panel. This side of the tumour is then separated from brain tissue with the laser. After isolating the lesion from surrounding brain tissue it may then be vaporized by laser as described above.

RESULTS

Between August 1984 and August 1989, 374 consecutive patients underwent computer assisted stereotactic craniotomies. Lesion locations are illustrated in Figure 6.9, and histologies, mortality and morbidity are listed in Table 6.1. The average age was 46.8 years (range 2–78 years).

Normal preoperative neurological examinations were recorded in 181 patients, including 63 patients who presented with seizures. The remaining 193 patients had a preoperative neurological deficit. Neurological examinations were performed at the time of discharge from the hospital or 2 weeks following surgery. These revealed that 116 of the 193 patients with preoperative deficits had improved from their preoperative levels. In addition, all of the 63 patients presenting with seizures were seizure free on medication at the 3 month follow-up examination.

The number of patients who were neurologically unchanged postoperatively was 167. Of

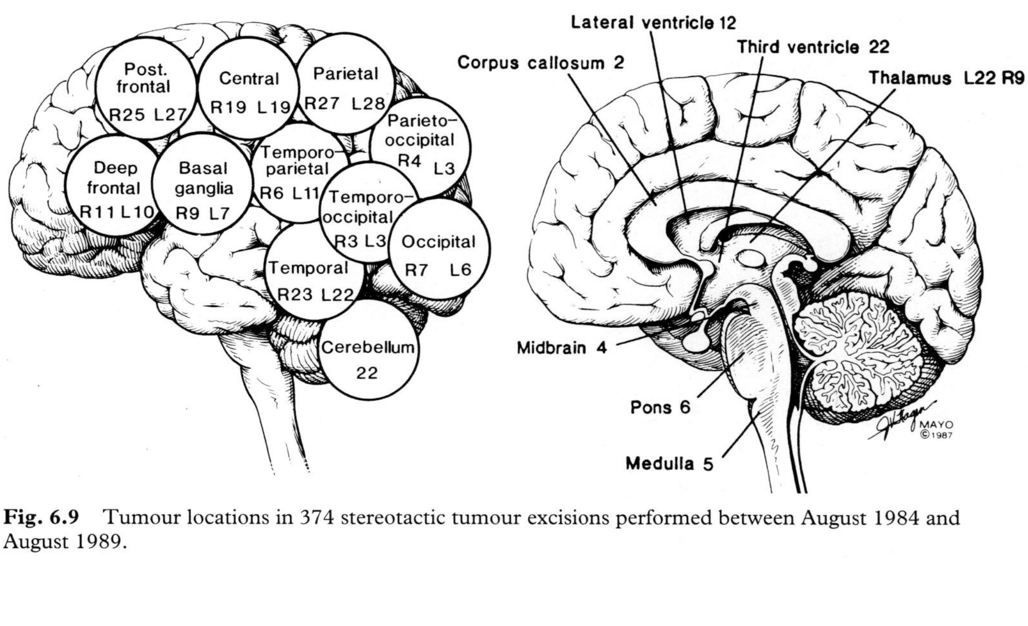

Fig. 6.9 Tumour locations in 374 stereotactic tumour excisions performed between August 1984 and August 1989.

Table 6.1 Histological findings in 374 stereotactic craniotomies

			Mortality (%)	Morbidity (%)
Glial Neoplasms		205		
Astrocytomas	151			
Grade IV	71		1.4	8
Grade III	15		—	13
Grade II	15		—	33
Grade I	5		—	—
Pilocytic astrocytomas	45		2.0	8
Oligodendrogliomas	32			
Oligoastrocytoma	13		—	3
Subependymoma	2		—	—
Ependymoma	4		—	—
Medulloblastoma	1		—	—
Neurocytoma	2		—	—
Non-glial tumours		113		
Metastatic	65		—	6
Meningioma	15		13.0	6
Lymphoma	7		—	—
Choroid plexus papilloma	1		—	—
Ganglioglioma	4		—	—
Colloid cyst	18		—	—
Haemangioblastoma	2		—	—
Teratoma	1		—	—
Non-neoplastic mass lesions		56		
Vascular lesions	36		—	12
Abscess	3		—	—
Cysticercosis	1		—	—
Haematoma	2		—	—
Tuberous sclerosis	4		—	—
Glial scar (epilepsy)	5		—	—
Radiation necrosis	5		—	—
Total		374		

these 167 patients, 110 had been normal preoperatively, and remained normal postoperatively; 57 patients had preoperative neurological deficits which did not improve postoperatively.

Morbidity and mortality

Following surgery, 28 patients were neurologically worse: nine patients were neurologically normal preoperatively and had deficits postoperatively; 16 additional patients experienced worsening of a deficit noted on the preoperative neurological examination. Postoperative deficits were thought to be due to the surgical approach or local perilesional trauma. In 12 of these 28 patients, postoperative neurologic deficits were consistent with neuronal injury along the surgical approach; eight patients with medial temporal or posterior ventral thalamic lesions sustained a permanent contralateral superior quadrantopsia and two others had a homonymous haemianopsia following the temporo-occipital approach necessary to resect their lesions. A trans-Sylvian exposure of a left subinsular metastatic tumour produced a contralateral arm dyspraxia in another patient. Finally, a transvermian exposure of a midline cerebellar thrombosed arteriovenous malformation resulted in increased gait apraxia.

Deficits consistent with surgical trauma to perineoplastic tissue or disruption of brain parenchymal blood supply was seen in 16 additional patients. This most commonly occurred in high grade glial neoplasms with peritumoral tumour cell infiltration or in highly vascular neoplasms. Three deaths occurred within 1 month following surgery in this series of 374 patients: one from massive brain stem oedema following resection of a ventral thalamic astrocytoma with brain stem infiltration apparent on MRI, and two from massive pulmonary embolization: one 2 weeks following resection of a large left lateral ventricle meningioma and the other 6 days following resection of a thalamic glioblastoma.

Specific lesion types

Based on this overall experience, we have been able to draw certain conclusions about the appropriateness of computer assisted stereotactic laser microsurgery in specific lesions. In addition, we have derived certain technical manoeuvres which are useful in the stereotactic removal of various lesions depending on their histology and anatomic location.

High grade glial tumours

Computer assisted stereotactic resection can remove all CT defined contrast enhancing portions of high grade glial neoplasms from neurologically important subcortical areas with acceptable levels of mortality and morbidity (Kelly et al 1986, Kelly 1987, 1988). Postoperative CT studies usually demonstrate absence of contrast enhancement around the surgical defect (Fig. 6.10). Nevertheless, mean postoperative survival of our patients harbouring grade 4 astrocytomas (Kernohan classification),

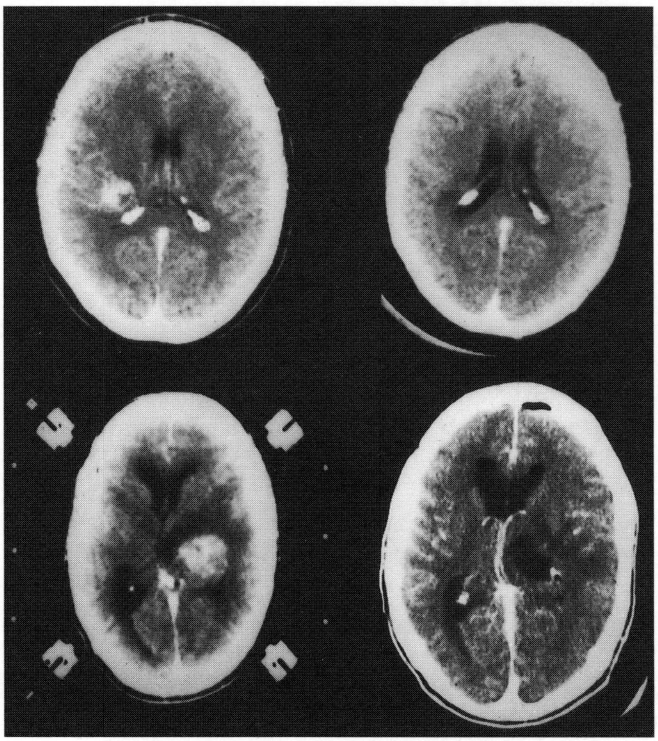

Fig. 6.10 Preoperative (left) and postoperative (right) contrast enhanced CT scans in patients with grade IV astrocytomas who underwent stereotactic resection of lesions from the right medial parietal area (top) and left posterior thalamus (bottom).

treated with postoperative external beam radiation therapy (50–65 Gy) was 42 weeks (average survival 47 weeks). In the typical case, new areas of contrast enhancement on CT scanning developed within low density areas surrounding the surgical defect within 6–9 months following the procedure (Kelly 1987, 1990). Death in the majority of these cases was therefore due to tumour 'recurrence' and progression. However, we are discussing length of survival here only; not quality of survival, which in general is better following resection of the lesions and radiation therapy, than following biopsy alone and radiation.

The mean survival time of 42 weeks in our group of patients all having grade 4 astrocytomas in central and deep-seated locations (historically associated with poor survival and high surgical morbidity and mortality) is similar to survival times of 37 weeks quoted in other series in the literature (Frankel & German 1958, Hitchcock & Sato 1964, Jelsma & Bucy 1967, Gehan & Walker 1977). However, there are two major reasons why our results cannot be compared to historical controls. First, a high percentage of the patients in these other series harboured lesions in the frontal and temporal lobes which are more amenable to radical surgical resection by lobectomy (Jelsma & Bucy 1967, Behan & Walker 1977). Secondly, in the above, the author is considering survival following stereotactic resection of grade 4 astrocytomas only and would caution the reader in comparing these survival statistics to those reported in other series for 'glioblastomas' (Coffey et al 1988). In most histological grading schemes for astrocytomas, the presence or absence of necrosis separates 'glioblastomas' from 'anaplastic astrocytomas', respectively. But in the Kernohan classification scheme (used at the Mayo Clinic), necrosis can be found in grade 3 and 4 astrocytomas. Endothelial proliferation and frequency of mitoses are used to differentiate between grade 3 and 4 tumours. Therefore, in most histological classification schemes, 'glioblastomas' can contain some Kernohan grade 3 tumours mixed in with grade 4 neoplasms. The point here is that mean survival in a series of 'glioblastomas' which contain grade 3 and 4 astrocytomas should be longer than mean survival in a series of pure grade 4 astrocytomas.

Preoperative stereotactic MRI (especially the T_2 weighted image) in high grade glial tumours always demonstrates much larger areas of abnormality than indicated by contrast enhancement on CT scanning (Kelly et al 1987a,b). However, examination of stereotactic serial biopsy specimens obtained from regions of CT contrast enhancement, CT hypodensity and MRI defined abnormality in patients with high grade gliomas reveal that a large area of intact oedematous brain parenchyma infiltrated by aggressive isolated tumour cells surrounds the mass of tumour tissue represented by CT contrast enhancement (Burger et al 1983, Kelly et al 1987a,b, Daumas-Duport et al 1989). In fact, this oedematous infiltrated parenchyma usually extends as far as, and in some cases beyond, the area of signal prolongation abnormality on the T_2 weighted MRI scan (Kelly et al 1987a,b).

It would be technically possible utilizing volumetric stereotaxis to resect the volume defined by the MRI abnormality. This in theory would substantially prolong postoperative survival (Hoshino et al 1972, Hoshino 1984). However, unacceptable neurological deficits would result from removal of the intact, albeit infiltrated, parenchyma.

Therefore, in grade 4 astrocytomas, it is practical to resect the volume of tissue defined by contrast enhancement on CT scanning only. This permits the most aggressive reduction in tumour burden possible and preservation of neurological function in the majority of patients with grade 4 astrocytomas. Radiation therapy and chemotherapy are then administered in attempts to kill the isolated tumour cells which reside in the intact parenchyma left behind. However, until we have a means for selectively and safely targeting these isolated tumour cells, we can expect few significant changes in the survival of these patients.

Although the cellular elements within grade 3 astrocytomas, mixed gliomas and oligodendrogliomas are not as mitotically active as in the grade 4 tumour, isolated tumour cells also infiltrate intact and surrounding oedematous parenchyma (Kelly et al 1987a) and defy surgical attempts to cure them. In contrast to grade 4 astrocytomas, grade 3 gliomas, particularly astrocytomas, tend to have larger volumes of tumour cell infiltrated parenchyma in comparison to the volume of tumour tissue than grade 4 lesions. Thus, the benefit of resecting a relatively small tumour tissue mass in the face of a large volume of infiltrated parenchyma is questionable; so that in most grade 3 lesions surgeons tend to recommend biopsy over stereotactic resection. Recent studies which combine grade 4 and 3 astrocytomas into a group of 'malignant gliomas' in order to study the effect of biopsy versus resection on survival have not taken into consideration the fact that many grade 3 astrocytomas are infiltrating tumours and not appropriate for resection, whereas many grade 4 astrocytomas present a contrast enhancing mass lesion which can be resected. Such studies claim that there is no difference in survival of 'malignant astrocytomas' in groups undergoing biopsy, and those undergoing resection (Coffey et al 1988). However, in our experience, a higher percentage of grade 4 gliomas undergo resection than grade 3 tumours. Grade 4 astrocytomas have a worse prognosis than grade 3 tumours. Thus, studies comparing biopsy and resection which do not stratify for tumour grade are not valid.

In grade 3 gliomas which can be stereotactically resected, tumour recurrences are seen later in the patient's postoperative course than with grade 4 astrocytomas. However, these lesions generally 'recur' in the same spatial pattern as described for grade 4 tumours. Nevertheless, as with the grade 4 astrocytomas, the procedure can remove all of the solid tumour tissue component of selected neoplasms having significant contrast enhancing volume on stereotactic CT scanning.

Low grade astrocytomas

In adults, low grade astrocytomas are usually manifest by an area of low density on CT scanning and prolongation of signal on MRI (18). Neurological deficits are very rarely noted and the usual presenting problems are seizures. Stereotactic serial biopsy studies of low grade fibrillary astrocytomas, mixed gliomas and oligodendrogliomas reveal that most of the 'tumour' is comprised of infiltrated intact parenchyma with little tumour tissue proper (Kelly 1987). Resection of the 'tumour' by CT stereotactic craniotomy is, in fact, resection of intact but infiltrated parenchyma. In important brain areas, this results in a postoperative neurological deficit and stereotactic resection is therefore rejected as an option (Kelly et al 1986, Kelly 1988). In some cases, though, the lesion is confined to expendible brain tissue such as the posterior portion of the superior frontal convolution. These lesions can then be resected in their entirety.

Pilocytic astrocytomas, on the other hand, which tend to occur in children and young adults, are histologically circumscribed. In spite of the fact that many are located in the thalamus and other important subcortical locations, they can be completely resected by the computer assisted stereotactic technique with excellent postoperative results (Kelly et al 1986, McGirr & Kelly 1987, Kelly 1988) (Fig. 6.11). These lesions exhibit prominent enhancement on CT or on MRI with gadolinium, and the borders of these lesions are accurately defined by the contrast enhancement.

Metastatic tumours

It is generally thought that metastatic tumours are histologically circumscribed and that there is usually no problem in identifying the plane between tumour and oedematous brain. This is frequently true. In some cases, however, this interface may not be so clear, especially when bleeding is encountered. In fact, reported surgical series of metastatic tumour removed at non-stereotactic craniotomy admit to a certain percentage of patients with incomplete resections (Van Eck et al 1965, Raskind et al 1971, Haar & Patterson 1972, Yardini et al 1984). However, with volumetric stereotaxis and intraoperative

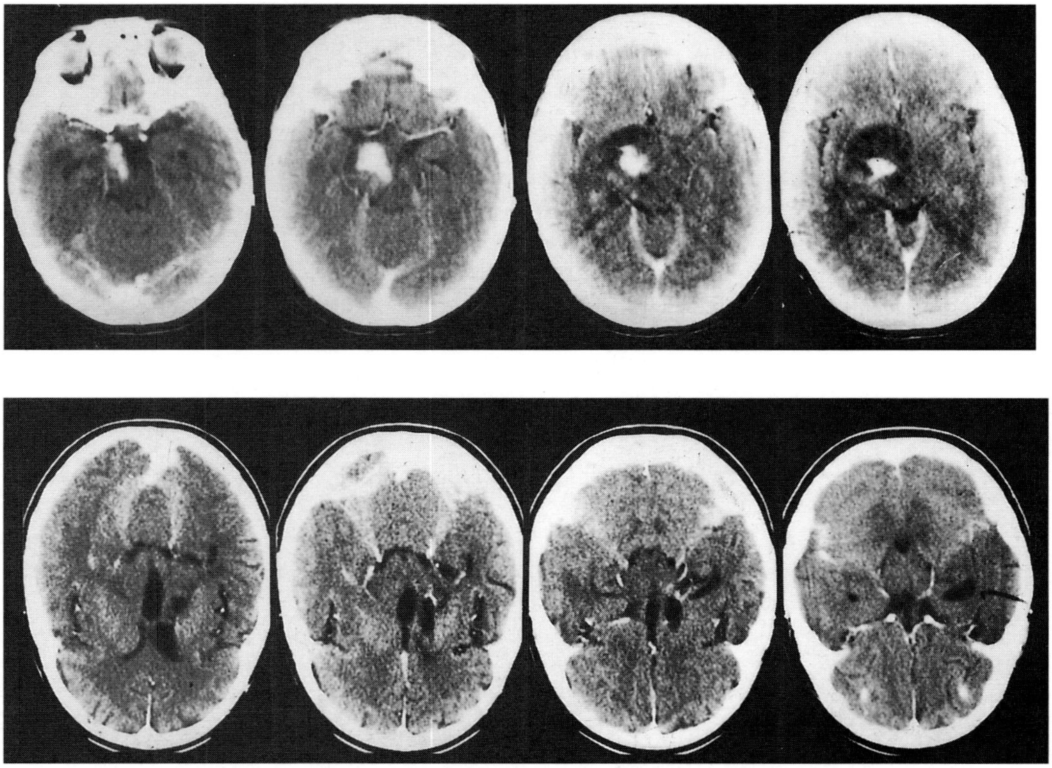

Fig. 6.11 Preoperative (top) and postoperative (bottom) contrast enhanced CT scan in a 16-year-old girl with a right thalamic partially cystic pilocytic astrocytoma which extended from the right ventral thalamus into the midbrain and optic tract. An anterior approach was utilized. The patient had a haemiparesis preoperatively which was improved on her postoperative examination.

image displays, identification of the plane between tumour and brain is straightforward and, in fact, simple. These lesions can be completely resected by computer assisted stereotactic craniotomy (Fig. 6.12).

Stereotactic resection techniques can be advantageous in superficial metastases as well as deeply situated lesions. First, stereotactic point localization helps centre small cranial trephines directly over superficial lesions (the trephine need be no larger than the cross-sectional area of the neoplasm). The approach is therefore selective, direct and no more brain than absolutely necessary need be exposed. In addition, a deep seated metastasis can be located by a stereotactically directed probe which guides the surgeon to the lesion.

Postoperative morbidity for stereotactic resection of centrally located and deep seated metastatic tumours is 6% (mortality 0%) (Kelly et al 1988a). This compares favourably with that associated with conventional craniotomy for these lesions in the past (mortality 11%) (Van Eck et al 1965, Raskind et al 1971, Haar & Patterson 1972, Yardini et al 1984). External beam radiation therapy has followed surgery in most of our patients. The rationale for this is to treat possible microscopic metastatic lesions not visible on CT scanning.

Vascular malformations

Cryptic arterio-venous malformations and cavernous haemangiomas are well circumscribed lesions which can be completely removed stereotactically with relatively low risk. A by-product of

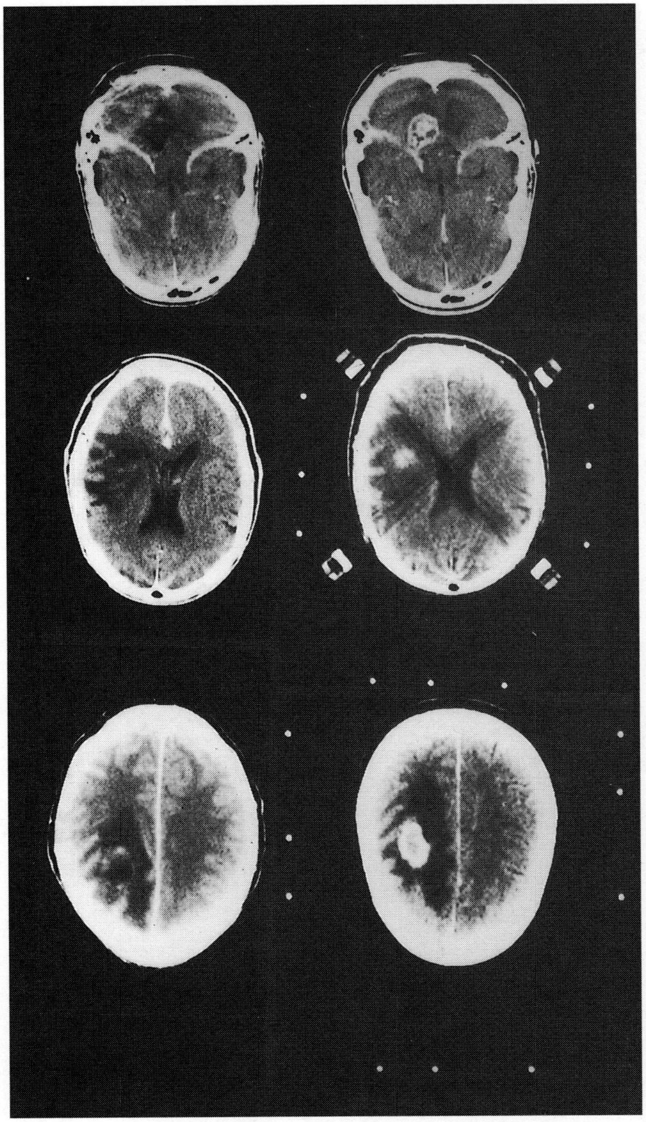

Fig. 6.12 Preoperative (left) and postoperative (right) CT scans on three patients who underwent stereotactic resection for metastatic adenocarcinoma from the left precentral convolution (top), metastatic adenocarcinoma from under the insular cortex, utilizing a transSylvian approach (middle), and metastatic adenocarcinoma from the middle cerebellar peduncle, which employed a transcerebellar approach. (From Kelly et al (1988a).)

establishing the histology is that a cessation or significant reduction of seizures, when present, usually results (Kelly 1988).

Small deep seated active AVMs may also be resected utilizing similar techniques. The position of the feeding vessels is established in the three dimensional surgical planning matrix and approached and clipped or coagulated first, before the remainder of the lesion is dissected away from the surrounding parenchyma.

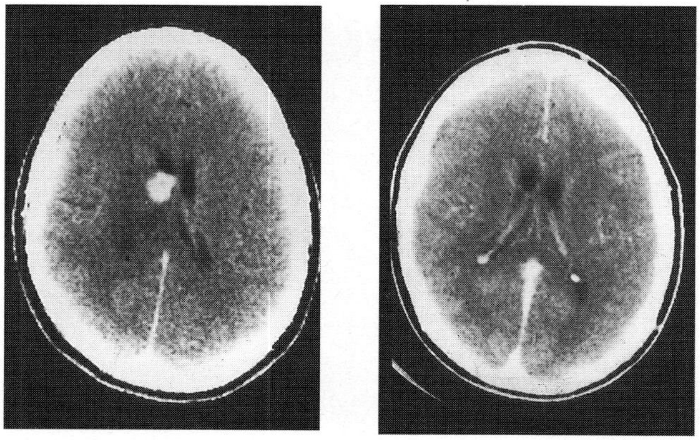

left **right**

Fig. 6.13 Preoperative (left) and postoperative (right) CT scans in a 27-year-old male with small meningioma attached to choroid plexus posterior to the foramen of Monro.

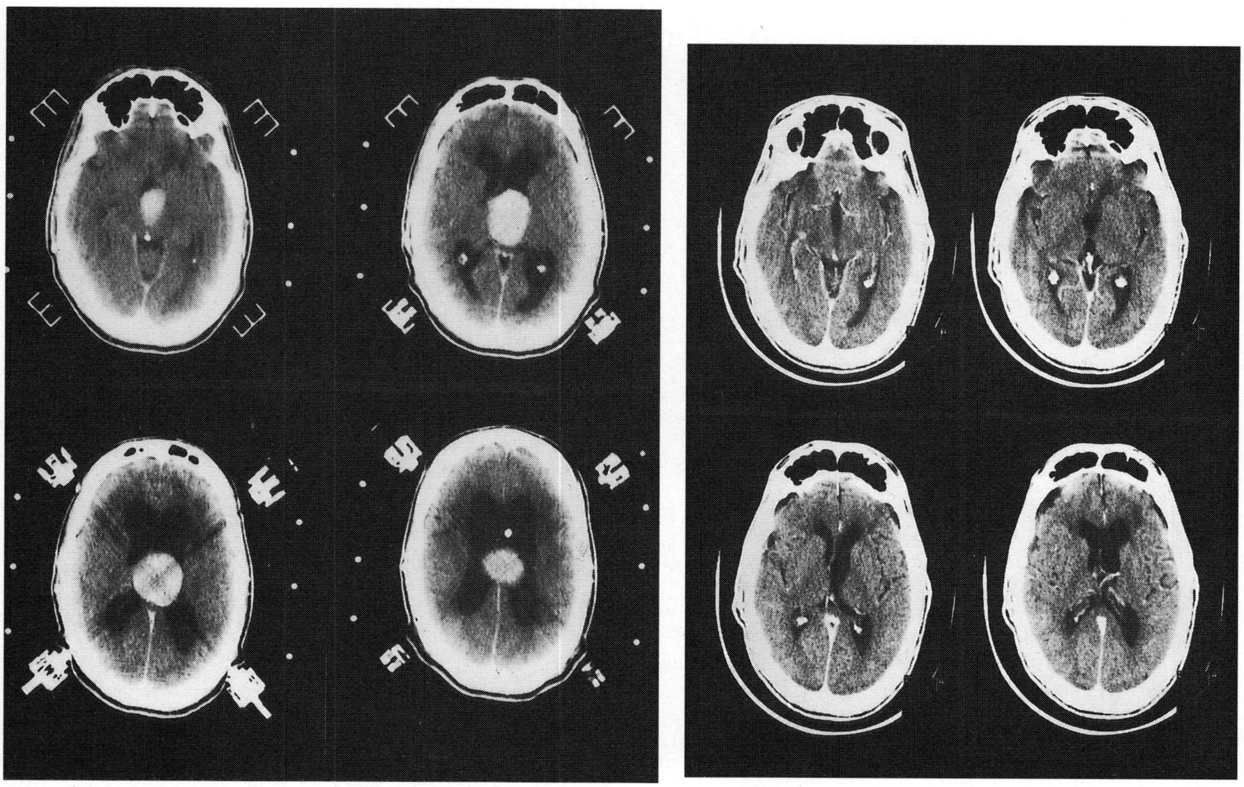

a **b**

Fig. 6.14 **a** Giant colloid cyst which fills the third ventricle. The contents of the cyst were viscous and partially calcified. The lesion was approached through the left lateral ventricle, sacrificing the left fornix. **b** The postoperative CT scan. The patient had a preoperative recent memory deficit which had improved 3 months following surgery.

Intraventricular lesions

A limited direct approach to and exposure of intraventricular lesions can be made utilizing the stereotactic resection technique described in this chapter. Brain and ventricular incisions need to be only large enough to remove the lesion. Thus, intraventricular lesions such as meningiomas, neurocytomas, subependymomas and colloid cysts are removed through a $1\frac{1}{2}$" (40 mm) trephine and a 2 cm cylindrical retractor (Figs. 6.13 and 6.14). In general, lesions located in the frontal horn, foramen of Monro or anterior portion of the body of the lateral ventricle are approached by means of a trephine made at the patient's hairline, and a surgical pathway which employs a microsurgically opened superior frontal sulcus and stereotactically directed white matter incision to the intraventricular lesion. Lesions in the posterior body of the ventricle or atrial region are approached through a cortical/white matter incision made in the superior parietal lobule.

Large third ventricular lesions are usually approached anteriorly through the right lateral ventricle and foramen of Monro. One fornix can be incised in order to extend the stereotactic retractor into the third ventricular lesion. The thalamostriate vein is preserved. An internal decompression of the lesion is performed until only a thin rim of the capsule remains. The computer display of the cross-sections of the digitized tumour volume is extremely useful in this step as the surgeon knows where tumour stops and third ventricular wall begins with respect to the walls of the retractor. One can be quite aggressive within the tumour with reduced risk of extending through the capsule and damaging the walls of the third ventricle. Following this internal decompression, the retractor is withdrawn to the level of the roof of the third ventricle and the capsule is carefully dissected from the walls of the third ventricle. The tumour capsule can be contracted utilizing a defocused carbon dioxide laser or bipolar forceps, which facilitates the dissection of the capsule from the wall of the third ventricle.

CONCLUSION

The volumetric stereotactic resection technique provides a means for maintenance of three dimensional surgical orientation in subcortical procedures. This allows a surgeon to not only find the lesion but also stay oriented within it. Furthermore, the intraoperative CT and MRI based tumour slice images help the surgeon find and develop a plane between tumour and surrounding brain tissue. Preoperative computer based surgical planning allows one to choose the safest possible surgical approach to a lesion, taking the location of normal anatomical structure into account. Tumours in important subcortical areas are approached through non-essential brain tissue and this does not necessarily have to be the shortest route to the lesion. The resection of the lesion is precise and monitored not only by visualization of the surgical field by the surgeon but also by the CT and MRI based rendition of the surgical field displayed by the operating room computer system.

With the computer assisted volumetric stereotactic method described, it is theoretically possible to resect all tumours detected by CT or MRI. The procedure has been found to be most effective for the resection of histologically circumscribed lesions from deep seated intra-axial locations. For instance, pilocytic astrocytomas can be removed with minimal morbidity from any subcortical location, including the thalamus, by this method. In addition, patients harbouring other circumscribed glial tumours, metastatic tumours, and thrombosed vascular malformations can derive significant benefit from this procedure.

In high grade gliomas, adjuvant therapy directed at neoplastic cells remaining in the hypodense zone surrounding the area of contrast enhancement resected by the stereotactic procedure is administered with the greatest surgical reduction of tumour burden possible. In selected cases, a significant reduction of tumour cell burden in high grade glial neoplasms may favourably influence survival and response to external radiation and chemotherapy.

REFERENCES

Boethius J, Bergstrom M, Greitz T, Ribbe T 1980 CT localization in stereotactic surgery. Applied Neurophysiology 43: 164–169

Brown R A 1979 A computerized tomography–computer graphics approach to stereotaxic localization. Journal of Neurosurgery 50: 715–720

Burger P C, Dubois P J, Schold S C Jr, Smith K R Jr, Odom G L, Crafts D C, Giangaspero F 1983 Computerized tomographic and pathologic studies of the untreated, quiescent, and recurrent glioblastoma multiforme. Journal of Neurosurgery 59: 159–168

Coffey R J, Lunsford L D, Taylor F H 1988 Survival after stereotactic biopsy of malignant gliomas. Neurosurgery 22(3): 465–473

Daumas-Duport C, Monsaingeon V, Szenthe L, Szikla G 1982 Serial stereotactic biopsies: a double histological code of gliomas according to malignancy and 3-D configuration, as an aid to therapeutic decision and assessment of results. Applied Neurophysiology 45: 431–437

Daumas-Duport C, Scheithauer B W, Kelly P J 1987 A histologic and cytologic method for the spatial definition of gliomas. Mayo Clinic Proceedings 62: 435–449

Frankel S A, German W J 1958 Glioblastoma multiforme: review of 219 cases with regard to natural history, diagnostic methods, and treatment. Journal of Neurosurgery 15: 489–503

Gehan E A, Walker M D 1977 Prognostic factors for patients with brain tumours. National Cancer Institute Monograph 46: 189–195

Goerss S, Kelly P J, Kall B, Alker G J Jr 1982 A computed tomographic stereotactic adaptation system. Neurosurgery 10: 375–379

Goodenough D J, Weaver K E, Davis D O 1975 Potential artifacts associated with the scanning pattern of the EMI scanner. Radiology 117: 615–620

Haar F, Patterson R H Jr 1972 Surgery for metastatic intracranial neoplasm. Cancer 30: 1241–1245

Hitchcock E, Sato F 1964 Treatment of malignant gliomata. Journal of Neurosurgery 21: 497–505

Hoshino T 1984 A commentary on the biology and growth kinetics of low grade and high grade gliomas. Journal of Neurosurgery 27: 388–400

Hoshino T, Barker M, Wilson C B, Boldrey E B, Fewer D 1972 Cell kinetics of human gliomas. Journal of Neurosurgery 37: 15–26

Jelsma R, Bucy P C 1967 The treatment of glioblastoma multiforme of the brain. Journal of Neurosurgery 27: 388–400

Kelly P J 1987 Stereotactic technology in tumor surgery. Clinical Neurosurgery 35: 215–253

Kelly P J 1988 Volumetric stereotactic surgical resection of intra-axial brain mass lesions. Mayo Clinic Proceedings 63: 1186–1198

Kelly P J 1989 Stereotactic biopsy and resection in thalamic astrocytomas. Neurosurgery 25: 185–195

Kelly P J 1990 Stereotactic imaging, surgical planning and computer assisted volumetric resection of intracranial lesions: methods and results. Advances and Technical Standards in Neurosurgery 17: 77–118

Kelly P J, Alker G J Jr 1980 A method for stereotactic laser microsurgery in the treatment of deep seated CNS neoplasms. Applied Neurophysiology 43: 210–215

Kelly P J, Alker G J Jr 1981 A stereotactic approach to deep seated CNS neoplasms using the carbon dioxide laser. Surgical Neurology 15: 331–334

Kelly P J, Olson M H, Wright A E 1978 Stereotactic implantation of Iridium^{192} into CNS neoplasms. Surgical Neurology 10: 349–354

Kelly P J, Olson M H, Wright A E, Giorgi C 1979 CT localization and stereotactic implantation of Ir^{192} into CNS neoplasms. In: Szikla G (ed) Stereotactic cerebral irradiation, Elsevier/North Holland, Amsterdam, pp 123–128

Kelly P J, Alker G J Jr, Goerss S J 1982 Computer assisted stereotactic laser microsurgery for the treatment of intracranial neoplasms. Neurosurgery 10: 324–331

Kelly P J, Alker G J Jr, Zoll J G 1982b A microstereotactic approach to deep seated arteriovenous malformation: Case report and technical note. Surgical Neurology 17: 260–262

Kelly P J, Alker G J Jr, Kall B, Goerss S 1983 Precision resection of intra-axial CNS lesions by CT-based stereotactic craniotomy and computer monitored CO_2 laser. Acta Neurochirurgica 68: 1–9

Kelly P J, Kall B A, Goerss S J 1984 Transposition of volumetric information derived from computed tomography scanning into stereotactic space. Surgical Neurology 21: 465–471

Kelly P J, Kall B, Goerss S, Earnest F 1986 Computer-assisted stereotaxic resection of intra-axial brain neoplasms. Journal of Neurosurgery 64: 427–439

Kelly P J, Daumas-Duport C, Kispert D B, Kall B A, Scheithauer B W, Illig J W 1987a Imaging-based stereotactic serial biopsies in untreated intracranial glial neoplasms. Journal of Neurosurgery 66: 865–874

Kelly P J, Daumas-Duport C, Scheithauer B W, Kall B A, Kispert D B 1987b Stereotactic histologic correlations of computed tomography- and magnetic resonance imaging-defined abnormalities in patients with glial neoplasms. Mayo Clinic Proceedings 62: 450–459

Kelly P J, Kall B A, Goerss S J 1988a The results of CT-based computer assisted stereotactic resection of metastatic intracranial tumours. Neurosurgery 22: 7–17

Kelly P J, Goerss S J, Kall B A 1988b Evolution of contemporary instrumentation for computer-assisted stereotactic surgery. Surgical Neurology 30: 204–215

Kelly P J, Goerss S J, Kall B A 1988c The stereotactic retractor in computer assisted stereotactic microsurgery: a technical note. Journal of Neurosurgery 69: 301–306

MacGee E E 1971 Surgical treatment of cerebral metastases from lung cancer: the effect on quality and duration of survival. Journal of Neurosurgery 35: 416–420

McGirr S J, Kelly P J, Scheithauer B W 1987 Stereotactic resection of juvenile pilocytic astrocytomas of the thalamus and basal ganglia. Neurosurgery 20: 447–452

Moore M R, Black P McL, Ellenbogen R, Gall C M, Eldredge E 1989 Stereotactic craniotomy: methods and results using the Brown–Roberts–Wells stereotactic frame. Neurosurgery 25: 572–578

Perry J H, Rosenbaum A E, Lunsford L D, Swink C A, Zorub D S 1980 Computed tomography guided stereotactic surgery: conception and development of a new stereotactic methodology. Neurosurgery 7: 376–381

Raskind R, Weiss S E, Manning J J, Wernuth R E 1971 Survival after surgical excision of single metastatic brain tumours. American Journal of Radiology 111: 323–328

Van Eck J H M, Go K G, Ebels E J 1965 Metastatic tumours of the brain. Psychiatria Neurologia Neurochirurgia 68: 443–462

Yardeni D, Reichenthal E, Zucker G, Rubenstein A, Cohen M, Israeli J, Shalit M N 1984 Neurosurgical management of single brain metastasis. Surgical Neurology 21: 377–384

7. Development of ultrasound guided brain tumour surgery

J. Koivukangas

BACKGROUND

Image guided brain surgery has traditionally been synonymous with stereotactic surgery, which was originally based on mechanical frames and anteroposterior and lateral skull films. With the development of computerized tomography (CT), many stereotactic frames were adapted to the new digital imaging technology, often using computers for calculations and graphics. Within the last 5 years or so, electromechanical devices called neuronavigators have been developed to connect digital imaging data flexibly to the surgical field. Since ultrasound is the only real time imaging method available for the operative theatre, various methods for adapting this imaging mode to image directed brain surgery have been described.

The application of ultrasound to brain tumour surgery began about 40 years ago in Minneapolis in the USA. In 1950, French et al reported on the first experimental attempts to use ultrasound for the localization of a cerebral tumour. The first actual 'clinical use of ultrasound in localization of brain tumours in operating room' was recorded in 1951 by the neurosurgeon William Peyton and reported 2 years later (Wild & Reid 1953). This cross-disciplinary work was made possible by the application by neurosurgeons of early research in the Department of Electrical Engineering, University of Minnesota. Since then, the focus of research in intraoperative ultrasound has been in the localization of brain tumours, first with A scan and then with non-real time B scan technology.

Real time B ultrasonography was developed for clinical use only about a decade ago. Its application to brain and spinal surgery began around 1980 at several centres more or less independently (for reviews, see Koivukangas 1984, Chandler & Rubin, 1986). Originally the technology was rather crude, but it was soon realized that the key to intraoperative applications was transducer design and system user friendliness. The Oulu experience with application of ultrasound imaging to image guided brain surgery began in 1980 with basic laboratory investigations in collaboration with the Department of Electrical Engineering, University of Oulu. It has passed through several stages to the concept of multimodality image guided brain tumour surgery.

LABORATORY INVESTIGATIONS

Image guided brain surgery begins with a stable, preferably rigid, connection between the images and the brain. In early laboratory investigations, the tissue specimen was placed in a water tank and a single element ultrasound transducer passed above the specimen, sending and receiving pulses at uniform intervals. A, B, holographic B and C images were analysed (Fig. 7.1). The images showed that the sulci, fissures, ventricular walls, choroid plexus, falx, tentorium and skull could be identified as hyperechogenic (bright) features. In rigid laboratory conditions even the configuration of associative white matter bundles could be discerned. Grey matter was clearly more echogenic than white matter. Various tumours such as gliomas and meningiomas were usually at least partially hyperechogenic, while infarcts were hypoechogenic. These experiments formed the basis of clinical ultrasound imaging which began in 1981. More importantly, the rigid experimental set-up served as the model for our later work towards three dimensional image guided brain surgery (Koivukangas et al 1986).

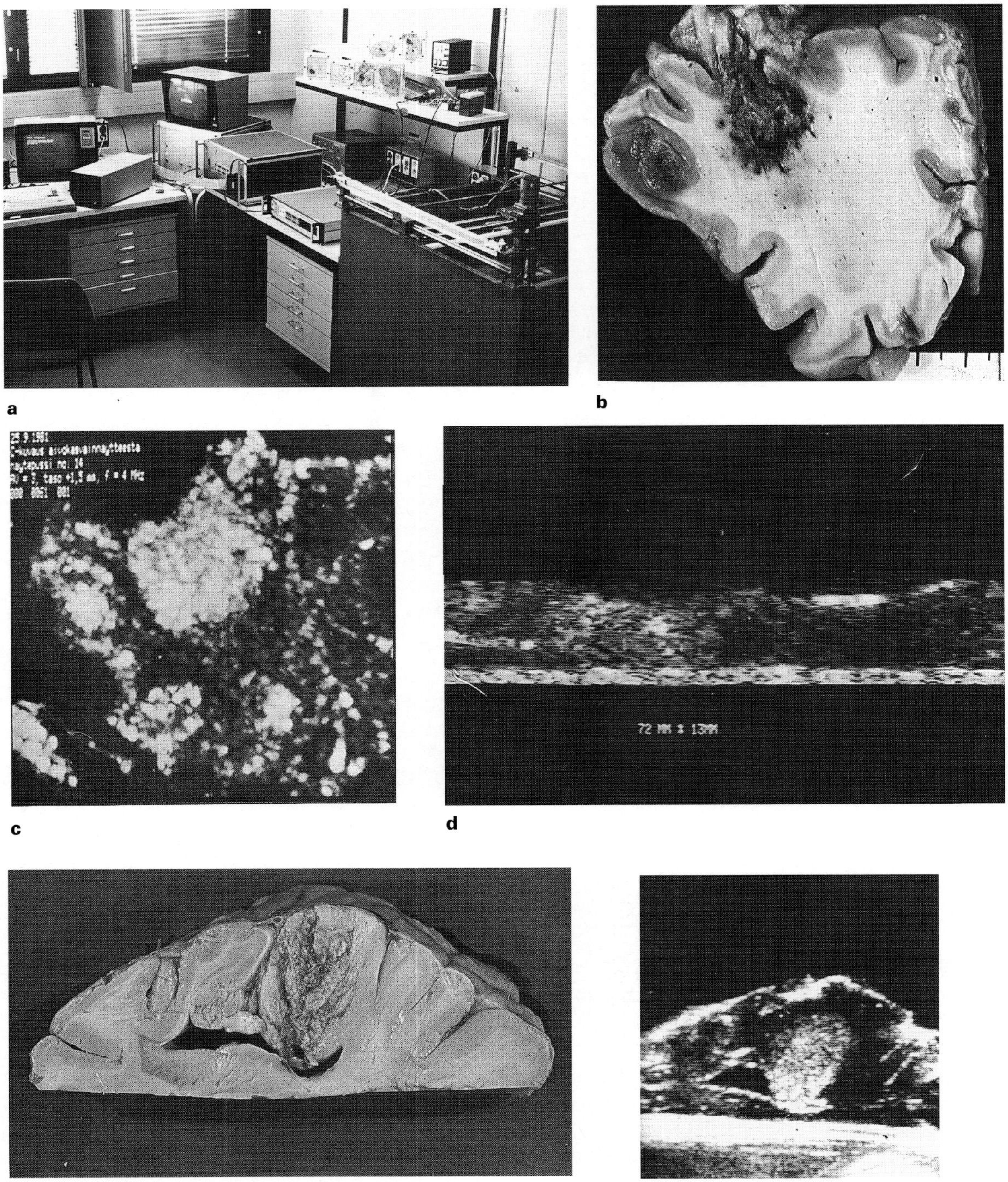

Fig. 7.1 **a** Early laboratory for the study of tissue specimens in a water tank (right), where brain tumour ultrasound properties were examined and the principles of volumetric ultrasound guidance developed. **b** Frontal lobe specimen showing subcortical astrocytoma. **c** C scan of the specimen showing highly echogenic tumour extending from the surface into hypoechogenic white matter, associative white matter fibres and relatively high echogenicity of cortical grey matter. **d** Ultrasound holographic B scan of the same specimen showing hyperechogenic tumour within white matter. **e** Brain specimen showing subcortical low grade astrocytoma extending into the cerebral ventricle. **f** B scan of the specimen displays the small low grade astrocytoma as a hyperechogenic tumour relatively well demarcated within a gyrus.

EARLY CLINICAL STUDIES

The first real time ultrasound imagers were developed for general soft tissue examination. The probe, in particular, was usually fairly large and employed mechanical sector technology (Fig. 7.2). Soon Rubin and Dohrmann (1982) reported on a scanner designed to accommodate neurosurgical operations and Tsutsumi et al (1982) described a needle guide mounted rigidly on the ultrasound probe. This facilitated image guided brain tumour biopsy. It was soon realized that ultrasound images gave supplementary data that could be compared with that of X-ray CT to give a more comprehensive picture of the tumour. The chief advantages of ultrasound guided biopsy have been that the biop-

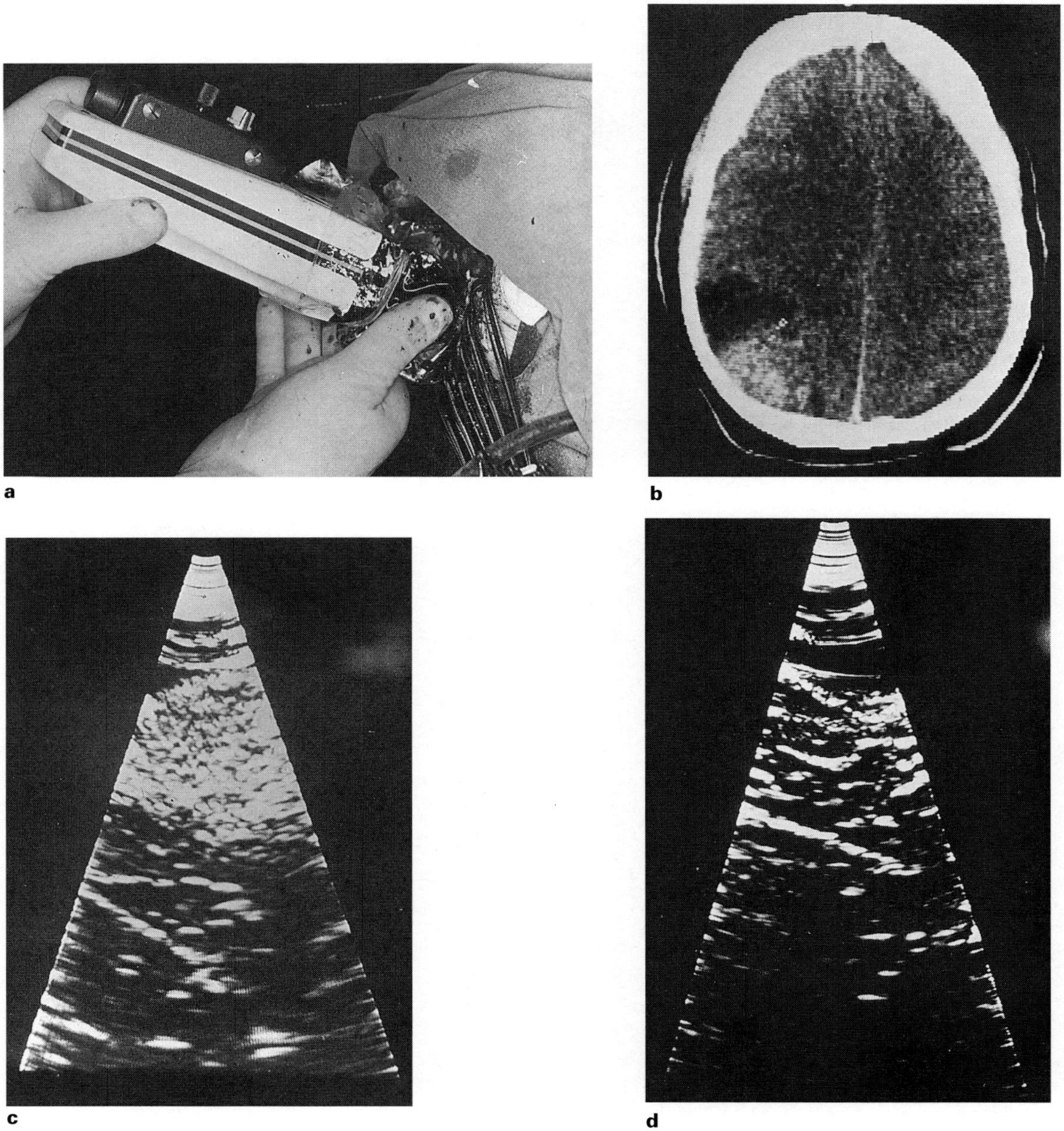

Fig. 7.2 First experiences with real time ultrasound imaging using **a** one of the first available probes demonstrated the possibility of following the removal of high grade astrocytoma (**b** contrast enhanced CT image), with **c** hyperechogenic tumour **d** grossly totally removed.

sy site can be determined during surgery, several biopsy trajectories can readily be chosen and the effects of biopsy can be checked to rule out haemorrhage.

The present series consists of 70 brain tumour patients operated on between 1981 and 1990 with ultrasound control. Most of the patients (76%) operated on during this first decade of application had cerebral glioma, almost all of them (92.7%) supratentorially situated. The most common locations were subcortically in the frontal, temporal and parietal lobes. Of the astrocytomas, 61% were 2–4 cm in maximum diameter on CT and magnetic resonance imaging (MRI) scans. In 10 cases, ultrasound control was used during operation for recurrent glioma. 11 of the glioma patients underwent biopsy procedures, 34 partial resection and 10 gross total removal of tumour (Koivukangas & Koivukangas 1986).

During this first decade of experience with real time B ultrasound, the imager and probe technology continually improved (Fig. 7.3). Because of the academic nature of our ultrasound programme (Koivukangas 1984), six different ultrasound scan-

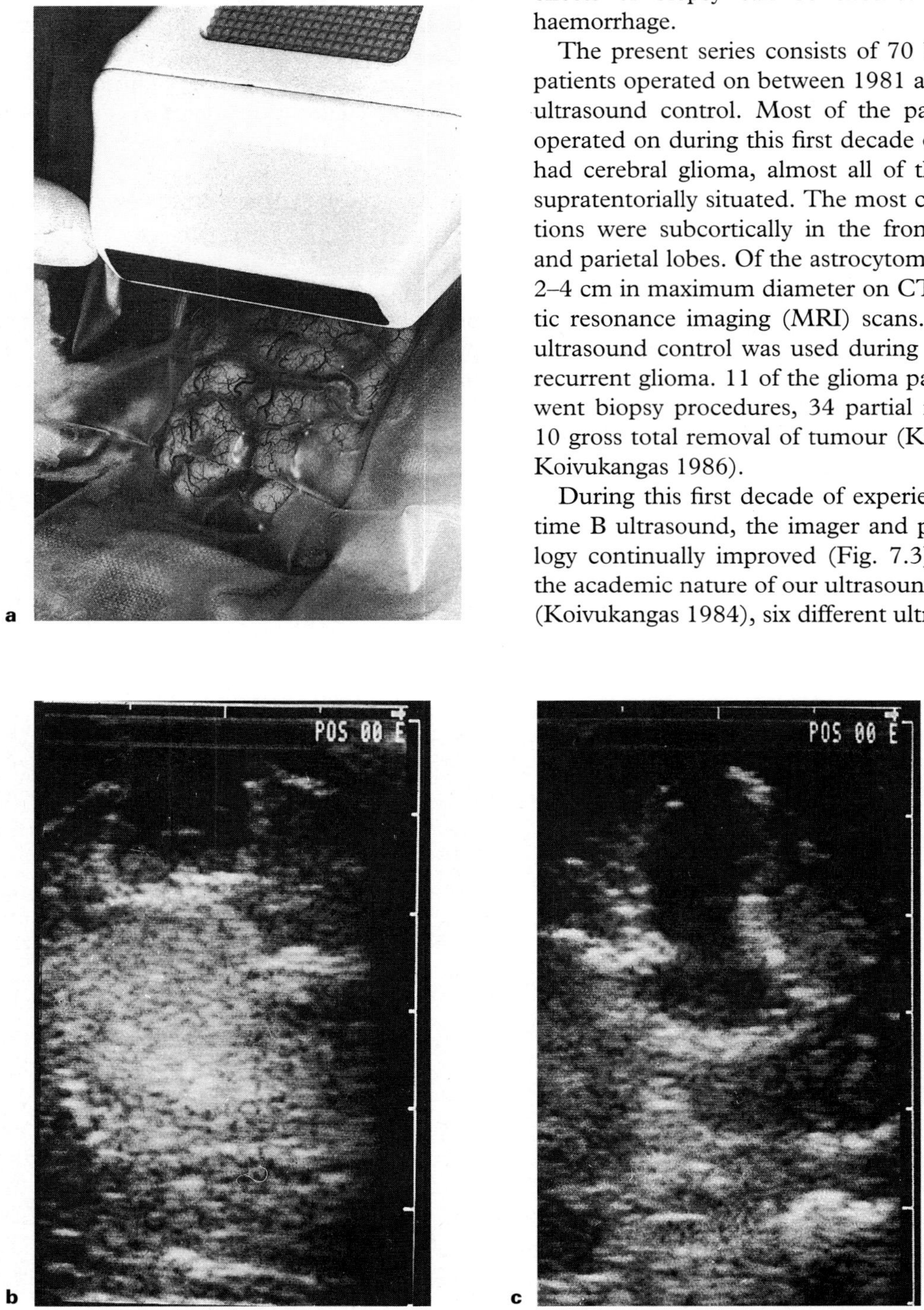

Fig. 7.3 **a** Modern linear array probes (38 mm in width) can be used during craniotomy to **b** follow approach to subcortical hyperechogenic low grade astrocytoma and **c** resection of the tumour.

ners with 11 transducers were used and rigorously evaluated in the neurosurgical setting and for imaging nervous tissue in general (Alasaarela & Koivukangas 1990). Currently, biopsy of subcortical masses is routinely performed with ultrasound control in our clinic. During the last 2 years, ultrasound has further been incorporated in the development of a neuronavigator, as described below.

MECHANICAL FIXATION OF THE ULTRASOUND PROBE

In 1982 Tsutsumi et al had already described a lockable 'fixation apparatus' for holding the ultrasound probe. This was a simple mechanical probe holder connected to the surgical table that could be locked into the desired position. There was also a biopsy needle guide tunnel connected to the ultrasound probe. Later, self-retaining retractor arms were used to fix the ultrasound probe in place once the site for the burr hole and biopsy had been chosen. These methods allowed the neurosurgeon to place the probe on the surface of the dura or brain, search for the tumour and a suitable trajectory, lock the probe in that position and introduce a biopsy needle or forceps using the guide apparatus. The biopsy instrument could be followed as it passed in the plane of the real time ultrasound image to the tumour for biopsy.

A multijointed arm that could be used for ultrasound guided biopsy, but could also repeatedly and exactly be repositioned during brain tumour resection was designed by Koivukangas and Noponen for Bruel and Kjaer in 1985 (Fig. 7.4). The ultrasound probe could also be rotated along its longitudinal axis at desired degree intervals to produce a three dimensional set of ultrasound images.

Berger (1986) described a simple fixation device, which could be screwed into an enlarged burr hole. An ultrasound probe could be placed in the probe holder and locked into position. Then, following removal of the ultrasound probe, a biopsy needle could be passed along the 'central vector' of the ultrasound image to the selected depth within the tumour. The passage of the biopsy needle could not be followed by ultrasound, but following withdrawal of the biopsy sample, the track of the needle could be examined with ultrasound for haemorrhage.

Heilbrun et al (1983) mentioned briefly the rigid connection of the ultrasound probe to a stereotactic frame for biopsy. The obvious advantages were supplementary information about diffuse intracerebral tumours and the possibility of checking the biopsy site for haemorrhage. Koivukangas and Kelly (1986) described early experience with this method in tumour resection control (see Fig. 7.4). Problems with the method were transducer size and difficulties in interpretation of images during resection using tubular brain retractors. By connecting the ultrasound probe to the Laitinen frame it was found that biopsy and even resection could be followed (Fig. 7.4), but the frame was not able to accommodate true open stereotactic resection: although the ultrasound probe could be connected to the frame there was no connection between the means of tissue removal and the frame.

THE ULTRASOUND SURGICAL ADAPTER

An effort to rigidly connect three dimensional ultrasound imaging to the surgical field and the means of tissue removal resulted in the development of the ultrasound surgical adapter in 1985 (Koivukangas & Louhisalmi 1990). The idea was based on the principle of volumetric ultrasound imaging (Fig. 7.5). The adapter (Fig. 7.6) guides the movement of the ultrasound probe above the brain during surgery and then, following removal of the probe, the adapter orients the surgical laser to the imaged brain. The adapter was attached to the craniotomy in a watertight fashion, because water is required as a coupling medium. Furthermore, the lid of the adapter holding the ultrasound probe is also watertight, so the craniotomy site does not need to be parallel with the floor in order to hold the coupling water. Another advantage of the system is that the tip of the transducer is held 1–2 cm above the brain or dura, so near-field artefacts occurring within the first centimetre in many types of probes do not interfere with the image of brain. Thus, the dura and most superficial regions of the brain are also well visualized.

The surgical adapter allows either sequential parallel images or sequential radial images at

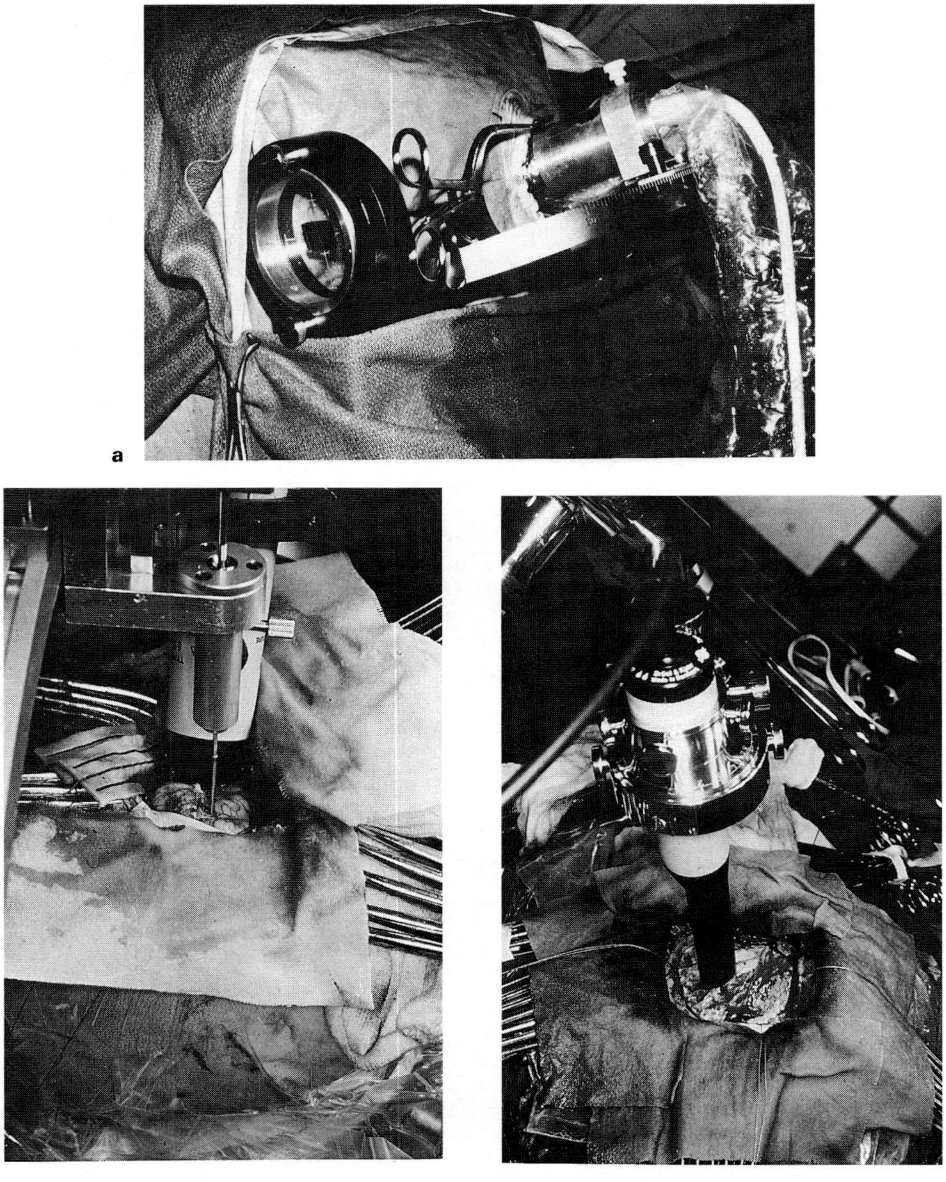

a

b

c

Fig. 7.4 **a, b** The ultrasound probe can be placed directly on various conventional stereotactic frames with customized holding pieces to control tumour resection or biopsy. **c** Alternatively, an ultrasound probe holder clamped to the surgical table or Mayfield headholder can repeatedly and exactly reposition the probe during resection of tumour. This apparatus also allows rotation of probe at even intervals to obtain three dimensional information about a tumour.

specified uniform intervals. The images are transferred to the computer, and the tumour is then outlined on each image. Because the images are rigidly related to the adapter, a truly stereotactic graphic representation of the tumour is produced. Similar to the method described by Kelly (1988), tumour outlines are then reconstructed perpendicularly to the axis of the surgical laser. The microscope is rigidly aligned to the adapter, with the central optical axis of the microscope, and the laser beam, passing through the centre point of the adapter. At the desired measured depth, the first tumour outline is called for, and the laser removes that layer line by line. The laser first draws the reconstructed outline on the presenting surface, using the visible pilot laser

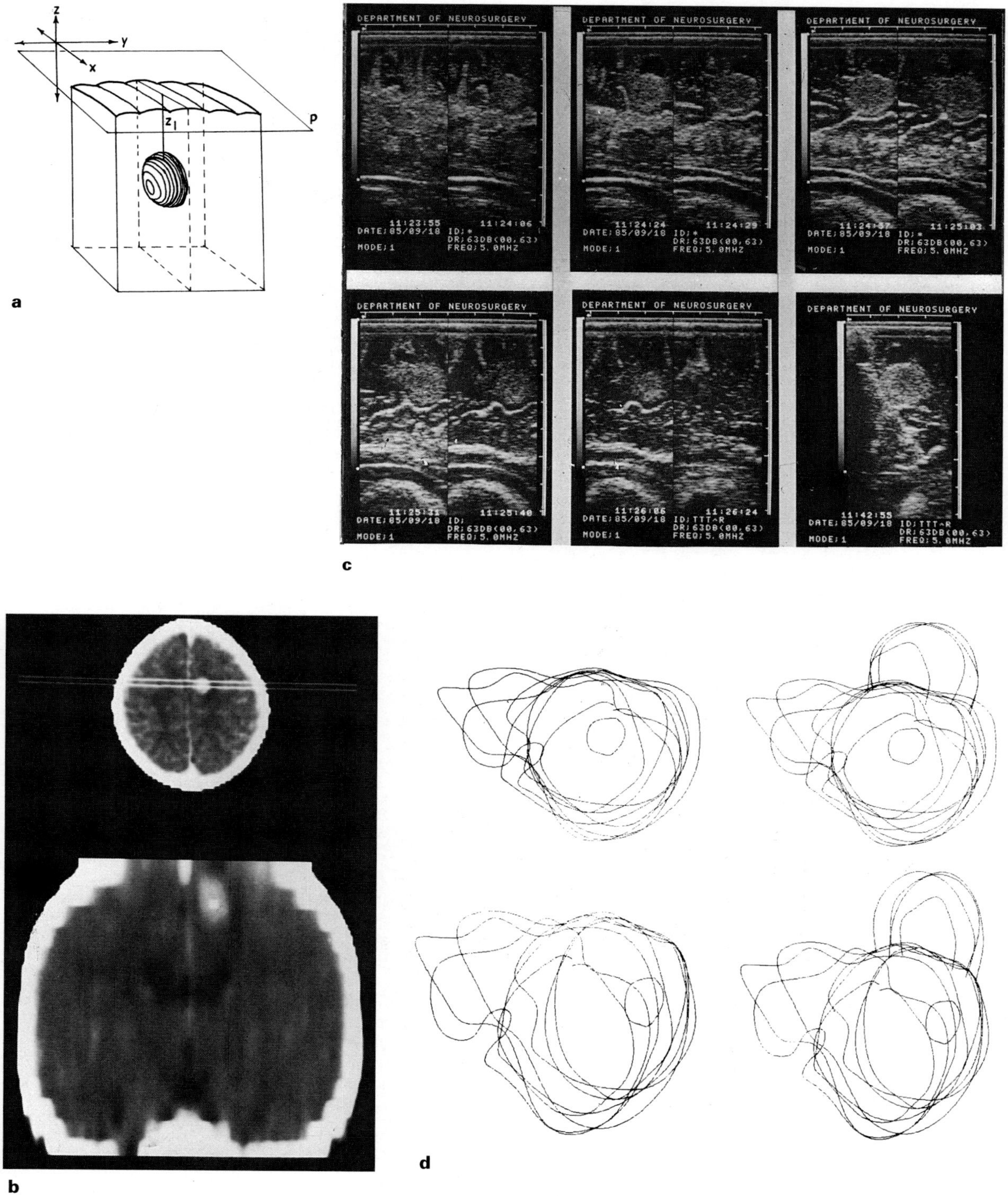

Fig. 7.5 **a** The principle of volumetric ultrasound imaging for the brain surgery adapter: the ultrasound probe moves along plane P, the most direct approach to the tumour is indicated by z_1. A small low grade astrocytoma (**b** contrast enhanced CT) adjacent to the lower extremity motor strip caused monoplegia in a young boy. **c** A series of 10 linear array ultrasound images taken at 2 mm intervals shows the cystic tumour within one gyrus, extending along associative fibres to the adjacent gyrus (top right). **d** Three dimensional line drawings of the tumour seen back to back (upper) and rotated 30° (lower).

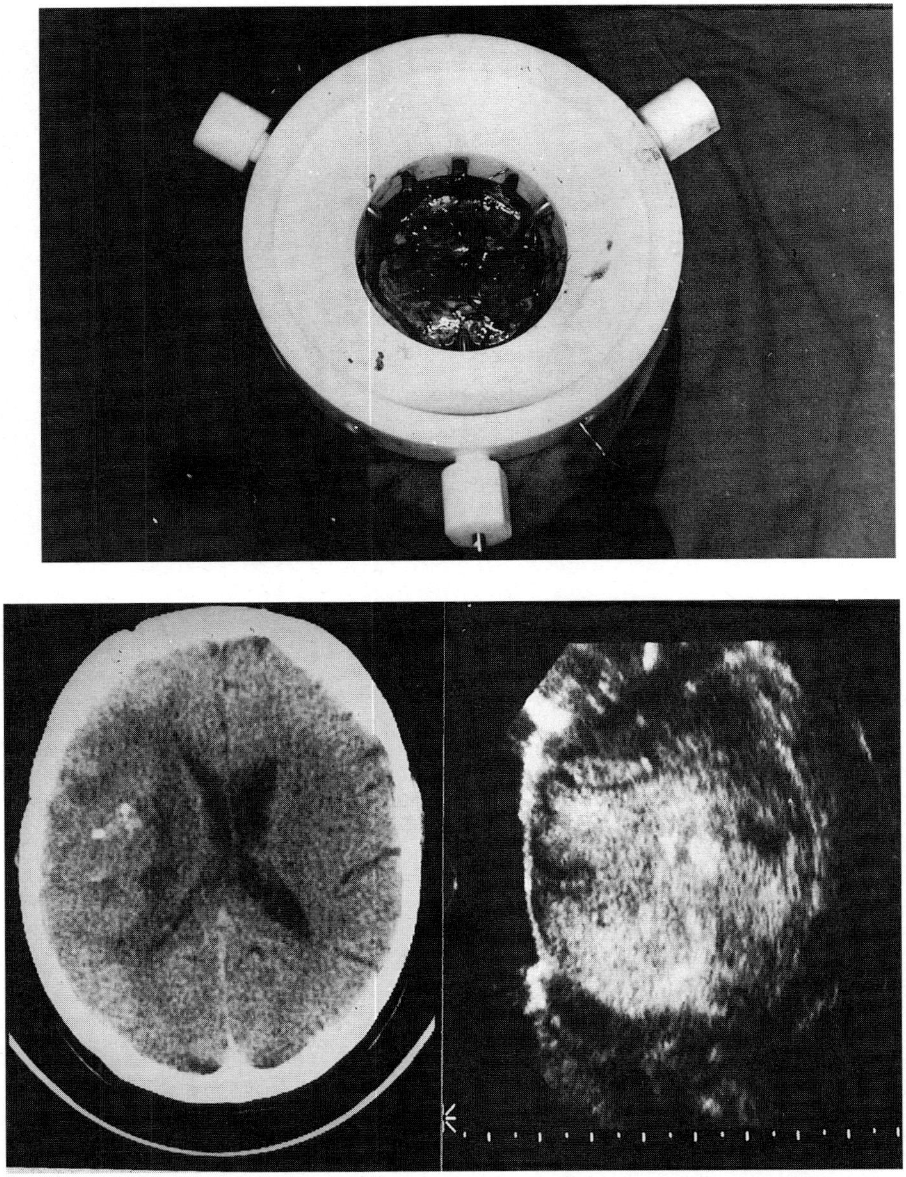

Fig. 7.6 **a** The brain surgery adapter is clamped to the edge of the craniotomy with silicone sealer to give a watertight fit. The ultrasound probe is attached to the adapter with a watertight lid, so the probe can be situated in Ringer's solution 1–2 cm above the dura or brain. **b** CT scan (left) of partially calcified temporal lobe astrocytoma and ultrasound scan (right) of tumour with probe well above dura, the tumour being seen in at least two gyri and extending near lateral ventricle. For laser resection of the tumour, the surgical microscope is rigidly connected to adapter (see text), here **c** laser evaporation of a small low grade astrocytoma is being performed. The outlines of the tumour are drawn using the computer 'mouse' and visualized on a flat monitor screen, all placed under **d** a sterile plastic draping for surgeon interaction.

mode, and upon approval by the neurosurgeon observing the outline through the microscope, the combined carbon dioxide/neodymium-yttrium aluminium garnet (CO_2/Nd-YAG) laser is then activated. At certain intervals, the surgical field is imaged with the ultrasound probe to check the progress of tumour resection.

Seven cases of radical laser resection of glioma have been performed by the author. The chief indication for the adapter at present appears to

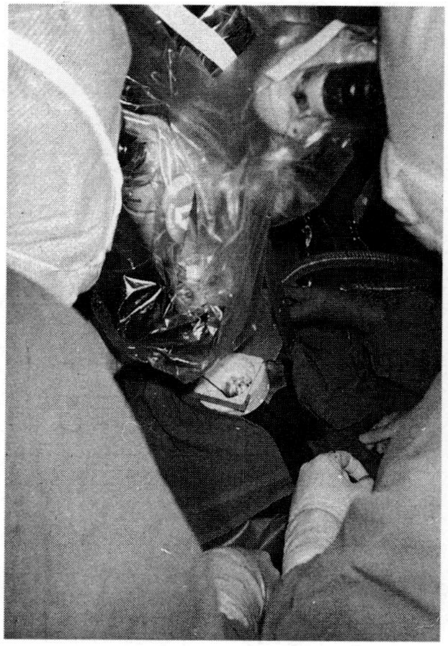
c

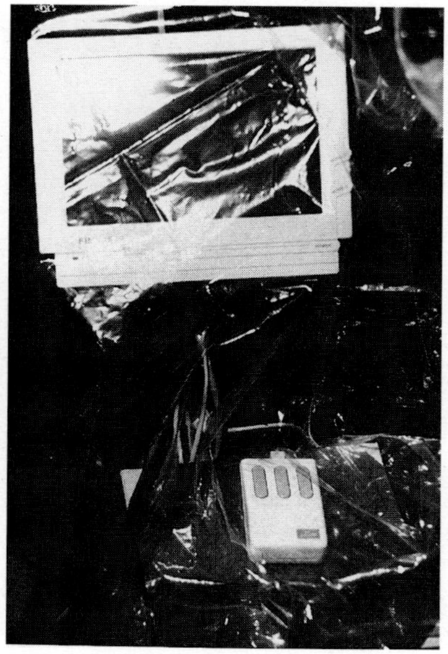
d

Fig. 7.6 *(Contd)*

be resection of a small subcortical astrocytoma or of a metastasis, when these tumours can be adequately delineated with ultrasound. Since the procedure is performed under the surgical microscope, haemostasis can be assured readily and the extent of tumour removal can be modified. Thus the method can also be used to debulk larger tumours whose edges can then be further dissected and removed with bipolar coagulation and irrigation–suction. The main disadvantage of the system in terms of stereotactic requirements is that presently, preoperative CT and MRI scans have not been rigidly oriented with the adapter.

THE ULTRASOUND GUIDED NEURONAVIGATOR

Conceptually, neuronavigators that give spatial accuracy in the 1–3 mm range and are rigidly lockable are really electromechanical extensions of the conventional mechanical stereotactic frames. Whereas the conventional stereotactic frames have been originally based on the anteroposterior and lateral plain skull films, neuronavigators are based on interactive computer manipulations of digital imaging data. Here, the neuronavigator is more than a pointer; it is an electromechanical precision instrument that serves to hold various instruments in desired positions (Fig. 7.7).

The neuronavigator was first described by Watanabe et al in 1987. It has served as a pointer for purposes of orientation within the brain in most reports. Hence the name 'neuronavigator'. In the present system, the principle of a common central axis has been employed to make the neuronavigator more versatile. The present neuronavigator (Koivu Kangas et al 1992) is a six jointed mechatronic arm with high precision optical encoders measuring the movement of each joint. It is connected to the Mayfield headholder which also fixes the patient's head during surgery. The neuronavigator is connected to the UNIX workstation (Hewlett-Packard 700 series) whose memory contains the preoperative CT/MRI data, including the fiducial points, either fatty vitamin or aluminium spheres. The workstation also contains the customized three dimensional image software. Before surgery the CT/MRI data is transferred to the workstation via an Ethernet data line. The procedure can be rehearsed in the treatment planning room, which is also connected to the surgical theatre via the Ethernet data line. At our hospital, between February 1990 and April 1992, 13 procedures have been performed during the development of neuronavigator hardware and software (Table 7.1).

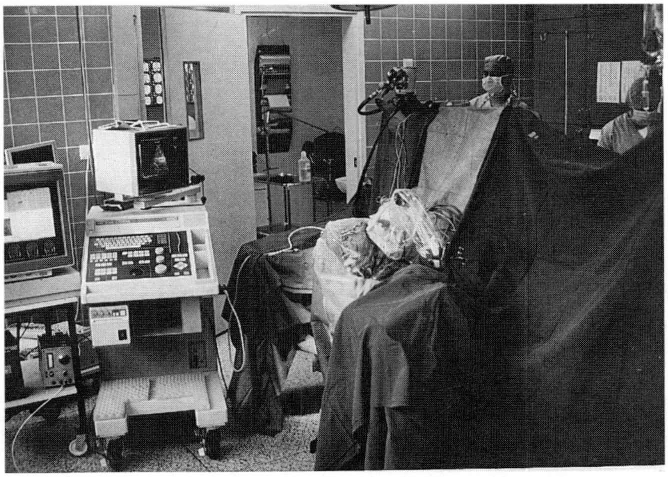

a

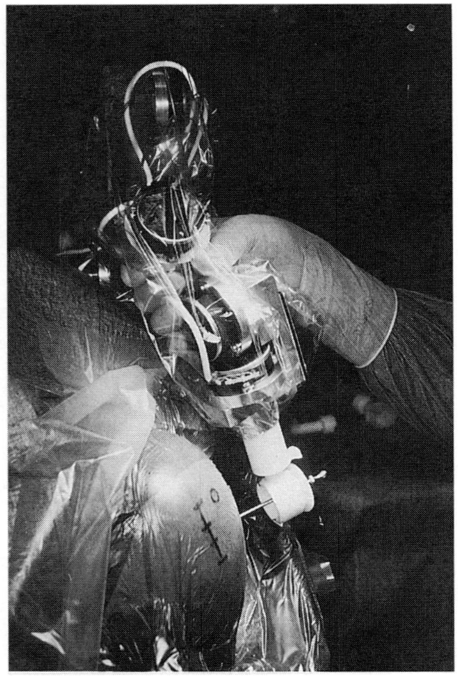

b

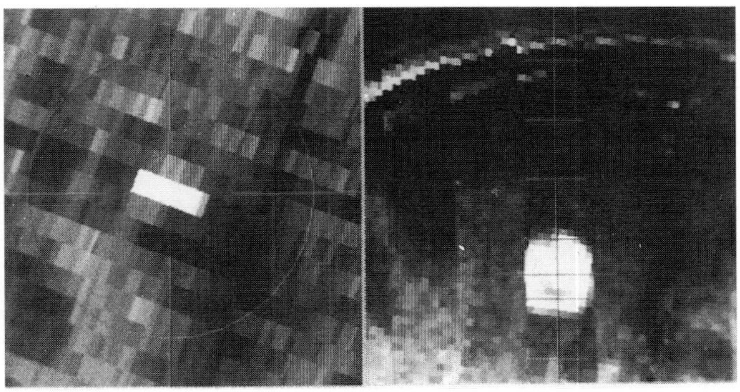

c

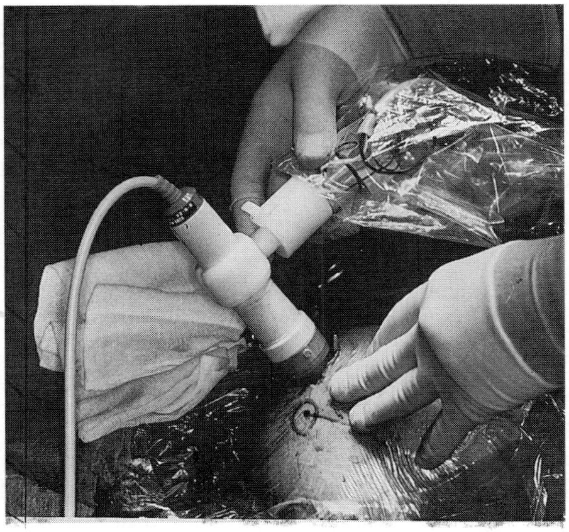

d

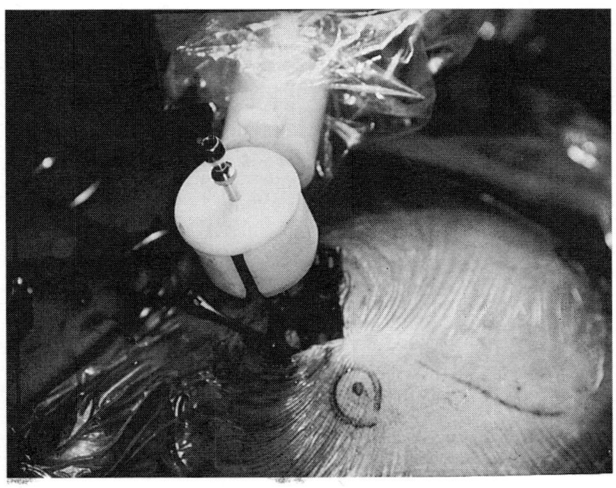

e

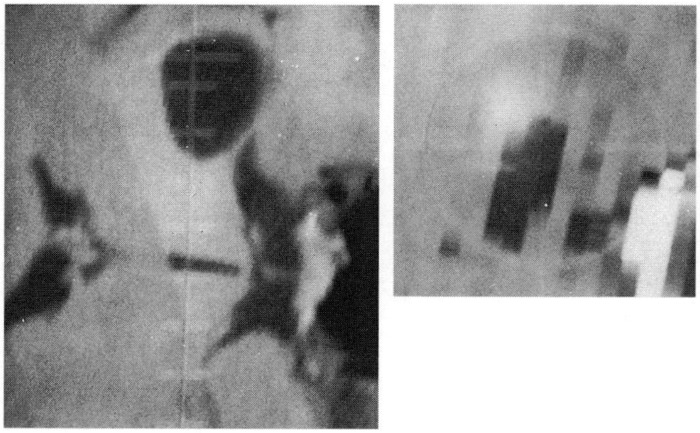

f

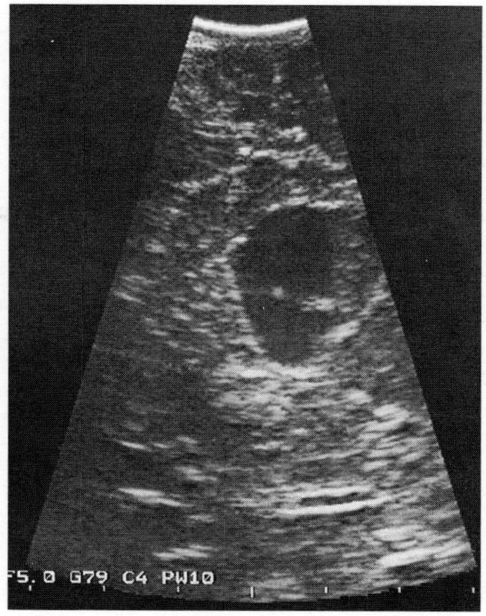

g

Fig. 7.7 **a** The neuronavigator is clamped to the Mayfield headholder (right), the ultrasound scanner (centre) and computer workstation (left) showing images. **b** First, the neuronavigator is calibrated to fiducial points on the scalp and then the burr hole site (as drawn) and trajectory are planned. **c** As the neuronavigator pointer is moved on the scalp, pertinent CT/MRI reconstructions are shown on the workstation monitor: (right) the reconstruction along the axis of the pointer. with the axis of the pointer shown extending into brain as a graduated line through contrast enhanced low-grade astrocytoma; (left) the reconstruction in the perpendicular plane at the level of the tumour. **d** After burr hole and dural incision, the ultrasound probe is aligned with the neuronavigator, giving an image in same plane as the CT/MRI reconstructions. **e** The biopsy needle guide is then aligned with the neuronavigator and a biopsy is taken. In another case, the MRI reconstructions show **f** a cystic lesion, with **g** the corresponding ultrasound image. Note that the central axis of the MRI reconstruction on the left coincides with the central axis of the ultrasound image, because both images are from the same plane.

During surgery, the neuronavigator is first calibrated using the fiducial markers, i.e. the tip of the pointer is touched to 4 minute tattoo spots on the scalp where the spheres were situated during imaging. These points are also indicated on the respective images on the workstation display. Calibration is carried out by voice control of the computer within 1 minute. Then, the pointer is touched to the scalp and the workstation monitor displays the reconstructed image in the plane of the pointer, with a graduated red line indicating the extension of the pointer axis in the image plane. Another reconstructed image is simultaneously shown in the plane perpendicular to the axis of the pointer, at the desired depth. As the pointer is moved on the scalp, the reconstructions appear on the monitor in almost real time, within 2 seconds.

The principle of the common central axis means that the important axes of all instruments attached to the neuronavigator are aligned along the same axis (see Fig. 7.7 and Table 7.1):

1. The axis of the pointer described above (all patients in Table 7.1).
2. The biopsy forceps guide needle is also aligned along the same axis, i.e. the forceps will pass along the red line in the reconstructed image to the prescribed depth (patients KS, HJ, MP, HN, NS, LH).
3. The neuroendoscope will also be passed along the same line (patient SS).
4. The ultrasound probe is connected to the neuronavigator in such a way that the central axis of the probe, i.e. the midline of the ultrasound images corresponds to the same red line in the CT/MRI reconstructions (all patients in Table 7.1).
5. The optical axis of the surgical microscope also coincides with the common central axis.

Table 7.1 Patient series operated with ultrasound guided neuronavigator

Patient	Sex	Age (years)	Tumour site[a]	Diagnosis[b]	Comments[c]
AK	F	32	L-FP	Agr4	Laitinen stereoguide, recurrent tumour resection
PK	F	36	R-P	LGA	Laitinen stereoguide, laser resection
KS	M	56	L-T	Agr4	5 MHz sector, CT/16–22 mm, biopsy
HJ	M	34	L-FP	LGA	5 MHz sector, deep diffuse tumour, MRI/45–65 mm, biopsy
MP	M	46	R-FP	LGA	5 MHz sector, CT–MRI/30–40 mm, large deep diffuse lesion, biopsy
HN	F	53	R-P	ICH	5 MHz sector, EEG–SEP, microscope alignment, CT/30 mm, drainage and biopsy
NS	M	67	R-FT	LGA	5 MHz convex, burr hole, CT/20–40 mm, large diffuse lesion, biopsy
LH	F	43	R-FT	LGA	5 MHz sector, MRI/20–35 mm, large diffuse lesion, biopsy
SS	F	44	R-T	Cyst	5 MHz convex, burr hole, endoscope alignment and examination, MRI/35 mm, biopsy and drainage
RA	M	31	L-T	LGO	5 MHz convex, EEG depth electrode alignment, microscope alignment, MRI/15 mm, 22 mm diameter, total removal
EN	M	35	R-P	Cavernous haemangioma	5 MHz convex, microscope alignment and pilot laser alignment, MRI–CT/28 mm, 15 mm diameter, total removal
KK	M	27	L-TP	ICH	5 MHz convex, microscope alignment, MRI/30 mm, 25 mm diameter, drainage
IK	F	45	L-F	Meningioma	5 MHz convex, microscope alignment, MRI/convexity, 10 mm diameter, total removal

[a] L,left; R,right; F,frontal; FP,frontoparietal; P,parietal, FT,frontotemporal; T,temporal lobe; TP,temporoparietal.
[b] LGA,low grade astrocytoma; Agr4,astrocytoma grade IV; ICH,chronic intracerebral haematoma; LGO,low grade oligodendroglioma; cyst,porencephalic cyst with reactive gliosis.
[c] 5 MHz sector and convex transducers, EEG-SEP (somatosensory evoked potentials) control intraoperatively, MRI and/or CT data were used as indicated, with depth of biopsy or distance to presenting surface of lesion. Microscope, endoscope, depth electrode alignment—these were aligned with the neuronavigator so that the central optical axis of the microscope and endoscope and the depth electrode corresponded to the common axis in reconstructed images (see text). Patients AK and PK: the neuronavigator was calibrated with a non-invasive Laitinen stereoguide—in all other cases four scalp fiducials.

When the microscope is aligned to the surgical field with the neuronavigator, the neurosurgeon looking at the centre of the surgical field will look along the common axis (patients HN, RA, EN, KK, IK).

6. The surgical laser passes along the same common axis when it is aligned with the central optical axis of the microscope (patient EN).

Thus, the neuronavigator has been used as a pointer and rigid instrument holder. Obviously, it can also be used in dissection by connecting the ultrasound aspirator handpiece or suction tip to the neuronavigator, the axis of these instruments also being aligned along the common central axis of the system. The location of the tip of these instruments can be shown on the original CT/MRI scans and in the reconstructions.

In biopsy procedures, the burr hole can be placed in such a way that the trajectory of the biopsy probe will pass into the desired region while avoiding critical brain centres. After making the burr hole, the ultrasound probe is attached to the neuronavigator. The ultrasound images can be compared with the corresponding CT/MRI reconstructions because their planes are identical. The optimum site for biopsy can be chosen, since the ultrasound scan shows significant cerebral arteries on the basis of their pulsation on the real time image. The biopsy forceps can be passed under ultrasound control and any complications such as haemorrhage can be ruled out.

At present the neuronavigator has been used for ultrasound controlled biopsy procedures, neuroendoscopy, haematoma drainage and microscope and laser alignment (see Table 7.1). Laser treatment as well as the use of the neuronavigator during actual microdissection have been planned. Already the neuronavigator has been helpful in

Table 7.2 Applications of ultrasound in image directed brain tumour surgery (University of Oulu)

1. General surgical orientation and delineation of intracerebral lesions
2. Biopsy procedures:
   - Freehand with or without ultrasound probe needle guide
   - Stereotactic (conventional frame)
   - Neuronavigator
3. Resection of tumour:
   - Freehand use of ultrasound probe during resection
   - Surgical adapter–laser resection
   - Neuronavigator

planning small craniotomies for tumour resection, allowing the use of the intergyral approach to the tumours. The sulci can be visualized with both MRI and ultrasound and they often extend close to subcortical and even deep lesions. Repeated ultrasound imaging guides the dissection directly to the tumour.

CONCLUSION

The 1980s has seen tremendous progress in ultrasound and other imaging technology. Simultaneously, the development of the surgical microscope, laser and ultrasound aspirator has given the neurosurgeon new instruments with which to treat brain tumours. Based on the experience outlined in this chapter, it seems that in the future there is a need to further integrate these advances in imaging and treatment in a meaningful practical fashion to aid the neurosurgeon. Ultrasound imaging fills one requirement: real time intraoperative imaging that can supplement other imaging methods and guide the biopsy, dissection and removal of brain tumours. The present strategy for the use of ultrasound imaging in the author's clinic is summarized in Table 7.2.

ACKNOWLEDGEMENTS

This work has been generously funded during two large multidisciplinary projects, the so-called UHB project and the neuronavigator project, by the Academy of Finland, the Technological Development Center of Finland and several foundations, particularly the Inari and Reijo Holopainen Foundation. The neuronavigator project has been awarded Eureka status. Figures 7.1a–d and 7.2b–d were originally published in the author's doctoral thesis and are republished with permission of *Acta Universitas Ouluensis*. Figures 7.3a and 4a are republished with permission of the *Annals of Clinical Research*.

I have had the unique opportunity to collaborate with several academic engineering fellows, including E. Alasaarela PhD, J. Ylitalo PhD, K. Tervonen PhD, Y. Louhisalmi MSc, J. Alakuijala MSc and J. Oikarinen MSc.

REFERENCES

Alasaarela E, Koivukangas J 1990 Evaluation of image quality of ultrasound scanners in medical diagnostics. Journal of Ultrasound in Medicine 9: 23–34

Berger M S 1986 Ultrasound-guided stereotaxic biopsy using a new apparatus. Journal of Neurosurgery 65: 550–554

Chandler W F, Rubin J M 1986 Intraoperative use of real time ultrasound in neurosurgery. Contemporary Neurosurgery 8(8): 1–8

French L A, Wild J J, Neal D 1950 Detection of cerebral tumours by ultrasonic pulses. Pilot studies on postmortem material. Cancer 3: 705–708

Heilbrun M P, Mukuno D H, Lee T G 1983 Intraoperative ultrasound assisted stereotaxic brain surgery. Radiology 148: 576–577

Kelly P J 1988 Volumetric stereotaxis and computer-assisted stereotactic resection of subcortical lesions. In: Lundsford L D (ed) Modern stereotactic neurosurgery. Marinus Nijhoff, Boston

Koivukangas J 1984 Ultrasound imaging in operative neurosurgery: an experimental and clinical study with special reference to ultrasound holographic B (UHB) imaging. Doctoral dissertation. Acta Universitatis Ouluensis Series D. University of Oulu Printing Center, Oulu

Koivukangas J, Kelly P J 1986 Application of ultrasound imaging to stereotactic brain tumour surgery. Annals of Clinical Research 18(Suppl 47): 25–32

Koivukangas J, Koivukangas P 1986 Treatment of low-grade cerebral astrocytoma: New methods and evaluation of results. Annals of Clinical Research 18(Suppl 47): 115–124

Koivukangas J, Louhisalmi Y 1990 Computer-guided laser for neurosurgery. Annales Chirurgiae et Gynaecologiae 79: 192–196

Koivukangas J, Ylitalo J, Alasaarela E 1986 Three-dimensional ultrasound imaging in neurosurgery. Annals of Clinical Research 18(Suppl 47): 65–72

Koivukangas J, Louhisalmi Y, Alakuijala J, Oikarinen J 1992 Ultrasound controlled neuronavigator guided brain surgery. Journal of Neurosurgery (accepted for publication)

Rubin J M, Dohrmann G J 1982 The surgeon's eye into the brain. Diagnostic Imaging Sept: 26–30

Tsutsumi Y, Andoh Y, Inoue N 1982 Ultrasound guided biopsy for deep-seated brain tumours. Journal of Neurosurgery 57: 164–167

Watanabe E, Watanabe T, Manaka S et al 1987 Three-dimensional digitizer (neuronavigator): new equipment for computed tomography-guided stereotaxic surgery. Surgical Neurology 27: 543–547

Wild J J, Reid J M 1953 The effects of biological tissues on 15-ms pulsed ultrasound. Journal of the Acoustical Society of America 25: 270–280

8. Interstitial irradiation treatment of low grade gliomas

Ch. B. Ostertag

INTRODUCTION

The optimal therapy for low grade cerebral gliomas, i.e. supratentorial differentiated gliomas World Health Organization (WHO) grades I and II and moderately anaplastic gliomas, remains equivocal. Some neurosurgeons advocate total resection, others believe in subtotal resection and subsequent radiation therapy. Many neurologists question any kind of invasive therapy. Their argument is that surgery can never be an appropriate treatment for gliomas because surgery aims at localized lesions and gliomas are in general poorly localized (Cohadon 1990). The effectiveness of external beam radiotherapy, although questioned for differentiated gliomas in younger age groups, is clear in prolonging life in adults (Bloom & Walsh 1975, Leibel & Sheline 1987). External beam radiotherapy is based on a differential effect of radiation on healthy and neoplastic brain tissues (therapeutic ratio). The tolerance of the surrounding healthy brain poses a serious limitation to the tumour destructive dose (Jellinger 1977). To achieve tumour destruction without damage to the surrounding brain, either by surgical dissection or by radiation, interstitial radiation treatment (IRT) techniques were conceptualized and have been used since 1900 for a variety of brain tumours (Bernstein & Gutin 1981).

Several groups recognized the usefulness of the stereotactic methodology for the precise placement of radioactive sources into brain tumours. With the availability of artificial low energy gamma ray sources such as iodine-125 (^{125}I) and the advent of new imaging techniques, such as computerized tomography (CT) and magnetic resonance imaging (MRI), the treatment modality has again stimulated new interest. The following retrospective review of patients who were selected during a 10 year period for stereotactic biopsy and interstitial irradiation of differentiated supratentorial cerebral gliomas is undertaken in an attempt to define the place and usefulness of the method.

CLINICAL MATERIAL

In the period 1979–1991, 430 consecutive patients with differentiated gliomas, i.e. pilocytic astrocytomas, astrocytomas WHO grade II, oligoastrocytomas and oligodendrogliomas, in inaccessible or functionally critical locations in the brain were treated with IRT using ^{125}I implants. Patients treated with iridium-192 (^{192}Ir) implants are not included in this report. The tumours were delineated either on CT or MRI and histologically verified with the help of serial stereotactic biopsies. Diffusely infiltrative tumours, tumours crossing the midline, and malignant, non-delineated tumours were excluded on grounds of their invasiveness and growth pattern. Also excluded were patients with a rapidly deteriorating neurological status or major mass effect with imminent brain herniation. After IRT, consecutive CT/MRI control scans were performed at 2 days, 6 weeks and every 3 months following IRT. The patients were closely followed by neurological examination including Karnofsky performance status and compared with previous examinations.

METHOD OF STEREOTACTIC BIOPSY

For all stereotactic procedures, i.e. biopsy and interstitial irradiation, a modified Riechert stereotactic system was used (Ostertag et al 1980, Ostertag 1988a). The headring is fixed to the cranium with vertical plastic posts with changeable steel pins (Mayfield) and is worn under local anaesthesia throughout the scanning and stereotactic procedures.

Digital imaging (CT, MRI) provides an internal coordinate system which corresponds to the right angle coordinate axis of the Riechert stereotactic system. All coordinates are defined in relationship to the headring fixed after the image cross-hair is centred with the x and y axes of the headring. The z coordinate corresponds to the indicated table incrementation. This method avoids the imprecision of multiple measurements of external fiducial points, which is necessary when the patient's head is freely movable in the CT/MRI gantry during the scanning procedure.

After CT/MRI scanning, the patient is transferred to the operating theatre. The headring is fixed to a stand, which allows orthogonal anteroposterior and lateral plain radiography and angiography to be carried out. Since the angiographic studies are carried out following a CT/MRI scan examination with the headring fixed to the patient's skull, coordinates of any point on the CT/MRI scans obtained from the standard software of the CT/MRI scanner can be made to coincide with those measured on the radiographic films. In the presence of a pathological vascularization the outline of the lesion is easily transposed on the angiographic films by simply marking on the angiograms the coordinates of the borders of the lesion, read on the graduated cross-hair of the CT scan images.

For stereoscopic viewing an oblique projection can also be obtained by an exact 6° rotation of the headring (Moringlane et al 1988).

The patient is normally kept under mild sedation (midazolam) and the procedure itself is carried out under local anaesthesia. After the patient's head is prepared and draped, a 2 cm skin incision is made over the appropriate entry point under local anaesthesia. A 5 mm burr hole is made oriented in the line of transit of the biopsy probe. After the opening of the dura a biopsy forceps is introduced under fluoroscopic control, guided through a guide cannula. With the mouth of the forceps closed, the instrument is advanced. The mouth is opened at the predetermined site and in cases of solid tumours tissue specimens are taken stepwise at 1–5 mm intervals (serial biopsy). The guide cannula can also be used to aspirate the contents of cystic lesions or to introduce radioactive material for interstitial irradiation.

The optimum tract for serial biopsies is selected using CT/MRI data, including computer reformations, which provide an estimate of the shape and geometry of the lesion and taking into consideration the stereotactic angiographic data. Usually only one tract of serial biopsies is carried out. For the spatial definition of infiltrative gliomas further tracts and serial biopsies can be helpful. The patient is kept in a supine position for a standard stereotaxic biopsy procedure using a precoronal paramedian approach. However, for lesions in the parietal, occipital or cerebellar location a lateral position of the patient is preferred. The potential and accuracy of serial stereotactic biopsy have been described elsewhere (Ostertag 1988b).

METHOD OF INTERSTITIAL IRRADIATION

^{125}I seeds (provided by Amersham Buchler, Braunschweig, Germany) were used either as permanent (lost) (1979–1985) or removable (temporary) implants (1985–1991). The clinical dosimetry for ^{125}I implants was carried out with respect to the physical and biological properties: ^{125}I emits primarily low energy X-radiation of 27–35 kV. According to several investigators, the relative biological efficiency is in the range 1.2–1.4 (Anderson et al 1981). According to Sondhaus (1981) the specific dose rate factor is 1.32 cGy/h and 1 mCi at 1 cm in tissue (Fig. 8.1). For a clinical situation the calculated accumulated dosage for permanent or temporary implants ranged between 3000 and 7000 cGy. This dose was calculated to accumulate within 90 days on the outer radius of a tumour when permanent implants were used (mean dose rate 3 cGy/h). Since 1986 only temporary implants, i.e. seeds in Teflon catheters, have been used, with a mean dose rate of 10 cGy/h (Fig. 8.2). Before implantation each seed was calibrated in a burr hole ionization chamber (Curiementor, PTW,

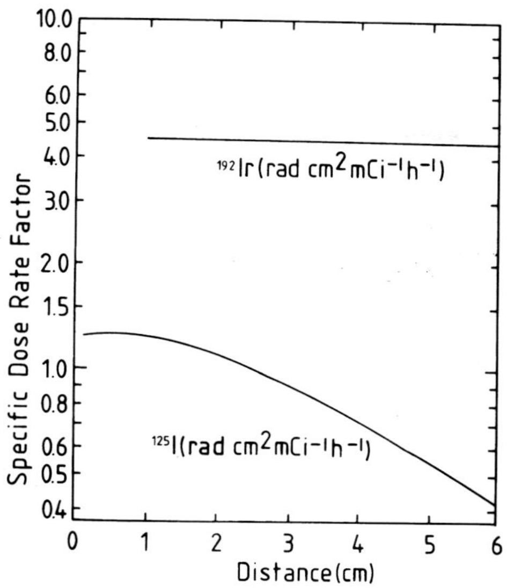

Fig. 8.1 Comparison of specific dose rate factors of the gamma ray emitters ^{192}Ir and ^{125}I. Note that the gamma energy of ^{125}I is rapidly absorbed by the tissue. (Modified after Itilaris, 1975.)

Freiburg, Germany). Because of the seed configuration, i.e. a titanium rod with welded ends (Fig. 8.3), the dose distribution is non-isotropic, which makes the calibration difficult (Krishnaswamy 1978, Anderson et al 1981). The non-isotropic dose distribution is, however, more or less irrelevant for the biological effect, as demonstrated experimentally (Ostertag et al 1983). Using temporary ^{125}I seeds makes

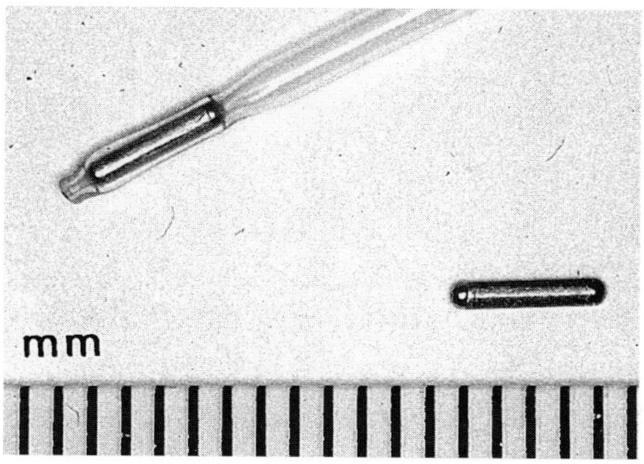

Fig. 8.2 Temporary ^{125}I seed implantation is carried out with the seed fixed in the tip of a Teflon catheter cut to an appropriate length. The catheter is fixed at the dura with a titanium clip.

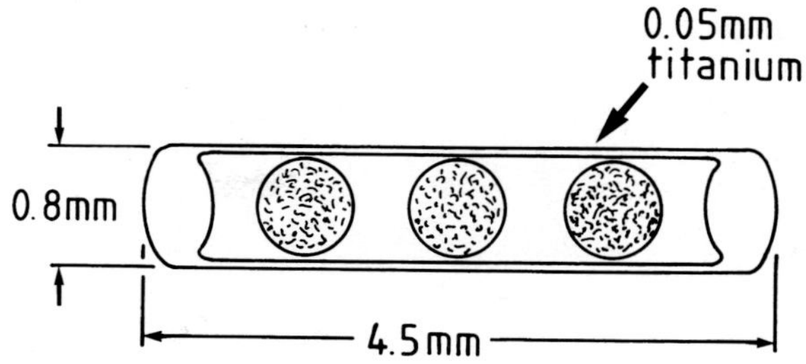

Fig. 8.3 ^{125}I seeds (model 6702) consist of a welded titanium capsule containing ^{125}I absorbed on anion exchange resin spheres.

interstitial irradiation rather more cost effective since the seeds can be reused two to four times.

The definition of the treatment volume is carried out using CT and/or MRI, cerebral angiography under stereotactic conditions, and serial biopsies in one or more tracts establishing a morphological diagnosis, including the delineation and invasiveness of the tumour. In patients in whom the stereotactic intraoperative tissue diagnosis, delineation and classification was unequivocal, the implantation of one or more iodine seeds was carried out in one procedure. When doubts remained regarding the diagnosis and grading, a second procedure was required. Target coordinates for interstitial implants were usually chosen in the centre of the tumour volume or along a suitable axis through the tumour using a best fit method. In exceptional cases, multiple targets and tracts were chosen. The number and activities of the iodine seeds were selected according to the tumour shape and volume with special reference to the anatomical site. Radiation protection regulations limit the level of radiation discharge of the patient to less than 1 μSv/h at a distance of 1 m. This level of radiation was rarely exceeded, and special isolation of the patient in a private room has not been necessary. The patients were hospitalized for 3–6 days (minimum 2 days). Temporary seeds require removal by reopening the skin incision under local anaesthesia after a calculated application time, i.e. 3–6 weeks after the implantation. The performance of various diagnostic and therapeutic steps within one stereotactic procedure takes $1\frac{1}{2}$ hours under local anaesthesia and mild sedation (except for children) and is undoubtedly of benefit to the brain tumour patient.

RESULTS

From December 1979 until March 1991, 430 patients harbouring primary low grade cerebral gliomas underwent a stereotactic diagnostic biopsy and were treated with ^{125}I interstitial irradiation. Among 430 patients were 34 patients who had undergone a previous partial resection of their tumour or had a local recurrence after resection. 14 patients had been subjected to radiation therapy before biopsy and IRT. All patients presented with progressive neurological deficits or showed evidence of CT/MRI confirmed tumour growth, or both. These included pilocytic astrocytomas (106 cases), astrocytic tumours WHO grade II (251 cases), oligoastrocytomas (44 cases) and oligodendrogliomas (29 cases) (Table 8.1). The location of the lesions included the basal ganglia and thalamus (85 cases), midbrain–upper pons (45 cases), hypothalamus (55 cases), insula and temporal lobe (103 cases), frontal lobe (104 cases) and parietal area (38 cases) (Table 8.2). 122 patients were aged 16 years or younger. At the time of implantation, 339 patients (79%) had a Karnofsky performance status of 70 or higher; 91 patients (21%) had a Karnofsky performance status lower than 70. The primary and presenting symptom in 240 patients (56%) was epilepsy, in 61 patients (14%) a paresis, in 60 patients (14%) increased intracranial pressure, in 38 patients (9%) ophthalmological symptoms and in 31 patients (7%) mental disturbances only. There was an operative morbidity without a mortality of 3.1% in this series due to the operative procedure of biopsy, together with implanting and removing the ^{125}I seeds. In 12 cases (2.6%), follow-up examination revealed functional defects in the vicinity of the implant, particularly in the hypothalamus and midbrain–thalamus, which were interpreted as due to local radiation damage.

Table 8.1 Interstitial radiation treatment for brain tumours

Histology (WHO grade)	Number of cases	Percentage
Pilocytic astrocytoma	106	
Astrocytoma (II)	251	
Oligoastrocytoma (II)	44	62
Oligodendroglioma (II)	29	
Ependymoma	20	
Anaplastic astrocytoma (III)	75	19
Glioblastoma (IV)	34	
Other	131	19
Total	690	100

Table 8.2 Interstitial radiation treatment for low grade gliomas

Tumour location	Number of cases	Percentage
Frontal lobe	104	24
Temporal lobe	103	24
Parietal–occipital lobe	38	9
Basal nuclei–thalamus	85	20
Hypothalamus–chiasm	55	13
Midbrain–pons	45	10
Total	430	100

Pilocytic astrocytomas

In all 106 patients with pilocytic astrocytomas the diagnosis was confirmed by stereotactic serial biopsies. The majority (76 patients) were 16 years of age or less, 30 patients were older than 16 years (mean age 14.3 years). The average preoperative Karnofsky performance status was 68. The tumour was located in 29 patients on the right side, in 30 patients on the left side and in 47 patients in the midline. The topographical distribution is given in Table 8.3. The mean treatment volume was 17.4 ml (SD ± 15.5 ml) The neurological status at follow-up examinations (median follow-up period 4.7 years) revealed an improvement of neurological function in 32 patients (30%), no change in 46 (43%) patients and worsening of preoperative noted

Table 8.3 Interstitial radiation treatment for pilocytic astrocytomas

Tumour location	Number of cases	Percentage
Frontal lobe	1	
Temporal lobe	9	9
Basal nuclei–thalamus	38	
Hypothalamus–chiasm	33	91
Midbrain–pons	25	
Total	106	100

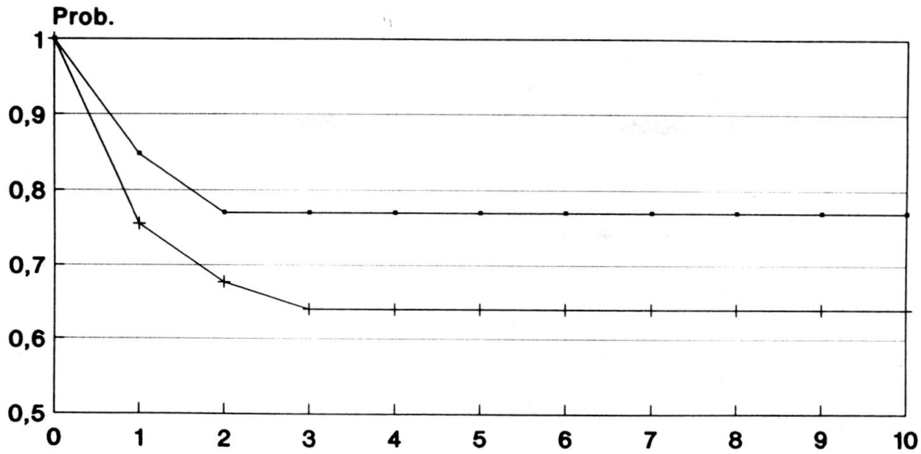

Fig. 8.4 Life table plot (Cutler & Ederer 1958) of the probability of survival in 106 patients who had pilocytic astrocytomas (black squares) and 251 patients who had astrocytomas (WHO grade II).

deficit in 28 patients (27%). Four patients received additional subsequent external beam radiation therapy. The median survival in all patients was more than 9 years. The 5 and 10 year survival rate was 77% (Fig. 8.4).

Astrocytomas WHO grade II

In 251 patients the stereotactic biopsy established the histological diagnosis of an astrocytoma WHO grade II. The mean age of patients with cerebral astrocytomas was 33.8 years (40 patients aged 16 years or less, 211 patients aged over 16 years). Astrocytomas were found in the right hemisphere in 100 patients, in the left hemisphere in 147 patients and in four patients in the midline. Of the lesions, 176 were found in functionally critical cortical areas of the hemispheres (70%) (Table 8.4).

Table 8.4 Interstitial radiation treatment for astrocytomas WHO grade II

Tumour location	Number of cases	Percentage
Frontal lobe	73	
Temporal lobe	72	70
Parietal–occipital lobe	31	
Basal nuclei–thalamus	36	
Hypothalamus–chiasm	19	30
Midbrain–pons	20	
Total	251	100

The mean preoperative Karnofsky performance status for all patients was 78%. The mean treatment volume was 21.2 ml (SD ± 17.5 ml). Follow-up examinations (mean follow-up period 3.5 years) revealed an improvement in 95 patients (38%), a stabilization of the disease in 87 patients (35%) and a progressive deterioration in 69 patients (Fig. 8.5). Additional subsequent external beam radiotherapy because of uncontrolled infiltrative tumour growth was instituted in 24 patients. Expanding tumour cysts were observed in 15 patients 2–10 months after the implantation which required internal or external drainage using a Rickham reservoir. Since these cysts are part of the natural history of astrocytomas and were never observed in the immediate vicinity of the implant, it remains unresolved whether the cause for this was the interstitial implants or not. The median survival for all 251 patients was more than 9 years, while the 5 and 10 year survival rate was 63% (see Fig. 8.4).

Oligoastrocytomas and oligodendrogliomas

Stereotactic serial biopsy revealed in 73 patients oligoastrocytomas (44 patients) or oligodendrogliomas (19 patients). The mean age was 41.7 and 32.2 years, respectively, seven patients with

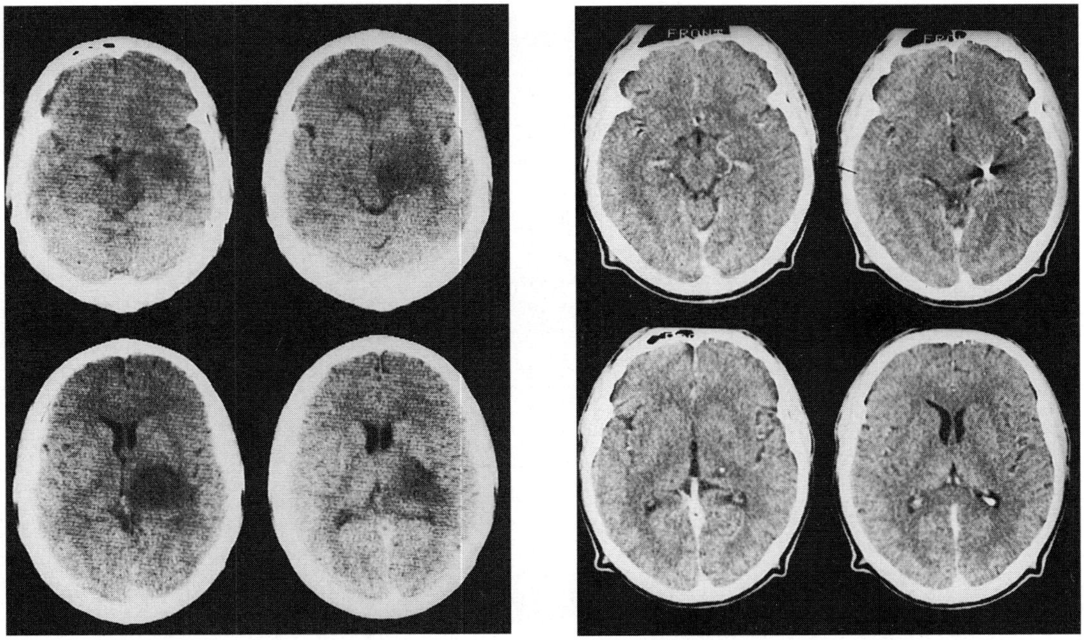

a **b**

Fig. 8.5 Interstitial irradiation of a fibrillary astrocytoma (WHO grade II) in the left thalamus (42-year-old male patient). **a** CT demonstrates a fairly delineated hypodense tumour which was verified as fibrillary astrocytoma by a serial stereotactic biopsy. One iodine seed in a catheter was implanted temporarily for 28 days (June 1986). The implanted activity was 16.8 mCi, the accumulated dose 6000 cGy, the dose rate 10 cGyh-1 and the treatment volume 21 cm3. **b** A CT control in March 1991 revealed an on-going local tumour control. The star shaped artefact is a metal marker which was placed during the stereotactic biopsy.

oligoastrocytomas were aged 16 years or less, 66 patients including all cases of oligodendrogliomas were in the adult age group. 32 tumours were found in the right hemisphere, 31 in the left hemisphere and four cases in the midline (Fig. 8.6). The mean preoperative Karnofsky performance status was 71 and 79, respectively.

The mean treatment volume was 16.9 and 24.9 ml, (SD ± 10.5 and 18.2 ml), respectively. The follow-up examination (mean follow-up period 3.0 and 3.4 years) revealed an improvement in 40 patients (53%), a stabilization of the disease in 21 patients (28%) and a progressive deterioration due to uncontrolled tumour growth in 14 cases. The median survival for the group of oligoastrocytomas and oligodendrogliomas was more than 8 and 5 years, respectively, with a 5 year survival rate of 81% for oligoastrocytomas and 59% for oligodendrogliomas (Fig. 8.7).

SUMMARY

The goal of resective surgery is to achieve a selective removal of a tumour. The goal of radiotherapy is to achieve selective destruction of neoplastic tissue. The emphasis is on selectivity. The treatment volume, target volume and tumour volume, which should all be identical, differ considerably in the practice of routine surgery and conventional radiotherapy, however. IRT is conceptually envisioned to sterilize an area of the brain selectively without producing substantial damage to normal brain. Ideally, the treatment volume, target volume and tumour volume are the same.

Using IRT, a high radiation dose is applied locally, with a rapid fall-off outside the target volume, thus sparing normal brain from radiation, while selectively irradiating a tumour volume.

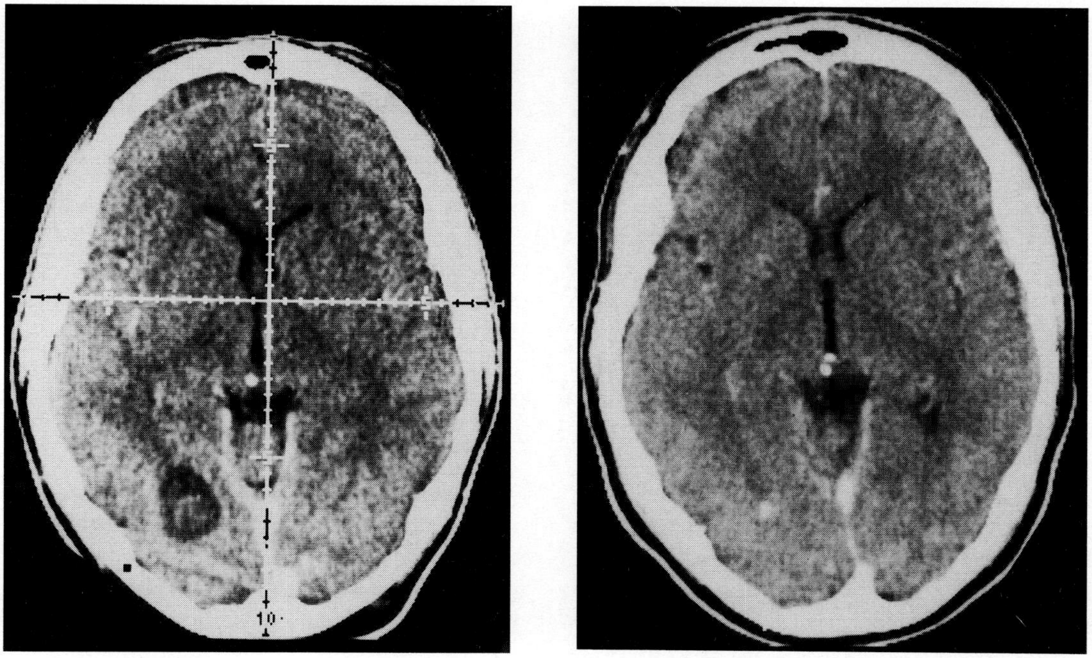

a b

Fig. 8.6 **a** Interstitial irradiation (^{125}I temporary implant) of a well delineated oligoastrocytoma in the right occipital lobe of a 19-year-old male patient (November 1987). The implanted activity was 7.4 mCi (temporary implant for 28 days), the accumulated dose 6000 cGy, the dose rate 9 cGyh-1, and the lesion volume 4 cm3. **b** CT control in August 1988 demonstrates a local tumour control without evidence of radiation side-effects or tumour progression.

Radiation from an interstitially implanted gamma ray source is delivered continuously at comparatively low dose rates compared with the high and intermittent dose rates delivered by external beam irradiation. The tumour destructive dose can be delivered in a relatively short period of time of 2–4 weeks when temporary implants are used, thereby avoiding hospitalization of the patient for 5–6 weeks and the side-effects of percutaneous radiation therapy. Continuous low

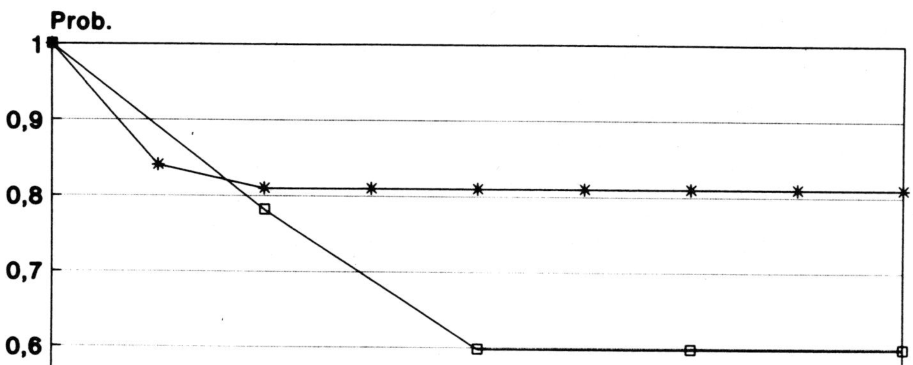

Fig. 8.7 Life table plot of the probability of survival in 44 patients who had oligoastrocytomas (asterisks) and 29 patients who had oligodendrogliomas (open squares).

dose rate irradiation seems to increase the effectiveness of radiation, possibly due to both cell kinetic interactions and oxygen dependency (Hall 1978). Using a low energy gamma ray emitter such as ^{125}I, the therapeutic ratio is enhanced as a result of the rapid dose fall-off in tissue within a distance in millimetre range. Since radiation from ^{125}I sources is effectively attenuated by surrounding tissue such as brain, bone and scalp, radioprotection no longer poses a serious problem (Hilaris 1975).

The low energy gamma radiation of ^{125}I and the absence of beta-radiation causes tissue reactions that are distinctly different from those caused by either beta ray emitting sources such as yttrium-90 or the high energy gamma ray emitters such as ^{192}Ir and gold-198 (beta energy yielded by platinum coating) (Kiessling et al 1984, Ostertag 1991). Depending on the energy range, application time, and dose rate, calcified or liquefied necrosis develops in normal brain surrounded by reactive glia and fibrinoid necrosis of endothelial cells. The response of neoplastic tissue to interstitial irradiation in terms of the volume of necrosis is 3–5 times greater when compared with ^{125}I radionecrosis in normal brain, indicating a differential effect of IRT between normal and neoplastic tissue (Ostertag et al 1984). The dose rate and energy determine the volume of the necrosis and the magnitude and duration of vasogenic oedema. The vasogenic oedema determines the extent of demyelination and reactive gliosis in the vicinity of the radionecrosis (Fike et al 1985, Janzer et al 1986, Groothuis et al 1987, Ostertag 1991). The oedema phase can be shortened by using temporary implants with moderate dose rates, in which case repair processes are free to take place after the removal of the radioactive source from the brain. For clinical application, it was concluded that temporary ^{125}I implants with a dose rate of approximately 10 $cGyh^{-1}$ might be the most favourable. ^{125}I was therefore preferred over ^{192}Ir and other sources for its relative biological effectiveness, its cost effectiveness and its ease of handling and radioprotection.

Astrocytomas and other low grade cerebral gliomas have variable topographic patterns (Burger 1987, Daumas-Duport & Scheithauer 1987). An application of a local therapy must be carried out in recognition of the morphological findings of the individual case. We therefore selected only a small subgroup of low grade gliomas for IRT, namely those which were circumscribed tumours with only limited extension of tumour cells into the periphery. These were only 35% of the total group of low grade gliomas (1290 cases) seen at the author's institution (Neurochirurgische Universitatsklinik, Freiburg) during the same time period. This subgroup of patients with low grade cerebral gliomas had a fairly good survival rate when compared with data from the literature (Laws et al 1984, 1985, Mahaley et al 1989, Soffietti et al 1989). In more than 70% of patients a neurological improvement or stabilization of the disease accompanied by a reduction or suppression of epilepsy was observed after IRT, and other workers in the field have corroborated these data (Mundinger 1966, Mundinger & Metzel 1968, Cooperative Study of the Stereotactic Group of Paris Sainte-Anne 1979, Rougier et al 1984, Gutin & Leibel 1985, Rossi et al 1985)

The neurosurgical literature generally supports the philosophy of radical surgery of low grade gliomas where possible (Laws et al 1984, Ciric et al 1987). The conclusion, however, is biased in that there is a tendency for the most favourable lesions to be treated with radical surgery and the less favourable, i.e. deep seated, non-cystic or infiltrative tumours, to be treated with more limited approaches (Laws et al 1985). The literature analysis shows that there is little justification for dogmatic statements concerning the relationship between increasing patient survival times and aggressive surgical management (Laws et al 1985, Morantz 1987, Nazzaro & Neuwelt 1990). For both surgery and IRT, the more delineated, non-infiltrative low grade gliomas are the preferred cases. By both methods a selective destruction and removal of the tumour bulk is undertaken. Using IRT a calculated radionecrosis is induced with consecutive removal by macrophage activity. IRT therefore is considered a radio surgical rather than a radiotherapeutic method. There is conflict between surgery and IRT for surgically accessible low grade tumours located superficially. Large, well delineated low grade gliomas at or close to the surface of the brain also underwent open surgery and resection at the author's institution. Small gliomas, however, in or close to functionally critical cortical areas were selected for IRT. As was shown in this series, IRT is capable of dealing effectively with low grade gliomas, however, with less invasiveness, dissection of normal brain and lower costs compared with open surgery. The highly sophisticated volumetric stereotactic resection of subcortical tumours developed by Patrick Kelly and coworkers seems to be equally effective. However, the amount of dissection of normal brain tissue is certainly larger and the morbidity higher (Kelly 1989).

The place of conventional fractionated radiotherapy for low grade gliomas is still undefined. The growth kinetics of differentiated gliomas makes the difference in radiosensitivity between neoplasm and normal brain small or nonexistent (Hoshino 1984). There is support for the view that postoperative radiation therapy is beneficial in patients with incompletely resected low grade gliomas, particularly in the older age groups (over 40 years old). In children and infants the conventional radiation dose is likely to lead to unacceptable late sequelae (Sheline 1985). Bloom and Walsh (1975) correctly cautioned against high dose and large volume brain irradiation in cases of low grade gliomas 'because of the possible risk of serious brain injury occurring before tumour recurrence'. In such patients, conventional radiation therapy should be delayed as long as possible. In this series, conventional beam radiotherapy was used at the time of recurrence when further IRT was not feasible. IRT, however, avoids large volume brain irradiation. IRT is therefore particularly preferred in the paediatric age group when local tumour control is needed without exposing normal brain tissue to radiation. In many patients of the younger age group the limited approach of IRT has produced median survival figures of more than 9 years, i.e. in some of those patients the curative effect of IRT might be considered.

CONCLUSION

Our results to date suggest that image based IRT is an effective treatment of primary and residual low grade gliomas. The local tumour control by stereotactic IRT is the least traumatic treatment modality for geographically confined low grade gliomas. Since only a small proportion of patients with low grade gliomas are suitable candidates, patient selection plays a crucial role in the treatment results. The response to IRT of an individual tumour is difficult to predict. A major deficiency is the present histomorphological classification of glial tumours, particularly astrocytomas. The risk:benefit ratio must be considered in each individual patient when decisions are made between alternative and potentially harmful treatment modalities. A controlled clinical trial defining prognostic factors and proving the efficacy of the available methods must be carried out before final conclusions can be drawn.

REFERENCES

Anderson L L, Hsin M K, Ing-Yuan D 1981 Clinical dosimetry with 125–I. In: George F W (ed) Modern interstitial and intracavitary radiation cancer management. Masson, New York, pp 9–15

Bernstein M, Gutin P H 1981 Interstitial irradiation of brain tumours: a review. Neurosurgery 6: 741–750

Bloom H J W, Walsh L S 1975 Tumours of the central nervous system. In: Bloom H J G, Lemerle J, Neidhardt M K (eds) Cancer in children. Clinical management. Springer, Berlin

Burger P C 1987 The anatomy of astrocytomas. Mayo Clinic Proceedings 62: 527–529

Ciric I, Ammirati M, Vick N, Mikhael M 1987 Supratentorial gliomas: surgical considerations and immediate postoperative results. Neurosurgery 21: 21–26

Cohadon F 1990 Indications for surgery in the management of gliomas. In: Symon L et al (eds) Advances and technical standards in neurosurgery, vol 17. Springer-Verlag, Berlin, pp 189–234

Cooperative Study of the Stereotactic Group of Paris Sainte-Anne, Bordeaux, Grenoble, Marseille, Rennes 1979 Combined interstitial and external irradiation of gliomas: a progress report. INSERM Symposium 12: 329–338

Cutler S J, Ederer F 1958 Maximum utilization of the life table method in analyzing survival. Journal of Chronic Diseases 8: 699–712

Daumas-Duport C, Scheithauer B W 1987 A histologic and cytologic method for the spatial definition of gliomas. Mayo Clinic Proceedings 62: 435–449

Fike J R, Cann C E, Philips T L et al 1985 Radiation brain

damage induced by interstitial 125-I sources: a canine model evaluated by quantitative computed tomography. Neurosurgery 16: 530–537

Groothuis D R, Wright D C, Ostertag C B 1987 Sequential changes of capillary permeability in normal canine brain associated with 125-I interstitial radiotherapy. Journal of Neurosurgery 67: 895–902

Gutin P H, Leibel S A 1985 Stereotactic interstitial irradiation of malignant brain tumours. Neurologic Clinics 3: 883–893

Hall E J (1978) Radiobiology for the radiologist. Harper and Row, New York, pp 123–129

Hilaris B S 1975 Handbook of interstitial brachytherapy. Publishing Sciences Group, Acton

Hoshino T 1984 A commentary on the biology and growth kinetics of low-grade and high-grade gliomas. Journal of Neurosurgery 61: 895–900

Janzer R C, Kleihues P, Ostertag C B 1986 Early and late effects on the normal dog brain of permanent interstitial iridium-192 irradiation. Acta Neuropathologica (Berlin) 70: 91–102

Jellinger K 1977 Human central system lesions following radiation therapy. Zentralblatt für Neurochirurgie 38: 199–200

Kelly P J 1989 Stereotactic biopsy and resection of thalamic astrocytomas. Neurosurgery 25: 185–195

Kiessling M, Kleihues P, Gassega E, Mundinger F, Ostertag C B, Weigel K 1984 Morphology of intracranial tumours and adjacent brain structures following interstitial iodine-125 radiotherapy. Acta neurochirurgica (suppl) (Wien) 33: 281–289

Krishnaswamy V 1978 Dose distribution around an 125-I seed source in tissue. Radiology 126: 489–491

Laws E R, Taylor W F, Marvin B C, Okazaki H 1984 Neurosurgical management of low grade astrocytoma of the cerebral hemispheres. Journal of Neurosurgery 61: 665–673

Laws E R, Taylor W F, Bergstralh E J et al 1985 The neurosurgical management of low grade astrocytoma. Clinics in Neurosurgery 575–588

Leibel S A, Sheline G E 1987 Radiotherapy for neoplasms of the brain. Journal of Neurosurgery 66: 1–22

Mahaley M S, Mettlin C, Natarajan N et al 1989 National survey of patterns of care for brain-tumour patients. Journal of Neurosurgery 71: 826–836

Morantz R A 1987 Radiation therapy in the treatment of cerebral astrocytoma. Neurosurgery 20: 975–982

Moringlane J R, Lippitz B, Ostertag C B 1988 Cerebral angiography under stereotactic conditions. Acta Neurochirurgica (Wien) 91: 147–150

Mundinger F 1966 The treatment of brain tumours with radioisotopes. Progress in Neurological Surgery 1: 101–257

Mundinger F, Metzel E 1968 Erfahrungen mit der lokalen Strahlenbehandlung inoperabler Zwischenhirn- und Basalganglientumoren mit der stereotaktischen Permanentimplantation von Iridium-192. Archiv für Psychiatrie und Nervenkrank 212: 70–90

Nazzaro J M, Neuwelt E A 1990 The role of surgery in the management of supratentorial intermediate and high-grade astrocytomas in adults. Journal of Neurosurgery 73: 331–344

Ostertag C B 1988a New head fixation for the Riechert stereotaxic system. Acta Neurochirurgica (Wien) 94: 88–92

Ostertag C B 1988b Reliability of stereotactic brain tumour biopsy. In: Lunsford L D (ed) Modern stereotactic neurosurgery. Martinus Nijhoff, Boston, pp 129–136

Ostertag C B 1991 Experimental central nervous system injury from implanted isotopes. In: Gutin P H, Leibel S A, Sheline G E (eds) Radiation injury of the nervous system. Raven Press, New York

Ostertag C B, Mennel H D, Kiessling M 1980 Stereotactic biopsy of brain tumours. Surgical Neurology 14: 275–283

Ostertag C B, Weigel K, Warnke P, Lombeck G, Kleihues P 1983 Sequential morphological changes in the dog brain after interstitial Iodine-125 irradiation. Neurosurgery 13: 523–528

Ostertag C B, Warnke P, Kleihues P, Bigner D 1984 Iodine-125 interstitial irradiation of virally induced dog brain tumours. Neurological Research 6: 176–180

Rossi G F, Scerrati M, Roselli R 1985 Epileptogenic cerebral low grade tumours: effect of interstitial stereotactic irradiation on seizures. Applied Neurophysiology 48: 127–132

Rougier A, Pigneux J, Cohadon F 1984 Combined interstitial and external irradiation of gliomas. Acta Neurochirurgica (suppl) (Wien) 33: 345–353

Sheline G E 1985 The role of radiation therapy in the treatment of low-grade gliomas. Clinics in Neurosurgery 563–574

Soffietti R, Chiò A, Giordana M T et al 1989 Prognostic factors in well-differentiated cerebral astsrocytomas in the adult. Neurosurgery 24: 686–692

Sondhaus C A 1981 I-125: physical properties, photon dosimetry and effectiveness. In: George F W (ed) Modern interstitial and intracavitary radiation cancer management. Masson, New York

9. Interstitial radiotherapy for high grade gliomas

P. K. Sneed   P. H. Gutin

INTRODUCTION

Two major factors form the basis for using interstitial radiotherapy in the treatment of high grade gliomas: the predominant pattern of failure is local (Hochberg & Pruitt 1980, Choucair et al 1986, Wallner et al 1989) and radiation therapy is the single most effective treatment modality (Walker et al 1978, 1979). The dose which can safely be delivered with conventional external beam therapy is limited by the tolerance of normal brain tissue (Sheline et al 1980 Marks et al 1981). Interstitial brachytherapy, that is, the placement of radioactive sources directly into the tumour to deliver radiation continuously at short range, makes it possible to give a very high dose of radiation to a tumour while limiting the dose to surrounding normal tissue.

Brachytherapy has a well established role in the treatment of gynaecological and head and neck cancers and has also been applied to a wide variety of other tumours (Hilaris 1975). Radioactive sources were first implanted in parenchymal brain tumours in 1914 (Frazier 1920). Since then, a large number of authors have reported on the use of brachytherapy for brain tumours (Bernstein & Gutin 1981). The largest series have concentrated on low grade gliomas (Talairach et al 1955, Mundinger 1964, Mundinger & Weigel 1984) but, at our institution, brain implants have been used predominantly for high grade gliomas.

The brain implant programme was established at the University of California, San Francisco (UCSF), in 1977. After initial experience with removable or permanent gold-198 (^{198}Au), iridium-192 (^{192}Ir) and low activity iodine-125 (^{125}I), high activity ^{125}I became the isotope of choice for temporary brain implants. Between December 1979 and June 1990, over 350 patients with high grade gliomas underwent interstitial radiotherapy with high activity ^{125}I at UCSF. This chapter presents relevant physical and radiobiological considerations and then discusses patient selection, implantation technique and results based on the UCSF experience.

PHYSICS AND RADIOBIOLOGY

The advantages of brachytherapy over teletherapy (conventional external beam radiotherapy) stem from both physical and radiobiological factors.

Physical considerations

^{125}I and ^{192}Ir are the isotopes most commonly used for interstitial brachytherapy. ^{125}I emits characteristic X-rays with an average energy of 28.5 kV and has a half-life of 59.6 days (Weaver et al 1990b). ^{192}Ir has a half-life of 74.2 days and emits 0.67 MeV beta particles and gamma rays with an average energy of 0.37 MeV (Weaver et al 1990b). Because the dose intensity is inversely proportional to the square of the distance away from a radioactive source and because there is attenuation of radiation by tissue, the radiation dose falls off very rapidly away from an individual source or outside of an array of sources. Arrays of either ^{125}I or ^{192}Ir sources implanted within a brain tumour can produce isodose contours of 40–60 cGy/h, which conform well to the tumour volume. We prefer to use ^{125}I for brain implants because its low energy simplifies radiation protection. ^{125}I is easily shielded with a 0.5 mm thickness of lead in contrast to the considerable thickness of lead required for ^{192}Ir. Furthermore, there is a more rapid fall off of the radiation dose in normal tissue outside the prescribed isodose line with ^{125}I as opposed to ^{192}Ir.

Radiobiological considerations

In addition to the advantageous dose distribution, there are radiobiological advantages to brachytherapy.

Hypoxic cells, which may make up a significant portion of the cells in a malignant glioma, are approximately three times more resistant to acute doses of radiation given at ≥ 100 cGy/min than are normally oxygenated cells. However, this effect is much less during low dose rate irradiation, probably because of inhibition of repair of sublethal radiation damage under hypoxic conditions (Hall et al 1966, Ling et al 1985). In addition, there is increased tumour cell killing as a fraction of previously hypoxic cells becomes oxygenated during brachytherapy in a process called reoxygenation (Hall 1988).

During low dose rate irradiation, proliferating tumour cells tend to accumulate in G_2, a radiosensitive phase of the cell cycle, whereas the non-cycling neuronal cells remain in G_1, a radioresistant phase (Hall 1985). However, if the radiation dose rate is too low and the tumour cells repopulate more rapidly than tumour cells are killed, brachytherapy will be ineffective (Hall 1985). For this reason, temporary implants of high activity ^{125}I sources are used at UCSF, instead of temporary or permanent implants of low activity ^{125}I, in order to treat high grade gliomas at dose rates of about 40–60 cGy/h.

Rationale for hyperthermia

There is a strong radiobiological rationale for combining hyperthermia with brachytherapy. Heat is known to kill cells exponentially as a function of time and temperature above about 41–42°C (Dewey et al 1980). Heat inhibits the repair of sublethal and potentially lethal radiation damage (Dewey et al 1980). Furthermore, radioresistant S phase cells and nutrient deprived, low pH hypoxic cells are particularly susceptible to heat damage (Dewey et al 1980). Numerous non-randomized clinical trials for extracranial superficial squamous cell carcinomas, adenocarcinomas and melanomas have demonstrated improved complete response rates and tumour control with combined radiation therapy and hyperthermia in comparison with radiation alone (Overgaard 1990). It is hoped that similar improvement in local control will be achieved when interstitial hyperthermia is used in conjunction with interstitial implants of brain tumours.

PATIENT SELECTION

Brain tumours considered to be suitable for temporary interstitial implants are unifocal, well circumscribed supratentorial lesions less than 5 cm in diameter. Evidence of tumour dissemination, as shown by subependymal spread or corpus callosum involvement, is considered to be a contraindication to brachytherapy. Infratentorial tumours and those invading deep white matter are not implanted because of the potentially disastrous consequences of radiation necrosis in these regions. In general, a Karnofsky performance status (KPS) of at least 70 is required because a KPS below 70 is associated with very poor survival.

INITIAL TREATMENT

Surgery

Tumours are maximally resected at the initial diagnosis. Depending on the tumour site, surgery may consist of biopsy, gross total resection or, most commonly, subtotal resection. A reoperation is performed after external beam radiation therapy or at the time of recurrence, prior to the brain implant, for those tumours producing a significant mass effect or oedema.

External beam radiation therapy

Newly diagnosed malignant gliomas are treated with external beam radiation therapy prior to brachytherapy. Focal radiation fields are used, including the tumour with a margin of approximately 3 cm, and treating at 1.8 Gy per fraction, five fractions per week, to a total dose of 59.4 Gy. Recurrent, implantable gliomas are treated with brachytherapy only.

Chemotherapy

Brain implant protocols for previously untreated malignant gliomas include hydroxyurea (HU) as a radiosensitizer given orally at a dose of 300 mg/m^2 at 6 hour intervals every Monday, Wednesday and Friday during external beam radiation therapy (Leibel et al 1987, Gutin et al 1991).

Following brachytherapy, previously untreated malignant gliomas have generally been treated with six cycles of PCV combination chemotherapy which includes lomustine (CCNU) (110 mg/m^2 orally on day 1), procarbazine (60 mg/m^2 orally on days 8–21), and vincristine (1.4 mg/m^2 intravenously on days 8 and 29) (Leibel et al 1987, Gutin et al 1991). After treatment failure, a variety of chemotherapeutic agents and regimens have been used.

IMPLANTATION TECHNIQUE

Preplanning

Within several days prior to the implant procedure, a contrast enhanced computerized tomography (CT) scan is performed to ensure that the lesion is visualized on CT and that it is technically implantable according to the criteria given above.

On the morning of the brain implant procedure, a Brown–Roberts–Wells (BRW) (Radionics, Burlington, Massachusetts, USA) stereotactic base ring is applied to the patient's skull under local anaesthesia in adults or under general anaesthesia in children. A graphite rod localizing system is mounted on the base ring and contrast enhanced CT is repeated with axial images obtained every 3 mm throughout the entire tumour volume.

Specialized treatment planning software for temporary brain implants was developed at UCSF and has been in use since 1986 (Weaver et al 1990a). This software is used prospectively to plan the locations of brain implant catheters and radiation sources on a VAX 11–780 or more recently, a VAX 4000, model 300 computer (Digital Equipment Corporation, Maynard, Massachusetts, USA). After the computer tape of the CT study has been loaded, CT images are displayed on a high resolution colour monitor. The target volume, encompassing the contrast enhanced tumour volume with a 0–5 mm margin, is marked on each CT image using a track ball. Positions of the nine localizing rods are digitized from a single CT image, establishing a correlation between CT space and BRW space. The programme permits CT image reconstruction and radiation isodose line display in any plane. Typically, sagittal and coronal as well as oblique views in the plane of and perpendicular to the direction of the implant catheters are viewed to help in the planning process. Catheter and source positions are specified empirically by the operator and adjusted in an iterative process until a satisfactory plan has been generated. Catheters are usually placed perpendicular to the skull surface, taking care to avoid the Sylvian fissure and sagittal and transverse sinuses. The programme does not require catheters to be parallel to each other or to conform to a grid, so that each catheter array is highly customized. Typically, 1–6 catheters are required with 1–4 ^{125}I sources per catheter. Sources within a given catheter are often separated by spacers 2 mm or more in length. Sources are chosen from a large stock, with a source strength ranging from about 3 to 40 mCi. In general, the 40–50 cGy/h isodose line is planned to encompass the target volume, conforming to the target volume as closely as possible. A dose–volume histogram, including information for normal tissue as well as the target volume, is available to help assess the adequacy of the plan. The time required to produce a plan is approximately 1–2 h.

Some centres prefer to implant a larger number of evenly spaced catheters throughout the target volume, creating a more homogeneous dose distribution within the target volume. We prefer to implant a smaller number of catheters to minimize the risk of cerebral oedema and bleeding. The two techniques yield very similar dose distributions outside of the target volume (Saw et al 1989).

At the end of the planning procedure, the program provides a print out of the BRW frame angles, target location for each catheter, source activities and spacer lengths. The ^{125}I sources are then calibrated, loaded into nylon catheters (1.04 mm inside diameter, 1.47 mm outside diameter), transported to the operating room in a lead lined covered tray, and sterilized.

Surgical procedure

When the preplanning process is nearing completion, the patient is transported to the operating room and the base ring is fixed to the operating room table with the patient in a semisitting position. Nafcillin 2 g is given intravenously preoperatively. The scalp is prepared with a povidone–iodine scrub.

Prior to implanting each catheter, the BRW arc-ring system is first mounted on a base frame. α, β, γ and δ angles are set on the arc-ring system and the phantom target (corresponding to the planned position of the catheter tip) is set according to x, y and z coordinates provided by the print out of the preplan. A probe is inserted through the guide on the arc to verify proper alignment with the target. Then the arc-ring system is released from the phantom base and attached to the base ring on the patient's head. The skin at the catheter site is anaesthetized, a small incision is made, and a twist drill inserted through the guide in the arc-ring assembly is used to make a 3.4 mm diameter hole in the skull. After penetrating the dura with a round ended metal K wire, the opening is dilated with a blunt probe. A 2.0 purse string suture is placed around the opening in the skin to later secure the loaded catheter and prevent cerebrospinal fluid leakage. For catheter sites near the midline or over the Sylvian fissure, a burr hole is made instead of a twist drill hole, in order to avoid injury to major blood vessels.

The arc-ring assembly is returned to the phantom base to determine the catheter insertion depth required to reach the target and then it is again mounted on the base ring on the patient's head. A Silastic catheter (1.57 mm inside diameter, 2.16 mm outside diameter) over a stylet is passed through a Silastic collar at the skin surface and through the twist drill hole in the skull, to the target depth (Fig. 9.1). The catheter and collar are glued together, the catheter is trimmed off about 1 cm from the scalp surface, and the collar is sutured to the skin. After all of the outer catheters have been inserted in this fashion, the inner catheters containing the ^{125}I sources are afterloaded and trimmed so that they protrude from the outer catheter by several millimetres. Figure 9.2 is a schematic diagram of the coaxial catheter system. The inner and outer catheters are fixed to each other with a haemostatic clip, the purse string sutures are tightened, and a

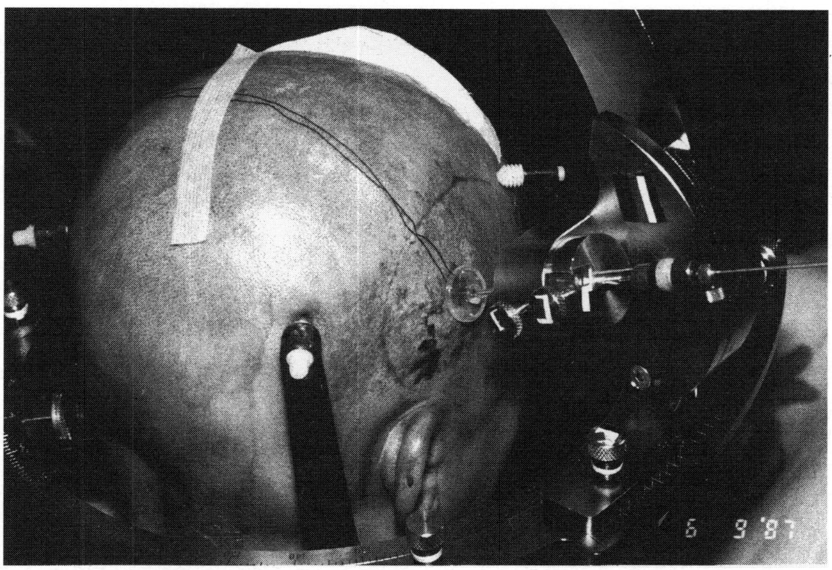

Fig. 9.1 Photograph of a brain implant procedure in progress, showing the implant catheter with an inner stylet passing through the guide on the arc-ring assembly and through a plastic collar on the scalp surface. The purse string suture is in place around the catheter entry site but has not yet been tightened.

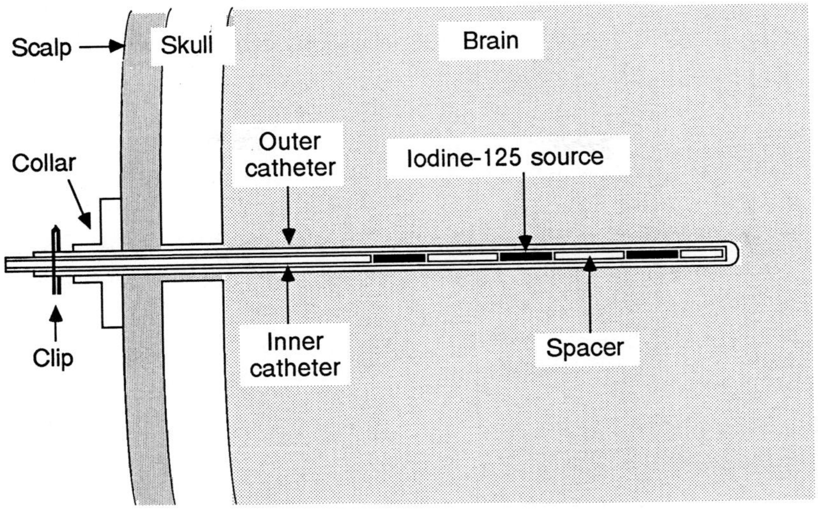

Fig. 9.2 Schematic diagram of the coaxial catheter system. The outer catheter passes through a plastic collar and a twist drill hole through the skull. The inner catheter houses the ^{125}I sources.

sterile gauze dressing is applied. Figure 9.3 shows the catheters in position at the conclusion of the implant procedure.

Source position verification

Immediately after the implant procedure, a localizing box with four fiducial markers on each face is mounted on the base ring on the patient's head. An anteroposterior and a lateral radiograph are taken through the localizing box in the operating room. The localizing box and base ring are removed from the patient's head and radiation precautions described below are instituted.

After digitizing into the computer the positions of the fiducial markers and the ^{125}I sources from the orthogonal radiographs, actual source positions and radiation isodose lines are calculated

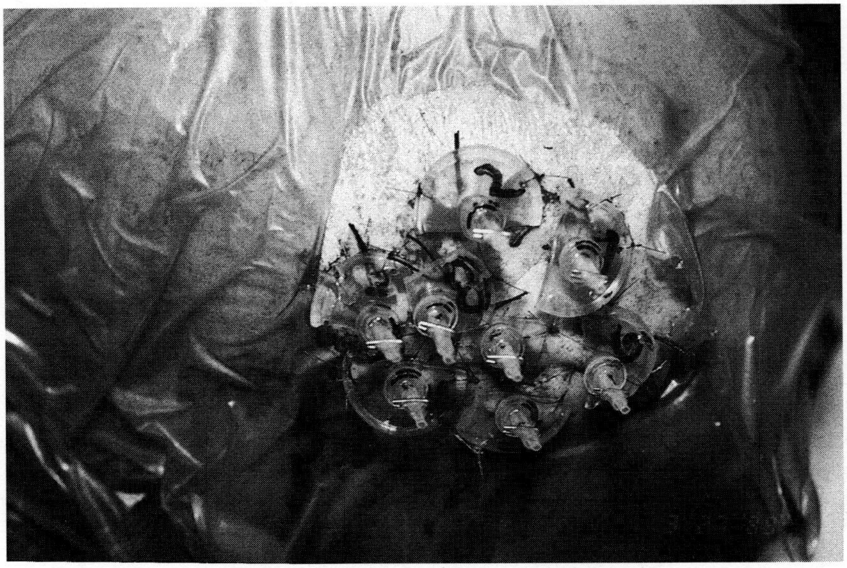

Fig. 9.3 Photograph of implant catheters and sources in place at the conclusion of an implant procedure.

and displayed on the preplanning CT images (Fig. 9.4) and an actual dose–volume histogram is generated. The software also calculates the parallel and perpendicular distance in millimetres between the actual and planned source positions. In the event of a significant miss, a new plan is created optimizing the source strengths and spacer lengths given by the actual catheter positions. Old inner catheters may be replaced with new, optimized inner catheters at the bedside.

Radiation protection

A major advantage of using ^{125}I is the ease of shielding. A small lead container or lead lined covered tray can be used to safely transport ^{125}I sources to and from the isotope safe.

While the ^{125}I sources are being afterloaded into the brain implant catheters, operating room personnel are protected by lead aprons and the surgeon is protected by leaded eyeglasses, a thyroid shield, a lead apron and non-disposable leaded surgical gloves.

Immediately after ^{125}I sources have been loaded, a radiation survey meter is used to measure exposure in milliroentgens per hour (mR/h) at various positions around the patient at a distance of 1 m, both without and with a protective hat. The hat is made of two layers of cloth divided into four triangular compartments into which 0.5 mm thick panels of flexible lead can be inserted. In most cases, the hat reduces radiation exposure to less than 0.1 mR/h at 1 m.

The patient is hospitalized in a single room while the radioactive sources are in place, usually for 4–7 days. The patient wears the protective hat only during visits from relatives or hospital personnel and visitors wear a lead apron while in the patient's room.

Implant removal

After the prescribed dose of radiation has been delivered, the sutures through the Silastic collar and the purse string sutures are removed and the inner and outer implant catheters are withdrawn as a unit. The skin at each catheter site is sutured and a sterile dressing is applied. Patients are generally discharged from the hospital on the day following implant removal.

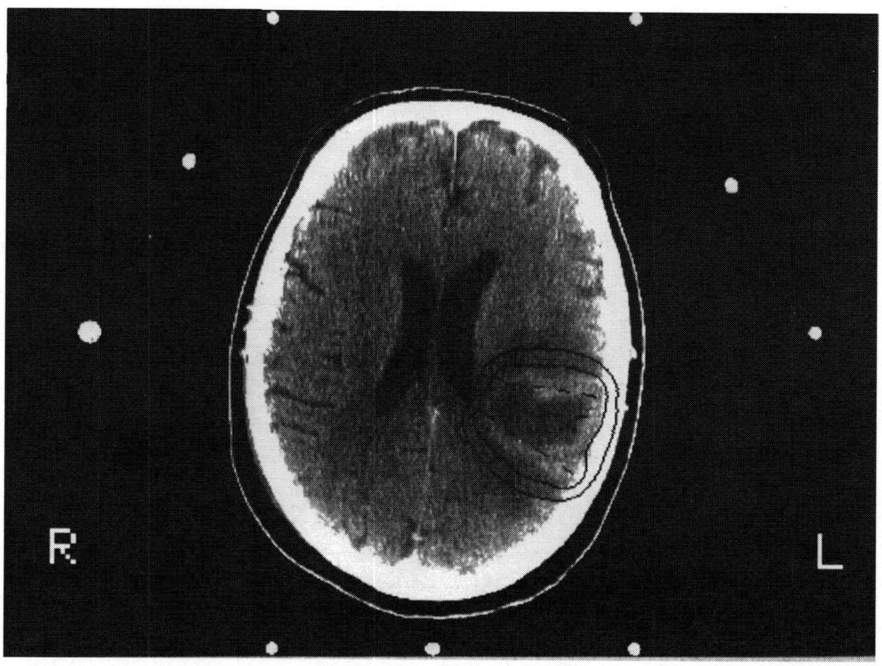

Fig. 9.4 CT scan showing actual ^{125}I source positions and resulting 20 and 40 cGy/h isodose lines for a glioblastoma multiforme implanted with four catheters. The radiation dose was prescribed at the 40 cGy/h isodose line.

Hyperthermia

When hyperthermia is combined with brachytherapy, the brain implant technique differs slightly from that used for brachytherapy alone. There is limited heating outside of an array of microwave antennae, requiring the brain implant catheters to be placed more peripherally, equally spaced about 1.2–2.0 cm apart from each other 3–5 mm inside the perimeter of the contrast enhancement on CT. One to three additional catheters are planned to house multisensor fibre optic thermometry probes, usually including one catheter at the centre of the tumour and one or two at the edge of the tumour.

After the outer catheters have been implanted stereotactically, inner catheters containing dummy radiation sources are loaded prior to source position verification. On the morning following surgery, the dummy sources are removed and the first hyperthermia treatment is given using 915 MHz helical coil microwave antennae (Satoh & Stauffer 1988 Satoh et al 1988) to heat as much of the tumour as possible to at least 42.5°C for 30 minutes. Antennae and thermometry probes are then removed and replaced with inner catheters containing the actual ^{125}I sources. A second hyperthermia treatment is given after a radiation dose of 60 Gy has been delivered. The hyperthermia technique is described in more detail elsewhere (Sneed et al 1991).

FOLLOW-UP EVALUATION

Patients are evaluated through the neuro-oncology service at UCSF, including assessment of clinical status, KPS, steroid requirement and contrast enhanced CT or gadolinium enhanced magnetic resonance imaging (MRI). Follow-up visits are scheduled at intervals of 2 months during the first year, intervals of 3 months for the next 2 years, and then at intervals of 6 months.

Approximately 50% of all brain implant patients later require reoperation for deteriorating clinical status and an increasing contrast enhancing lesion. Necrosis can mimic the appearance of progressive tumour on CT or MRI scans. Positron emission tomography (PET) using rubidium-82 to assess the integrity of the blood–brain barrier and [^{18}F]fluorodeoxyglucose to assess metabolic activity are helpful in distinguishing between recurrent tumour and radiation necrosis (Valk et al 1988).

STATISTICAL ANALYSIS

Actuarial survival is calculated using the method of Kaplan and Meier (Kaplan & Meier 1958), differences between survival curves are evaluated with the Mantel–Haenzel log rank test (Mantel 1966), and multivariate analysis of data is accomplished using the Cox proportional hazards linear regression model (Cox 1972, Breslow 1974).

RESULTS

The brain implant programme began at UCSF in 1977 with permanent or removable implants of ^{198}Au, ^{192}Ir or low activity ^{125}I. However, temporary implants of high activity ^{125}I have been used for high grade gliomas since December 1979. A review is in progress of over 350 consecutive patients with gliomas treated with high activity ^{125}I brain implants between December 1979 and June 1990. Results are currently available for three patient subgroups: 63 patients treated with external beam radiotherapy and a brain implant boost, 98 patients implanted for recurrent tumours, and 41 patients treated with thermoradiotherapy for recurrent malignant gliomas.

Implant boost for malignant gliomas

Between January 1982 and January 1990, 107 patients with previously untreated malignant gliomas were entered into a Northern California Oncology Group (NCOG) non-randomized trial of surgery, external beam radiotherapy (59.4–60.0 Gy at 1.8–2.0 Gy per fraction) with HU, followed by a brain implant boost, and then PCV chemotherapy for 1 year. There were 65 males and 42 females. At the time of the brain implant, the patient age ranged from 19 to 74 years and the KPS ranged from 70 to 100 (median 90). The mean age was 41 years for patients with non-glioblastoma multiforme anaplastic gliomas (NGM) and 51 years for patients with glioblastoma multiforme (GM) (Gutin et al 1991).

Of 101 evaluable patients, 63 actually had a brain implant, including 29 patients with NGM and 34 with GM. The most common reason for not proceeding with an implant boost was tumour progression or lack of regression such that the tumour was not deemed technically implantable after external beam radiotherapy. The median brachytherapy dose was 5500 cGy for patients with NGM (range 4600–7587 cGy) and 5193 cGy for those with GM (range 4200–6612 cGy) (Gutin et al 1991).

For all evaluable patients, the median survival from the date of diagnosis was 165 weeks for NGM (40 patients) and 67 weeks for GM (67 patients). For the 29 patients with NGM who actually underwent a brain implant boost, the median survival was 157 weeks. For the 34 patients implanted for GM, the median survival was 88 weeks, nine were alive 2 years after diagnosis and three were alive at 3 years (Gutin et al 1991).

There were no major surgical complications, 52% of patients implanted for NGM and 44% of those implanted for GM underwent reoperation at a median of 46 and 41 weeks, respectively, for tumour progression and/or necrosis (Gutin et al 1991).

There was a small decrease of the KPS with time after a brain implant. For patients with NGM, the mean KPS was 91 (range 90–100) 1 month after the implant and 78 (range 90–100) 30 months after the implant. For patients with GM, the mean KPS decreased from 86 (range 70–100) 1 month after the implant to 75 (range 60–100) 2 years after the implant (Gutin et al 1991).

Implant alone for recurrent malignant gliomas

Between January 1980 and January 1988, 98 patients were treated with high-activity ^{125}I brain implants for recurrent malignant gliomas. There were 95 evaluable patients including 50 with NGM and 45 with GM. There were 55 males and 40 females ranging in age from 5 to 66 years (median age 35 years for NGM and 50 years for GM). The median KPS was 90 (range 70–90). All patients had evidence of disease progression after previous external beam radiation therapy. 38 patients had also been treated with previous chemotherapy (Leibel et al 1989).

The mean brachytherapy dose delivered was 74.4 Gy for NGM and 70.2 Gy for GM (range 52.7–150.0 Gy) at a mean dose rate of 42 cGyh^{-h} (range 20–90 cGyh^{-h}) using 2–12 sources (mean 6.5) in 1–6 catheters (mean 2.7). Survival was measured from the date of the brain implant until death or last follow-up. The median survival was 81 weeks for patients with NGM and 54 weeks for those with GM. 14 patients with NGM and four with GM were still alive at least 3 years after the brain implant for recurrence (Leibel et al 1989).

Serious surgical complications included wound dehiscence requiring skin grafting (2), abscess in the tumour bed (1), meningitis (1), intracranial haemorrhage (1), and cerebral oedema requiring mannitol and steroid therapy (1). 47 patients (49%) were reoperated at a median of 29 weeks after the brain implant for clinical deterioration with increasing steroid dependency and mass effect at the implant site. CT scans showed ring enhancement around a central area of low attenuation corresponding to the high dose implant volume. Pathological findings generally included necrosis and residual tumour cells (Leibel et al 1989).

Implant with hyperthermia for recurrent malignant gliomas

Between July 1987 and September 1990, 42 recurrent malignant gliomas (16 NGM and 26 GM) in 41 patients were treated with interstitial thermoradiotherapy (Sneed et al 1992). There were 26 males and 15 females. The patient age ranged from 18 to 71 years (median 43 years) and the KPS from 40 to 90 (median 90). Prior therapy included external beam radiotherapy in all patients (median dose 59.4 Gy, range 44–80 Gy), a prior interstitial brain implant in three patients and chemotherapy in 24 patients.

Except for one patient with a KPS of 40 treated with only 32.4 Gy, the brachytherapy dose ranged from 47.6 to 63.3 Gy (median 59 Gy) given at a dose rate of 37–70 cGy/h (median 44 cGy/h). Tumours were heated with 1–8 antennae (median 4) and thermometry was accomplished using 1–3 dedicated thermometry

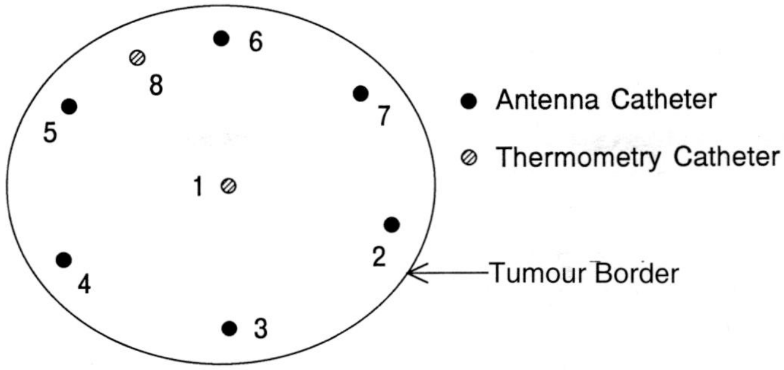

Fig. 9.5 Schematic diagram of a typical arrangement of antennae and thermometry probes for hyperthermia, including six antennae relatively equally spaced inside the perimeter of the tumour volume, and two additional thermometry catheters, one at the centre of the tumour and one near the tumour edge.

catheters (median 2). Figure 9.5 is a schematic diagram of a typical antenna and thermometry probe arrangement used to treat a recurrent GM. Figure 9.6 shows the resulting steady state temperature–depth profile for that patient treatment. For all 42 tumours treated, the steady state minimum tumour temperature for the best (or only) hyperthermia treatment ranged from 37.4 to 45.7°C (median 40.3°C), the average tumour temperature from 39.2 to 47.4°C (median 43.2°C) and the maximum tumour temperature from 40.3 to 51.7°C (median 45.6°C). T_{90} was defined as the temperature exceeded by 90% of the measured steady state tumour temperatures for any given patient treatment. Figure 9.7 shows the T_{90} calculation for the heat treatment depicted in Figure 9.6. T_{90} for the best treatment ranged from 38.0 to 45.8°C (median 41.2°C).

Actuarial survival was calculated from the date of the implant until death or last follow-up. The median survival was 47 weeks for patients with GM. The median survival time has not yet been reached for patients with NGM, with a median follow-up of 92 weeks in the living patients with NGM. The probability of survival at 12 and 18 months was 81 and 65%, respectively, for patients with NGM (Sneed et al 1992).

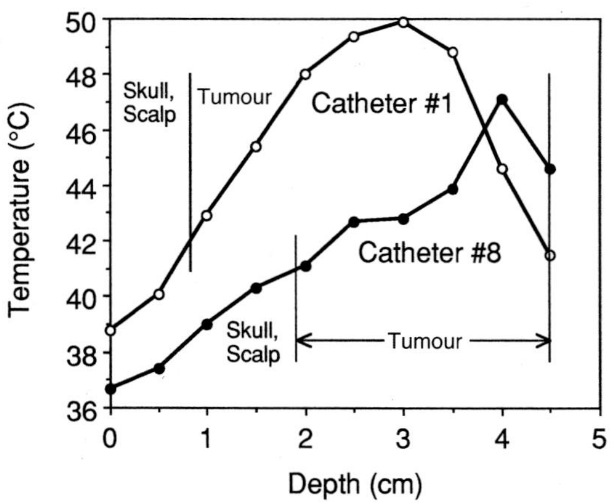

Fig. 9.6 Steady state temperatures versus depth in tissue for a recurrent GM treated with the catheter arrangement shown in Fig. 9.5. Tumour borders are indicated for both of the thermometry catheters.

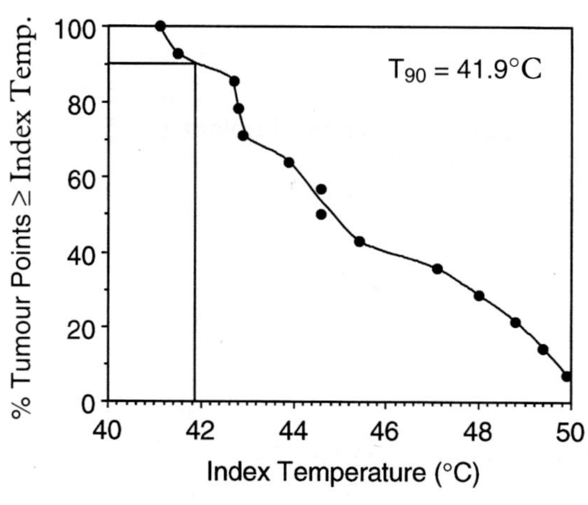

Fig. 9.7 The T_{90} for the patient treatment depicted in Figures 9.5 and 9.6 is determined by plotting the percentage of steady state tumour temperatures greater than or equal to the index temperature versus the index temperature. These data are fitted with a smooth curve to allow estimation of T_{90} by interpolation, the temperature exceeded by 90% of the measured intratumoural temperatures. For this particular patient treatment, T_{90} was 41.9°C.

Multivariate analyses were performed to assess the influence of age, KPS, histology, tumour volume, brachytherapy dose, subsequent reoperation, and various thermal parameters on survival and freedom from local tumour progression (FFP). Improved survival correlated with a higher KPS (p = 0.041) and with NGM as opposed to GM histological type (p = 0.067). A higher minimum tumour temperature and a higher T_{90} each correlated significantly with improved FFP (p = 0.000 9 and p = 0.001 46, respectively). The actuarial FFP was significantly better for $T_{90} \geq 41.5°C$ (n = 18) than for $T_{90} < 41.5°C$ (n = 24; p = 0.001) and for a minimum tumour temperature of at least 40.5°C (n = 20) than for a minimum tumour temperature less than 40.5°C (n = 22; p = 0.001). There was a trend towards improved actuarial survival for patients with $T_{90} \geq 41.5°C$ (n = 17) in comparison with those with $T_{90} < 41.5°C$ (n = 24; p = 0.083) (Sneed et al 1992).

Acute complications included reversible neurological changes in 13 patients, eight seizures, two infections and one case of deep venous thrombosis with pulmonary embolus. There were no treatment related deaths. 17 patients required reoperation for tumour and/or necrosis 5–51 weeks after thermoradiotherapy (median 19 weeks) (Sneed et al 1992).

SUMMARY

Primary GM

In a literature review spanning 1978–1985, the median survival ranged from 24 to 69 weeks for patients with newly diagnosed ('primary') GM treated with postoperative radiation and/or chemotherapy (Kornblith & Walker 1988). The median survival was 37 weeks for a total of 462 patients with GM treated on three randomized Radiation Therapy Oncology Group (RTOG) trials comparing radiation therapy with or without carmustine (BCNU) (Nelson et al 1985).

Patients treated with external beam radiotherapy followed by PCV or BCNU chemotherapy on NCOG protocol 6G61 had similar KPS (70–100), extent of resection, and age in comparison with patients who underwent a brain implant boost (Levin et al 1990a). For patients with primary GM, the median survival was 50 weeks for the PCV arm of NCOG 6G61 and 57 weeks for the BCNU arm of NCOG 6G61 (Levin et al 1990a), as opposed to 88 weeks for patients who had a brain implant boost after external beam radiotherapy (Gutin et al 1991).

Of course, the apparent improvement in survival with brachytherapy may be due in part to the circumscription, location and limited size of GM tumours eligible for a brain implant. A retrospective review of conventionally treated patients at the London Regional Canter Center in Toronto revealed that 40% of patients with GM had tumours suitable for a brain implant and had a KPS of at least 70. The median survival for this conventionally treated, brachytherapy eligible group was 13.9 months, as opposed to 5.8 months for the ineligible patients with GM (Florell et al 1992). The UCSF brain implant boost results compare favourably, with an actuarial median survival of 88 weeks (20.2 months) for patients with primary GM (Gutin et al 1991).

Other brachytherapy series have resulted in median survival ranging from 7 to 27 months for primary GM (Patchell et al 1988, Chun et al 1989, Kumar et al 1989, Bernstein et al 1990, Loeffler et al 1990, Selker et al 1991). The Brain Tumor Cooperative Group and the University of Toronto are conducting prospective randomized trials to evaluate interstitial brain implant boosts for malignant gliomas.

Recurrent GM

Reoperation for recurrent GM has been reported to result in a median survival of 29 or 36 weeks (Ammirati et al 1987, Harsh et al 1987) Single agent or combination chemotherapy has produced response or stabilization of recurrent GM in 29–75% of patients, with a median time to progression of 8–27 weeks (Levin 1985). In contrast, the use of brachytherapy at UCSF resulted in a median survival of 54 weeks for patients with recurrent GM (Leibel et al 1989). Encouragingly, some long term survivors were observed in the brachytherapy series. Therefore, an interstitial implant does seem to offer improved survival for patients with recurrent GM.

Other brachytherapy series for recurrent GM have yielded median survival ranging from 6 months to 58 weeks (Kumar et al 1989, Bernstein et al 1990, Larson et al 1990, Fass et al 1991, Selker et al 1991).

Primary NGM

The median survival achieved using brain implant boosts in our patients with primary NGM was 157 weeks (Gutin et al 1991). This result was very similar to results achieved without brachytherapy. RTOG protocols utilizing radiation therapy with or without BCNU yielded a median survival of 157 weeks in 94 patients with anaplastic astrocytoma (Nelson et al 1985). Patients with anaplastic astrocytoma treated on NCOG protocol 6G61 had a median survival of 157 weeks in the PCV chemotherapy arm and 82 weeks in the BCNU arm (Levin et al 1990a). On NCOG protocol 6G82–1, patients were treated with concomitant intravenous bromodeoxyuridine (BUdR) and external beam radiotherapy followed by PCV chemotherapy. Preliminary analysis revealed a median survival of 252 weeks for patients with anaplastic astrocytoma (Levin et al 1990b). Thus, for patients with primary NGM, brachytherapy does not appear to offer any advantage over treatment with external beam radiotherapy, radiosensitizers and chemotherapy.

Recurrent NGM

Other authors have reported median survival of 66 or 88 weeks for patients undergoing reoperation for recurrent anaplastic astrocytoma (Ammirati et al 1987, Harsh et al 1987). Chemotherapy has been reported to produce response or stabilization of disease in 50–84% of patients with recurrent NGM, with a median time to progression of 20–46 weeks (Levin 1985, Levin et al 1986). The use of brachytherapy at UCSF resulted in a median survival of 81 weeks (Leibel et al 1989). It is impossible to show a clear benefit of brachytherapy in these patients, given the lack of a randomized trial and the absence of a comparable patient population with which to correlate results. Our clinical impression is that brachytherapy does play a role in the treatment of recurrent NGM, along with judicious use of reoperation and a variety of chemotherapeutic regimens.

CONCLUSIONS AND CURRENT PRACTICE

The role of brachytherapy in the treatment of high grade gliomas cannot be well defined until results of high quality, prospective, randomized trials are available. Nevertheless, we feel that the UCSF results clearly demonstrate a favourable impact of high activity ^{125}I temporary interstitial implants on the survival of eligible patients with both primary and recurrent GM. Furthermore, the incidence of significant toxicity is quite low and the quality of life after treatment is very good, with only a modest decrement in the KPS over time.

Currently, brain implants are used at UCSF in the treatment of primary GM, recurrent GM, recurrent high grade NGM, and clinically aggressive recurrent low grade NGM.

Because brachytherapy boosts did not appear to improve survival for patients with primary NGM, we no longer perform brain implants in this group. Instead, these patients are entered on a new NCOG protocol, 6G90–3, which randomizes among three treatment arms: focal external beam irradiation alone (59.4 Gy at 180 cGy per fraction), irradiation plus intravenous BUdR and irradiation plus intravenous iododeoxyuridine (IUdR). PCV combination chemotherapy follows external beam radiotherapy for all three treatment arms.

Implant eligible patients with primary GM are currently entered on a randomized phase II study, NCOG protocol 6G90-2, for focal external beam radiotherapy to 59.4 Gy with HU followed by a 60 Gy brain implant boost with or without interstitial hyperthermia. A phase I trial is planned in patients with recurrent malignant gliomas combining an interstitial brain implant with intravenous BUdR or IUdR, in a continued search for strategies to improve survival and quality of life for patients with malignant gliomas.

REFERENCES

Ammirati M, Galicich J H, Arbit E, Liao Y 1987 Reoperation in the treatment of recurrent intracranial malignant gliomas. Neurosurgery 21: 607–614
Bernstein M, Gutin P H 1981 Interstitial irradiation of brain tumours: a review. Neurosurgery 9: 741–750
Bernstein M, Laperriere N, Leung P, McKenzie S 1990 Interstitial brachytherapy for malignant brain tumours: preliminary results. Neurosurgery 26: 371–380
Breslow N E 1974 Covariance analysis of censored survival data. Biometrics 30: 89–99
Choucair A K, Levin V A, Gutin P H 1986 Development of multiple lesions during radiation therapy and chemotherapy in patients with gliomas, Journal of Neurosurgery 65: 654–658
Chun M, McKeough P, Wu A, Kasdon D, Heros D, Chang H 1989 Interstitial iridium-192 implantation for malignant brain tumours. British Journal of Radiology 62: 158–162
Cox D R 1972 Regression models and life tables. Journal of the Royal Statistical Society 34: 187–220
Dewey W C, Freeman M L, Raaphorst G P et al 1980 Cell biology of hyperthermia and radiation. In: Meyn R E, Withers H R (eds) Radiation biology in cancer research. Raven Press, New York, pp 589–621
Fass D E, Malkin M G, Arbit E et al 1991 MSKCC brachytherapy results. Second Symposium on Stereotactic Treatment of Brain Tumours, New York, 28 February–1 March, p 29
Florell R C, Macdonald D R, Irish W D et al 1992 Selection bias, survival and brachytherapy for glioma. Journal of Neurosurgery 6: 179–183
Frazier C H 1920 The effects of radium emanations upon brain tumours. Surgery Gynecology and Obstetrics 31: 236–239
Gutin P H, Prados M D, Phillips T L et al 1991 External irradiation followed by an interstitial high activity iodine-125 implant "boost" in the initial treatment of malignant gliomas: NCOG study 6G82–2. International Journal of Radiation Oncology, Biology, Physics 21: 601–606
Hall E J 1985 The biological basis of endocurietherapy: the Henschke memorial lecture 1984. Endocurietherapy/Hyperthermia Oncology 1: 141–152
Hall E J 1988 Radiobiology for the radiologist. Lippincott, Philadelphia
Hall E J, Bedford J S, Oliver R 1966 Extreme hypoxia; its effect on the survival of mammalian cells irradiated at high and low dose-rates. British Journal of Radiology 39: 302–307
Harsh G R, Levin V A, Gutin P H, Seager M, Silver P, Wilson C B 1987 Reoperation for recurrent glioblastoma and anaplastic astrocytoma. Neurosurgery 21: 615–621
Hilaris B S (ed) 1975 Handbook of interstitial brachytherapy. Publishing Sciences Group, Acton, MA
Hochberg F H, Pruitt A 1980 Assumptions in the radiotherapy of glioblastoma. Neurology 30: 907–911
Kaplan E L, Meier P 1958 Nonparametric estimation from incomplete observations. Journal of the American Statistics Association 53: 457–481
Kornblith P L, Walker M 1988 Chemotherapy for malignant gliomas. Journal of Neurosurgery 68: 1–17
Kumar P P, Good R R, Jones E O, Patil A A, Leibrock L G, McComb R D 1989 Survival of patients with glioblastoma multiforme treated by intraoperative high-activity cobalt 60 endocurietherapy. Cancer 64: 1409–1413
Larson G L, Wilbanks J H, Dennis W S, Permenter W D, Easley J D 1990 Interstitial radiogold implantation for the treatment of recurrent high-grade gliomas. Cancer 66: 27–29
Leibel S, Gutin P, Phillips T et al 1987 The integration of interstitial implantation into the primary management of patients with malignant gliomas: results of a phase II Northern California Oncology Group trial. American Journal of Clinical Oncology 10: 106
Leibel S A, Gutin P H, Wara W M et al 1989 Survival and quality of life after interstitial implantation of removable high-activity iodine-125 sources for the treatment of patients with recurrent malignant gliomas. International Journal of Radiation Oncology, Biology, Physics 17: 1129–1139
Levin V 1985 Chemotherapy of primary brain tumours. Neurologic Clinics 3: 855–865
Levin V A, Phuphanich S, Liu H C et al 1986 Phase II study of combined BCNU and 5-fluorouracil, hydroxyurea and 6-mercaptopurine (BFHM) for the treatment of malignant gliomas. Cancer Treatment Reports 70: 1271–1274
Levin V A, Silver P, Hannigan J et al 1990a Superiority of post-radiotherapy adjuvant chemotherapy with CCNU, procarbazine and vincristine (PCV) over BCNU for anaplastic gliomas: NCOG 6G61 final report. International Journal of Radiation Oncology, Biology, Physics 18: 321–324
Levin V A, Wara W M, Gutin P H et al 1990b Initial analysis of NCOG 6G82–1: bromodeoxyuridine (BUdR) during irradiation followed by CCNU, procarbazine, and vincristine (PCV) chemotherapy for malignant gliomas. Proceedings of the American Society of Clinical Oncology 9: 91
Ling C C, Spiro I J, Mitchell J, Stickler R 1985 The variation of OER with dose rate. International Journal of Radiation Oncology, Biology, Physics 11: 1367–1373
Loeffler J S, Alexander E III, Wen P Y et al 1990 Results of stereotactic brachytherapy used in the initial management of patients with glioblastoma. Journal of the National Cancer Institute 82: 1918–1921
Mantel N 1966 Evaluation of survival data and two new rank order statistics arising in its consideration. Cancer Chemotherapy Reports 50: 163–170
Marks J E, Baglan R J, Prassad S C, Blank W F 1981 Cerebral radionecrosis: incidence and risk in relation to dose, time, fractionation and volume. International Journal of Radiation Oncology, Biology, Physics 7: 243–252
Mundinger F 1964 Die interstitielle Radio-Isotopen-Bestrahlung von Hirntumoren mit vergleichenden Langzeitergebnissen zur Rontgentiefentherapie. Acta Neurochirurgica 11: 89–109
Mundinger F, Weigel K 1984 Long-term results of stereotactic interstitial curietherapy. Acta Neurochirurgica, (suppl) 33: 367–371
Nelson D F, Nelson J S, Davis D R, Chang C H, Griffin T W, Pajak T F 1985 Survival and prognosis of patients with astrocytoma with atypical or anaplastic features. Journal of Neuro-Oncology 3: 99–103
Overgaard J 1990 The current and potential role of hyperthermia in radiotherapy. International Journal of Radiation Oncology, Biology, Physics 16: 535–549
Patchell R A, Maruyama Y, Tibbs P A, Beach J L, Kryscio R J, Young A B 1988 Neutron interstitial brachytherapy for

malignant gliomas: a pilot study. Journal of Neurosurgery 68: 67–72
Satoh R, Stauffer P R, Fike J R 1988 Thermal distribution studies of helical coil microwave antennas for interstitial hyperthermia. International Journal of Radiation Oncology, Biology, Physics 15: 1209–1218
Satoh T, Stauffer P R 1988 Implantable helical coil microwave antenna for interstitial hyperthermia. International Journal of Hyperthermia 4: 497–512
Saw C B, Suntharalingam N, Ayyangar K M, Tupchong L 1989 Dosimetric considerations of stereotactic brain implants. International Journal of Radiation Oncology, Biology, Physics 17: 887–891
Selker R G, Eddy M S, Arena V 1991 Pittsburgh brachytherapy experience. Second Symposium on Stereotactic Treatment of Brain Tumours, New York, 28 February–1 March, pp 23–24
Sheline G E, Wara W W, Smith V 1980 Therapeutic irradiation and brain injury. International Journal of Radiation Oncology, Biology, Physics 6: 1215–1228
Sneed P K, Stauffer P R, Gutin P H et al 1991 Interstitial irradiation and hyperthermia for the treatment of recurrent malignant brain tumours. Neurosurgery 28: 206–215
Sneed P K, Gutin P H, Stauffer P R et al 1992 Thermoradiotherapy of recurrent malignant brain tumours. International Journal of Radiation Oncology, Biology, Physics 23: 853–861
Talairach J, Ruggiero G, Aboulker J, David M 1955 A new method of treatment of inoperable brain tumours by stereotaxic implantation of radioactive gold — a preliminary report. British Journal of Radiology 28: 62–74
Valk P E, Budinger T F, Levin V A, Silver P, Gutin P H, Doyle W K 1988 PET of malignant cerebral tumours after interstitial brachytherapy. Journal of Neurosurgery 69: 830–838
Walker M D, Alexander E Jr, Hunt W E et al 1978 Evaluation of BCNU and/or radiotherapy in the treatment of anaplastic gliomas. Journal of Neurosurgery 49: 333–343
Walker M D, Strike T A, Sheline G E 1979 An analysis of dose-effect relationship in the radiotherapy of malignant gliomas. International Journal of Radiation Oncology, Biology, Physics 5: 1725–1731
Wallner K E, Galicich J H, Krol G, Arbit E, Malkin M G 1989 Patterns of failure following treatment for glioblastoma multiforme and anaplastic astrocytoma. International Journal of Radiation Oncology, Biology, Physics 16: 1405–1409
Weaver K, Smith V, Lewis J D et al 1990a A CT-based computerized treatment planning system for I-125 stereotactic brain implants. International Journal of Radiation Oncology, Biology, Physics 18: 445–454
Weaver K A, Anderson L L, Meli J A 1990b Source Characteristics. In: Anderson L L, Nath R, Weaver K A et al (eds) Interstitial brachytherapy: physical, biological, and clinical considerations. Raven Press, New York, pp 3–19

10. Stereotactic external beam radiotherapy

M. Brada J. D. Graham

INTRODUCTION

Localization of delivery of radiation is perhaps the most important factor responsible for the differential effect of radiation on tumour and normal tissue. This is particularly so with high dose radical treatment given with curative intent. Irradiation can be localized either by insertion of radioactive sources directly into the tumour — the technique of interstitial radiotherapy/brachytherapy (see Chs 8 and 9)—or with external beam radiotherapy. Two, three or more beams of high energy photons give a maximum radiation dose at the intersection of the radiation fields and define a volume which receives a high uniform dose of radiation ('target volume') with a lower dose given to the surrounding normal tissue. The target volume encompasses the tumour as seen on imaging and a surrounding border, which includes the estimate of microscopic spread with a further margin added for the inaccuracy of the technology of both imaging and treatment delivery. Modern linear accelerator (linac) systems deliver treatment with high precision, and most of the inaccuracy relates to patient movement during imaging and therapy. Routine use of computerized tomography (CT) and magnetic resonance imaging (MRI) and patient fixation with a plastic mask improve the accuracy of tumour localization and reduce movement during treatment.

Stereotactic radiotherapy further increases the precision of tumour localization and treatment, and increases the dose differential between the target volume and normal brain. Two major advances have allowed its development. Firstly, patient fixation with a stereotactic neurosurgical type frame which increases the precision of tumour localization and provides a firmer immobilization during treatment. The margin of inaccuracy is therefore considerably reduced with potentially less normal brain irradiated. The second advance has come with the development of high precision focused radiation by increasing the number of treatment fields, which increases the dose gradient between tumour and normal tissue.

In the initial attempts at stereotactic radiotherapy, multiple collimated orthovoltage X-ray beams and subsequently multiple cobalt sources were placed in a spherical distribution around the patient's head and focused on to a small central point (Leksell 1951). The number of individual sources increased (currently numbering over 200), and such commercially available equipment is described as a gamma unit or gamma knife. The technique developed further using modern linear accelerators. Moving a source of radiation around an isocentre is equivalent to multiple individual fields arranged in an arc. A number of arcs can be centred on a target volume resembling a spherical distribution of radiation sources. Alternatively, treatment can be given with multiple fixed fields sequentially during one therapy session. Stereotactic external beam radiotherapy or radiosurgery as it was originally described, encompasses both options — treatment with a gamma knife and with a linear accelerator using multiple arcs or multiple fixed fields. Although strict definitions have not been agreed, the term 'radiosurgery' should be reserved for single fraction treatment, while the term 'stereotactic radiotherapy' better describes fractionated stereotactic treatment. An alternative means of localized irradiation utilizes the property of the Bragg peak of heavy particles in the form of cyclotron generated protons or heavy charged particles. Whichever technique is used, stereotactic external beam radiotherapy in the treatment of central nervous system lesions is best described as stereotactically guided conformal radiotherapy.

Stereotactic radiotherapy of a small target volume irradiates less normal tissue to high dose than conventional radiotherapy, with a steep dose gradient between tumour and normal brain. In theory this should allow for a higher dose of radiation to the target while reducing or maintaining the dose to the surrounding normal tissue. These principles have been taken a step further by increasing the dose to the target volume beyond conventional radiation tolerance to further improve tumour control, assuming that the determinant of toxicity is the dose to normal tissue surrounding the target.

Single fraction stereotactic radiotherapy/radiosurgery has been successfully developed for the treatment of small inoperable intracranial arteriovenous malformations (AVMs), and certainly in this situation it has become accepted as the treatment of choice in defined circumstances. The role of stereotactic radiotherapy is under investigation in the treatment of a variety of intracranial tumours. In the following discussion we review the technical aspects of stereotactic radiotherapy and the currently available clinical information on its application in benign and malignant intracranial tumours.

TECHNIQUES

There are three separate methods for the delivery of stereotactic external beam radiotherapy. The gamma knife uses gamma rays (photons) from multiple cobalt sources, linear accelerators use multiple arcs of rotation to focus X-rays (photons) on a small volume and heavy particle accelerators use the distinct physical properties of helium ions or proton beams to achieve a sharply defined dose distribution. The first two techniques deliver ionizing radiation with identical physical characteristics. Heavy particle beams cause dense ionization over a short distance at a depth in tissue determined by the nature of the particles and the energy of the beam. The different physical properties of heavy particle beams make comparisons with photon techniques difficult since the distribution of the dose in tissues is different. Although the techniques of dose delivery differ, the methods of patient fixation and target localization are similar with each of the systems. The biological effects of charged particles and photons are also similar and can be compared in terms of equivalent radiation doses using photon irradiation as the standard.

Patient fixation

Radiotherapy to the brain has conventionally been given with the patient rigidly fixed during treatment. A head shell made from a plastic material such as acrylic fits over the face and head and is secured to the treatment couch. Each shell is individually moulded and requires a considerable degree of skill to achieve a good fit that will give reproducible positioning during fractionated radiotherapy.

For stereotactic radiotherapy the stereotactic frame, adapted from neurosurgical frames, acts both as a fixation and localization device. The commercially available gamma knife was developed using the Leksell frame (Bradshaw 1986) while linear accelerator based systems have used a variety of neurosurgical systems adapted for radiotherapy purposes, of which the Brown–Roberts–Wells (BRW) frame (Lutz et al 1988) is the most widely used. All these frames fix to the outer table of the skull with pins which are inserted under local anaesthesia. The frame acts as a baseline from which a three dimensional coordinate system is generated over the patient's head. Target localization and treatment must be performed in the same session since removal of the frame results in loss of the unique relationship between the frame and the head.

Attempts have been made to mark the positions of the pins in order to reproduce the set-up at a later time and so allow fractionated radiotherapy but repositioning of the frame is difficult and patient tolerance tends to be poor. Only two or three treatments have been given using this method (Colombo et al 1989). Other groups have developed lighter frames which have been left in position for periods of time (Houdek et al

1990, Souhami et al 1990). Despite concern over the risk of infection around the locating pins, the reported complications have been minimal. An elegant but invasive solution to the problem has been to implant markers under the skin of the patient's scalp. The head can then be placed in an identical position at each session using an electromagnetic system that generates three dimensional coordinates, so avoiding the need for an external frame (Jones et al 1990).

A major advance has come from the development of a relocatable stereotactic frame. Localization and treatment no longer need to be performed in a single session and it is possible to give multiple fractions of radiotherapy. To date, two relocatable systems have been developed. The frame developed by Leitinen et al locates by attachment to the external auditory meati and the bridge of the nose. A set of scales allows reproducible fixation based on individual anatomical relationships between these three points of fixation. Accuracy of relocation has been reported as ±1 mm and patient tolerance appears to be satisfactory (Hariz et al 1990).

The Gill–Thomas frame is based on the BRW system (Gill–Thomas–Cosman (GTC) localizer, Radionics, Burlington, Massachusetts, USA) and also uses a three point fixation (Gill et al 1991). The principal location is via the upper dentition. An individually moulded impression is taken of the upper teeth using a light cured acrylic impression material. Even in edentulous patients there is sufficient irregularity of the gums to allow an accurate fitting to be made. Stability is achieved by two other points of fixation. A head rest with an individually moulded silicon pad is positioned over the occiput using a graduated scale to mark the vertical and horizontal positions. Nylon straps over the top of the skull secure the entire device in position, allowing the patient free jaw movement. Initial fitting including the dental impression takes approximately 20 minutes. Subsequent fixation takes only a few minutes. The accuracy of relocation is greatest when the patient has a full set of teeth, when the frame can be refitted with less than 1 mm of variation, but even in edentulous patients the accuracy of relocation is less than 1.5 mm (Graham et al 1991a). The frame has been used to treat children as young as 3 years of age and is well tolerated. Intubation for anaesthesia can be performed with the frame fitted and location is secure enough to allow neurosurgery.

Localization and treatment planning

Target localization for radiotherapy involves the same steps used for neurosurgical biopsy. The frame acts as a base from which a three dimensional coordinate system is generated encompassing the head. The x and y coordinates lie in the axial plane and can be measured directly from CT or MRI scans. The z coordinate, which lies on the axis parallel to the couch top, is calculated from the separation of fiducial markers attached to the frame during scanning. For CT the accuracy with which any point can be defined is a function of the matrix on the axial slice and the slice thickness. Using the latest generation CT scanner with a 512 × 512 matrix and a frame of 35 cm width, the pixel size will be approximately 0.7 × 0.7 mm. Allowing for partial volume effects at the edge of a lesion the resolution cannot be better than 2.1 mm. A slice separation of 1.5–2.0 mm is commonly used. A similar fiducial system allows MRI and positron emission tomography (PET) to be used for target localization although problems of geometric distortion on MRI and the poor resolution of PET cameras need to be overcome (Peter et al 1987, Schad et al 1987).

For cerebral angiography a system of plates containing steel markers in orthogonal positions allows the calculation of the coordinates at any position on the film with an accuracy of ±0.5 mm (Serago et al 1991). For cerebral AVMs, angiographic localization of the nidus is more accurate than with CT but the coordinates have to be transferred to CT for dosimetric purposes. Care must be taken when using orthogonal angiography films to reconstruct in three dimensions. Inaccuracies of image projection may arise if only two views are taken (Bova & Friedman 1991). This may result in incorrect estimation of shape and size. For example, a horseshoe shaped lesion may appear as a cylinder on orthogonal films if only two views are taken. This will not affect the treatment volume if the target is being fitted within the smallest spherical dose volume but will result in overtreatment of normal tissue if some form of shaping of isodoses is being used. The target size may be underestimated if the long axis of a lesion lies at 45° to the orthogonal views. There may be up to a 41% reduction from the true length, resulting in significant undertreatment of a lesion.

A number of planning systems capable of carrying out dosimetry for stereotactic radiotherapy are commercially available. The most recent computer workstations carry out complex three dimensional reconstructions very rapidly. For stereotactic purposes the dose calculation algorithm must be able to cope with circular fields as small as 1 cm in diameter. Arcs are treated as a series of fixed beams usually at 10° increments; a simplification that speeds up the dose calculation without significant loss of accuracy. The patient outline and target volume are defined on each diagnostic image with additional images required to define the contours of the patient's skull. The target volume can be reconstructed in different planes so that the maximum diameter can be found and the appropriate circular field size, treatment isocentre and beam arrangement can be chosen. The aim is to encompass the target, which is often irregular, within the smallest spherical volume that will enclose it.

The appropriate target volume for external beam stereotactic radiotherapy of tumours has not been established. For malignant disease, the ring enhancing margin seen on contrast enhanced CT is encompassed with a margin of 2–5 mm, following the practice developed for interstitial implantation of radioactive sources. For cerebral AVMs the accepted practice has been to treat the lesion seen on angiography in the venous phase of filling. Most groups do not attempt to treat large feeding vessels.

Dose delivery

The prescribed dose

In conventional radiotherapy there are recommendations laid down by the International Commission on Radiation Units (ICRU) for an 'ideal' dose distribution which specify the maximum dose inhomogeneity within the target volume and the most appropriate isodose to which the treatment should be prescribed. There are no such criteria for dose definition in stereotactic radiotherapy and comparison of results between groups is difficult. For example, with the gamma knife the dose is usually prescribed to the 50% isodose line, which means that parts of the target volume will receive double the prescribed dose. Linear accelerator doses are prescribed to the 80 or 90% isodose lines, which results in less target volume dose inhomogeneity and a different dose distribution within the surrounding normal tissues. The use of multiple isocentres, to treat large or irregular volumes, results in even greater dose inhomogeneity within the target. It will be difficult to obtain a consensus on dose definition until treatment techniques, particularly for irregularly shaped targets, are established. However, we would recommend that ICRU practice is adopted with prescription to the 90% isodose line allowing for 10% dose inhomogeneity in the target volume.

The greatest experience with stereotactic external beam radiotherapy has been in the treatment of cerebral AVMs with large single fractions of radiation. Doses with the gamma knife have ranged from 20 to 40 Gy, usually to the 50% isodose lines. Linear accelerator doses are generally lower and have ranged from 18 to 25 Gy. The linear accelerator can treat larger lesions, and doses are commonly reduced as the target size increases. At the present time there seems to be little benefit from doses above 25 Gy given as a single fraction for the treatment of small AVMs (<3 cm in diameter). The results of treatment of large AVMs are less satisfactory.

Fractionated stereotactic radiotherapy has been used on small numbers of patients and a wide range of doses and fractionation schedules have been given. Patients with recurrent high grade glioma have been treated at The Royal Marsden Hospital with doses up to 45 Gy in nine fractions over 2 weeks following conventional radical radiotherapy. In the immediate post-treatment phase this dose was well tolerated although the long term toxicity is not defined and is likely to be considerable. A calculation by Brenner et al (1991) based on proven radiobiological parameters suggests that a dose of 50 Gy in nine fractions over 14 days is equivalent to a stereotactic interstitial radioactive implant of 70 Gy given over 1 week, which is known to be associated with a near 50% necrosis rate.

Dose optimization

When planning beam arrangements for stereotactic external beam radiotherapy it is necessary to consider three factors:

1. The target volume should be encompassed with a minimum inhomogeneity of dose
2. The dose to the surrounding normal tissues should be minimized
3. Critical structures should be avoided.

Intracranial tumours are seldom spherical yet the photon techniques of stereotactic external beam radiotherapy deliver the dose to an essentially spherical volume. The gamma knife does allow blocking of one or more of its sources, resulting in an ellipsoid distribution (Flickinger et al 1990), but irregularly shaped distributions are not possible with a single isocentre. The linear accelerator technique using multiple non-coplanar arcs and circular collimators suffers from the same inflexibility in terms of shaping of isodose curves. Weighting of arcs does not alter the shape significantly (Thomson1990).

For irregular target volumes the choice is either to use the largest circular collimator that will encompass the target and accept excessive normal tissue doses or to use multiple isocentres. The latter method is fraught with practical problems involved in encompassing an irregular volume within several spherical dose envelopes. It also results in considerable inhomogeneity of the dose within the target volume which appears to be associated with excessive late normal tissue damage (Nedzi et al 1991). The optimal technique for the treatment of irregular volumes will require the development of a dynamic multileaf collimator for the linear accelerator which can adjust during arcing, but this technology is not yet available. A more practical currently available conformal technique is to use multiple fixed non-coplanar fields with individually shaped shielding blocks.

A variety of beam arrangements have been used for linear accelerator based stereotactic radiotherapy, ranging from a single arc up to 11 arcs. A single arc treats a cylindrical volume and results in an excessive dose to surrounding normal tissue. It has been shown that 3–5 arcs give the best dose distribution for the treatment of spherical volumes in terms of minimizing the dose received by normal tissue within the 50% isodose (i.e. receiving 50% or more of the prescribed dose) (Graham et al 1991b). Larger, often irregular, volumes of 4–5 cm in diameter may be better treated by an arrangement of 6–8 static non-coplanar beams. A static beam arrangement, as used with heavy particle accelerators, allows conformal shaping of isodose curves using 'beam's eye view' facilities by which a target can be viewed in the plane of the radiation beam and customized blocking of the field performed. This is probably the best method currently available for the treatment of irregular volumes.

Critical structures such as the brain stem or optic chiasma should be avoided. Using a linear accelerator the positions of the arcs can be adjusted to alter the entry or exit paths. The gamma knife allows blocking of individual sources, so that the treatment volume can be changed from spherical to mildly elliptical, allowing a more rapid fall off in dose in one plane (Flickinger et al 1990). The scope for treating irregular target volumes is limited but beam blocking does allow the gamma knife to avoid treating sensitive structures within the brain.

Practical techniques

The gamma knife

The multisource cobalt radiosurgery unit — the gamma knife — was developed by Lars Leksell in Sweden in the 1950s and 1960s (Leksell 1983). Designed initially as a method of carrying out bloodless thalamotomy and similar stereotactic techniques for intractable pain, the bulk of clinical experience has been in the treatment of cerebral AVMs.

The commercially available unit consists of

201 highly collimated cobalt-60 sources in a hemispherical arrangement. A Leksell stereotactic frame is attached to the patient via pins to the outer table of the skull. Cerebral angiography is carried out in the frame and, with the frame still fitted, the patient then waits while radiotherapy planning is carried out. The target diameter is defined by a secondary collimator, which is a metal helmet drilled with appropriately sized holes. These are limited to a few sizes (usually 4,8,14 and 18 mm in diameter). The helmets are heavy and have to be winched into position on the couch each time a patient is treated. The stereotactic frame is secured within the helmet and, for treatment, the whole assembly, including the patient, is moved into the head of the machine, which contains the cobalt sources.

The linear accelerator

Most modern linear accelerators can be relatively easily adapted for stereotactic radiotherapy. Circular secondary collimators are fitted to the head of the machine to allow treatment of small target volumes. The stereotactic frame is attached either to the treatment couch or to a BRW stand fixed to the floor, which allows slightly higher precision in dose delivery by eliminating inaccuracies during rotation of the treatment couch. However, the floor stand is time consuming to set up and requires sophisticated interlocks to prevent vertical movement of the couch supporting the patient's body while the head is rigidly fixed.

Checks must be made before each treatment session to ensure that the position of the radiation isocentre (about which the radiation arcs rotate) can be accurately defined. If a floor stand is used the isocentre is found by direct measurement from this structure, which acts as a fixed reference point. If the stereotactic frame is fitted to the treatment table then the isocentre is located using alignment lasers fixed to the walls, and these must be calibrated (Tsai et al 1991). The linear accelerator can be converted from routine to stereotactic use in approximately 30-40 minutes.

A dose distribution very similar to the gamma knife can be achieved with an arrangement of multiple non-coplanar arcs. This requires a combination of gantry and table rotation, each of which results in a degree of inaccuracy in dose delivery. With careful adjustment, dose delivery should be within ±1 mm of the calculated isocentre. As with the gamma knife, the greatest inaccuracy arises when the target is defined on the diagnostic image.

Heavy particle beams

Heavy particle accelerators have tended to be available for medical purposes as an off-shoot of research programmes in particle physics. However, stereotactic radiotherapy has been one of the major uses. Most units are non-isocentric and the treatment set-up is complicated. Accuracy appears to be as good as with the linear accelerator technique. There are theoretical advantages to proton and helium ion beams in terms of dose delivery as the beams have a sharply defined stopping distance and distributions can be produced to encompass irregular volumes (Phillips et al 1990). The physical differences between heavy particles and photons make direct comparisons of the techniques difficult. The results of treatment, principally of AVMs, are comparable but, unless the capital and running costs can be reduced, heavy particle accelerators will remain limited to a few centres.

Comparison of techniques

The advantage of the gamma unit is its highly accurate dose delivery. There are relatively few moving parts and alignment of the collimator helmet to the hemispherical sources is very precise. The greatest inaccuracy remains the localization of the target from the diagnostic images. The disadvantages are the high capital cost and the radioactive shielding problems both at initial installation and at source replacement, which must be carried out every 4–5 years. The system is relatively inflexible compared to the linear accelerator, with field sizes limited to <2 cm in diameter and, with current fixation, treatment limited to single fractions. The gamma knife is a good method for treating small AVMs but is of limited use in the treatment of brain tumours.

The main advantages of the linear accelerator technique are its flexibility and low cost. There is no limitation in field size and beam shaping can be carried out for the treatment of irregular shapes. Treatment times of 30–40 minutes allow the technique to be performed with minimal disruption to the regular workload of the machine. There are more moving parts than the gamma knife and delivery is less precise (±1 mm compared with ±0.25 mm) although it is doubtful whether this results in any significant clinical difference.

Quality assurance

The delivery of high precision radiotherapy requires a rigorous programme of quality assurance. The linear accelerator demands greater time for quality assurance because of the larger number of moving parts.

For the linear accelerator there are two principle criteria that must be met:

1. The rotational axes of the gantry and table must intersect within a 1 mm diameter sphere at any position
2. The central axis of the collimated beam must intersect the above sphere at any gantry position.

In order to meet these criteria a sequence of exposures must be made with a metal ball approximately 1 cm in diameter placed at the isocentre with a circular collimator 2 cm in diameter in place. A film is exposed at a number of gantry and couch positions (usually 8–10) that reflect the usual range of movements during treatment. The film will demonstrate the amount of displacement of the metal sphere from the centre of the circular field and so geometric and beam alignment inaccuracies can be measured. This procedure should be undertaken regularly — some centres perform this check before each treatment session.

The positioning lasers must be aligned to the treatment isocentre before each treatment session within ±1 mm. If a floor stand is used to support the patient's head then the interlocks that prevent independent movement of the couch should be tested. The safety measures to prevent the gantry crashing with the patient support assembly must also be checked regularly. Less frequent measurements are made of the beam profile for each of the circular field sizes available and the dose rate during arcing (Tsai et al 1991).

With the gamma knife the problems of gantry and couch rotation are not encountered. Mechanical and beam alignment are checked in a similar way to that described above by placing a metal sphere at the isocentre and an unexposed film on the couch top beneath it within the exit path of the beams. The film will show any inaccuracy in alignment of the collimator helmet and the source channels through displacement of the circular shadow cast by the metal sphere from the centre of the circular field (Wu et al 1990).

For both techniques, dosimetric measurements should be made in a phantom to ensure accuracy of the treatment planning system. An ionization chamber can be used to measure the dose at the isocentre but the dose within the area of rapid fall-off around the target volume is best measured using standard sized (3×3×1 mm) lithium fluoride thermoluminescent dosimetry TLD chips.

The localization procedure should also be subjected to regular quality assurance. The accuracy of CT and angiographic localization can be checked by placing a steel sphere at a known coordinate position within the stereotactic frame and checking the calculated position with the true position.

THE PATHOPHYSIOLOGY OF STEREOTACTIC IRRADIATION

Radiobiology

Conventional radiotherapy seeks to exploit the greater sensitivity to radiation of tumour tissue compared to normal tissue. Unfortunately, for many relatively resistant tumours such as gliomas this difference is small and the maximum amount of radiation that can be delivered to a tumour is limited by the tolerance of the adjacent normal tissue. This problem may be overcome by fractionating the treatment rather than giving one or two large fractions (Berg & Lindgren 1963). Fractionation allows a higher tumour dose to be given for an equivalent level of late radiation damage to the brain. Another alternative is to reduce the volume of normal brain tissue treated, which is the basis of stereotactic radiotherapy. Any therapeutic advantage from stereotactic radiotherapy will rely on increased tolerance of normal brain tissue as a result of the volume reduction. A higher dose of radiation could then be given to the tumour for an equivalent level of late normal tissue damage.

What is the evidence for a volume effect in the brain? Spinal cord tolerance is volume dependent in animals. Experiments on rat spinal cord have shown that for equal doses of radiation the incidence of late radiation damage was higher when longer lengths of cord were treated (Hopewell et al 1987, van der Kogel 1987). Theoretical models suggest that the white matter of the brain should respond in a similar manner and a volume effect has been shown experimentally in the rabbit and monkey brains (Berg & Lindgren 1963, Kjellberg 1979). Kjellberg has produced an iso-necrosis line based on monkey and human data for stereotactic radiotherapy (Kjellberg et al 1983), but a recent review of the published literature has cast doubt on its validity. Marks & Spencer (1991) concluded that 'the influence of volume of irradiated brain on the tolerance of the brain to radiation is not well understood ... additional clinical and experimental data are needed'.

There is a theoretical advantage to using fractionated stereotactic radiotherapy for brain tumours. Damage to normal tissue will be lowest if multiple small fractions are used, but few centres can offer stereotactic radiotherapy on a daily basis over 5 or 6 weeks because of resource limitations. A compromise is to use fraction sizes of 4–5 Gy and rely on the reduced normal tissue volume with the stereotactic method more than off-setting any reduction in brain tolerance caused by the large fraction size. It has been estimated that a radical dose would be achieved by giving 50 Gy in nine fractions over 4 days (Brenner et al 1991).

The dose and fractionation schedule used for AVMs differs from that used for brain tumours. In the treatment of AVMs radiation is used to occlude blood vessels, an effect that occurs with late radiation damage in normal tissues. A schedule is required that causes maximum late radiation damage to the target but spares the surrounding normal tissues. Large single doses achieve such damage and the rapid dose fall-off with stereotactic radiation spares the normal brain. Problems arise with large lesions, which are often of irregular shape, where normal tissue may lie within the high dose envelope. In practice, larger lesions are usually treated with a reduced dose because of worries about the amount of normal brain tissue being irradiated, but reducing the dose results in a lower obliteration rate. The treatment of small AVMs of less than 3 cm in diameter with large (18–25 Gy) single fractions of stereotactic radiation gives excellent results with a low complication rate. The treatment of larger AVMs is at present unsatisfactory. Fractionated treatment would spare normal tissue but is likely to result in a lessened therapeutic effect. A few large fractions may prove to be the best compromise for the treatment of large AVMs.

Pathological effects

The effects of radiation on the brain can be classified as acute, early delayed and late reactions (Sheline et al 1980). Acute reactions are seen during or immediately after treatment and are thought to be the result of increased oedema. Corticosteroid medication often gives rapid relief of symptoms. The early delayed reaction occurs 6–8 weeks after irradiation as a transient deterioration seldom lasting more than 14 days. A more persistent course virtually always indicates progressive disease. There is some evidence that transient demyelination is the causative factor (Lampert & Davis 1964).

Late radiation damage occurs from about 4 months and, while most lesions appear within 2–3 years, the latent period may be up to 7 years (Sheline et al 1980). The principle factor is vascular damage. Focal radionecrosis results when an end arteriole is occluded and is rare at doses below 60 Gy and at fraction sizes of 2 Gy or less. The lesion is indistinguishable from tumour recurrence both on CT and MRI. Cerebral atherosclerosis is more common following irradiation, and moya moya disease, a rare vasculitis of the circle of Willis, has also been reported.

AVMs are obliterated as a result of the late

effects of radiation. Damage to the intima of blood vessels results in hyperplasia of the endothelial cells, thickening of the vessel wall and extravasation of fluid. The end result is often occlusion of the vessel, the desired result in the AVM but leading to necrosis if an end arteriole in normal brain tissue is occluded. Most late damage occurs within the first 2 years after treatment and the obliteration rate at 2 years is a widely quoted figure for the results of treatment of AVMs.

A dilemma exists over the use of a highly localized treatment such as stereotactic radiotherapy for the treatment of malignant brain tumours which may infiltrate widely. The poor results currently achieved in the treatment of high grade gliomas are manifest by our inability to control the tumour at the primary site. Recurrences at a distance from the primary site are unusual and virtually always associated with primary site recurrence (Wallner et al 1989). A number of pathological studies have shown tumour cells at a distance of 3–4 cm from the main bulk of tumour but small numbers of tumour cells should theoretically be controlled by lower doses of irradiation (Halperin et al 1989). The most logical treatment for high grade gliomas with radiation will involve two phases of treatment. The first phase, using conventional radiotherapy techniques, will give a dose of 55–60 Gy fractionated over 5–6 weeks to a generous volume and the second phase a stereotactic boost with either fractionated stereotactic external beam radiotherapy or a stereotactic interstitial implant to the enhancing volume seen on CT or MRI. This treatment strategy may possibly result in normal tissue damage within the high dose volume.

CLINICAL APPLICATIONS AND RESULTS IN BRAIN TUMOURS

Stereotactic external beam radiotherapy (SRT)/radiosurgery offers a technical advantage over conventional radiotherapy in the treatment of small lesions. Its application in the treatment of brain tumours is based on the premise that such high precision treatment with its technical advantages will be of clinical benefit. Theoretically, SRT may allow for a higher tumour dose without increased damage to normal brain, providing the limitation to conventional treatment is normal tissue damage outside the high dose volume. However, demonstrating improved dose distribution in small lesions is not sufficient as proof of benefit. To accept SRT as a better treatment it is necessary to demonstrate improved tumour control and survival for the same or lower toxicity for each tumour type studied. The following discussion will review the evidence for conventional and stereotactic radiotherapy. With the currently available systems, SRT is limited to tumours less than 5 cm in diameter.

In the absence of mature data examining the role of SRT, the results of interstitial radiotherapy are used as a model for the possible effect of localised irradiation. Low dose rate brachytherapy as practised with iodine-125(^{125}I) seeds and iridium-192 (^{192}Ir) wires is equivalent to fractionated SRT rather than single fraction radiosurgery. To enable an estimate of dose fractionation regimens for fractionated SRT, Brenner et al (1991) have published guidelines for choosing appropriate doses. These are based on experimentally derived radiobiological parameters using the equivalence for early effects to 70 Gy of ^{125}I low dose rate brachytherapy. Although such information may be of help in designing new treatment protocols, only detailed documentation of the effectiveness and side-effects of fractionated SRT will provide the guidelines for future treatment.

Gliomas

High grade gliomas

The most effective component of treatment of high grade gliomas is radiation therapy (Brada 1989). The role of surgery has not been tested in randomized studies, although it is generally accepted as valuable in alleviating initial symptoms largely by relieving pressure. Adjuvant chemotherapy with nitrosoureas also prolongs survival but the magnitude of benefit is limited (Stenning et al 1987). With optimum local and systemic therapy the overall results are poor, with a median survival of 40–60 weeks and few long term survivors (Shapiro 1986).

The rationale for high dose local irradiation

such as can be achieved with stereotactic radiotherapy comes from two sources: firstly, the evidence of a dose–response relationship in the control of glioma; and, secondly, the apparent localized nature of these tumours based on the recurrence pattern of treated tumours. An improvement in median survival has been demonstrated in non-randomized studies with increasing dose from 45 to 60 Gy (Walker et al 1979) and confirmed in a Medical Research Council (MRC) study comparing 45 Gy in 20 fractions to 60 Gy in 30 fractions (Bleehen & Stenning 1991). Using conventional radiotherapy there is no evidence that increasing the dose to a large volume beyond 60 Gy improves survival any further (Chang et al 1983).

The localized nature of glial tumours is a contentious issue. Tumour cells extend beyond the putative tumour margin as defined by current visualization with CT and MRI (Daumas-Duport et al 1987, Kelly et al 1987, Burger et al 1988). However, it is a common clinical experience that the majority of tumours recur locally, in close proximity to the residual tumour or directly as the extension of a residual mass (Hochberg & Pruitt 1980, Wallner et al 1989, Laing et al 1991). Although this may reflect a statistical phenomena with recurrence at the site of highest tumour cell density, an improvement in the control of the largest tumour mass may result in prolonged tumour control and possibly survival. Despite histological evidence for the infiltrative nature of gliomas and therefore the theoretical objection to an aggressive local treatment, attempts at high dose local radiation have been made both with interstitial and stereotactic radiotherapy.

Patients with recurrent supratentorial high grade gliomas selected by tumour size and performance status have been treated in phase II studies with high doses of interstitial radiotherapy ranging from 50 to 120 Gy (Leibel et al 1989). The reported median survival (86 weeks for patients with recurrent anaplastic astrocytoma and 53 weeks in patients with glioblastoma multiforme) is the best achieved with any form of treatment for recurrent glioma and points to a potential benefit for aggressive local treatment. However, patients were highly selected and a large proportion required reoperation due to necrosis at the irradiated site. At present it is not clear if the apparent benefit of interstitial radiotherapy is the result of focal high dose irradiation, the result of additional surgical excision or simply the consequence of selection (Florell et al 1992).

Based on the same rationale, small series of patients with recurrent high grade glioma have been treated with single fraction or fractionated stereotactic radiotherapy. Early results reported in abstract form show that median survival is similar to that achieved with interstitial radiotherapy (Loeffler & Alexander III 1991). As with interstitial treatment it is not clear if the encouraging results of stereotactic radiotherapy are due to the selection of patients with favourable prognoses. At The Royal Marsden Hospital we used fractionated SRT as part of phase I/II studies in patients with recurrent high grade astrocytomas. The median survival of the first 20 patients treated on a dose escalation schedule of 5 Gy per fraction was 7 months, with doses ranging from 20 to 45 Gy to previously irradiated tumours.

High dose localized irradiation has been incorporated as a boost in the initial treatment of high grade gliomas. Comparison of patients treated with an interstitial boost with historical controls suggested a survival advantage with a 2 year survival rate of 57% (Loeffler et al 1990a). The 2 year survival results of an interstitial boost following conventional therapy reported from San Francisco were 68% for anaplastic astrocytoma and 38% for glioblastoma multiforme (Gutin et al 1991). These patients were highly selected as they represent a population which is relatively young (median age 47 years), and with good functional status (mean Karnofsky score 91%). Although the reported results are encouraging, the value of an interstitial boost will only be proved in randomized studies which are currently underway in Canada (Bernstein et al 1990) and in the USA organised by Brain Tumour Cooperative Group, BTCG.

Selected patients with high grade glioma have been treated with single fraction stereotactic radiotherapy alone with high morbidity and unsatisfactory survival results (Sturm, personal communication). A few patients have received a stereotactic radiotherapy boost as an alternative to an interstitial boost and the results of such an approach are at present not possible to evaluate.

As with interstitial radiotherapy the role of SRT boost will have to be tested in large randomized studies.

In summary, the diagnosis of high grade astrocytoma carries a poor prognosis, and this is particularly so in patients with recurrent disease. In this situation there are few treatment options and it appears that localized treatment of small tumours with SRT offers some prolongation of survival. However, it is not possible to exclude patient selection as the main determinant of favourable outcome. Further investigation of stereotactic radiotherapy in recurrent tumours should continue, ideally in the form of randomized studies to define the optimum technique for best tumour control and least morbidity. The questions of appropriate total dose, fractionation and tumour size for stereotactic radiotherapy remain to be answered. In current phase II studies at The Royal Marsden Hospital in patients with recurrent high grade tumours fractionated SRT ranged from 30–50 Gy giving 5 Gy per fraction daily. The long term toxicity is not fully defined and is likely to be considerable. Five of 7 patients receiving doses ≥ 40 Gy on top of conventional radiotherapy and surviving more than 6 monthly developed late radiation damage (Laing et al 1993).

To establish the role of stereotactic radiotherapy in the primary treatment of high grade gliomas requires a randomized study, although some information on the potential role of local radiation boost will become available from randomized studies of interstitial radiotherapy which are currently underway.

Low grade gliomas

The role of localized treatment either in the form of surgery or conventional external beam radiotherapy is as yet unproven. Conventional radiotherapy is currently under investigation in randomized studies of the European Organization for Research and Therapy of Cancer (EORTC), MRC and BTCG. Nevertheless, radiotherapy appears to be an important independent prognostic factor as shown in two retrospective studies published in the last 10 years (Laws et al 1984, Shaw et al 1989). In addition, radiotherapy offers effective palliation in expanding tumours causing symptoms.

The overall 5 and 10 year survival probability of patients with low grade glioma is 40–50% and 10–20%, respectively, and depends on age, performance status and histology. In an attempt to improve the outcome, patients have been treated with interstitial radiotherapy. The reported 5 year survival of 121 patients with grade II astrocytoma was 65% (Ostertag 1989, Ostertag & Warnke 1991) with interstitial doses of 55 Gy (range 20–90 Gy) to small tumours ranging in diameter from 0.5 to 2.5 cm (mean 1.5 cm). The results are difficult to interpret because of the selection of patients for this procedure and, overall, they are not clearly superior to those for conventional treatment. A series of 55 patients with circumscribed brain stem and midbrain gliomas have been treated with interstitial radiotherapy with a 5 year survival rate of 55 and 27% for patients treated with ^{125}I and ^{192}Ir, respectively (Mundinger et al 1991).

14 patients with low grade astrocytoma have been treated with SRT (Pozza et al 1989), given in one or two fractions. During a short follow-up, one patient died. Although the 2 year survival rate was 100%, the 3.5 year survival rate was only 50%. Souhami et al (1991) reported early results on 15 patients with brain tumours treated with fractionated SRT to a dose of 38–46 Gy at 6.3–7 Gy per fraction using a conventional stereotactic frame. Seven patients had low grade astrocytomas measuring 17–25 mm in diameter and all were alive 12–37 months after treatment. Only four tumours were radiologically smaller after SRT. The Royal Marsden Hospital experience is limited to three cases of recurrent low grade glioma following conventional surgery and radiotherapy, and all remain alive 12–36 months after treatment.

In summary, SRT remains a treatment option in tumours of appropriate size. The long term benefits of such therapy are entirely undefined and on current evidence the role of stereotactic radiotherapy in the treatment of low grade glioma is not clear.

Brain metastases

The current treatment of multiple intracranial metastases, which represent 60–70% of patients with intracranial disease, is whole brain irradiation and, in chemosensitive tumours, chemotherapy. The median survival of patients with intracranial metastases is 3–4 months, and despite effective palliation with radiotherapy a third of patients recur with disease in the brain. Solitary brain metastases are seen on CT in 30–40% of patients although on gadolinium enhanced MRI the frequency of true solitary brain metastases is lower.

Patients undergoing excision of solitary metastases before radiation have a significantly better tumour control and survival compared to patients treated with external beam radiotherapy alone (Patchell et al 1990) and the optimum treatment at present should include surgery. Despite the improvement in local control, patients with solitary metastases, particularly those with uncontrolled disease elsewhere, have a poor overall prognosis. It is reasonable to consider a non-invasive radical local treatment as an alternative to surgery. Stereotactic radiotherapy offers such a possibility and has been used either alone or with whole brain irradiation in patients with solitary metastases. The use of single fraction stereotactic radiotherapy to doses of 20–30 Gy was reported in 12 patients (Sturm et al 1987). The study demonstrated a reduction in the size of enhancing lesions and temporary tumour control. However, the survival of these patients was poor and treatment of a large lesion with a high single dose was associated with significant morbidity. 18 patients with recurrent brain metastases (21 lesions) were treated with a single fraction SRT of 9–25 Gy (Loeffler et al 1990b). Such treatment was well tolerated and provided excellent control within the radiosurgery field except for two patients where the tumour recurred in the margin. Similar data was reported by Coffey et al (1991), who treated 24 patients with solitary metastases with single fraction radiosurgery of 16–20 Gy following conventional whole brain irradiation to 30–40 Gy. Again, the control of treated metastases was excellent. However, the survival of patients in all series was poor, with the median survival ranging from 5 to 10 months, and the disease recurring either elsewhere in the brain or systemically.

At The Royal Marsden Hospital we treated 19 patients (23 lesions) with fractionated SRT as a boost following whole brain irradiation in patients with solitary brain metastases. The median survival was 17 months and the control of metastatic lesions at the irradiated site was excellent, with a median progression-free survival at the irradiated site of 15 months.

Undoubtedly, stereotactic radiotherapy offers a non-invasive and well tolerated alternative to surgery. Patients with disease of poor prognosis are spared surgical intervention. Where SRT is used without whole brain irradiation, patients may retain hair unless tumour is close to the cranium. Although the dose/fractionation parameters for stereotactic radiotherapy have not been defined, our current recommendation for the treatment of solitary (one or two) brain metastases measuring less than 4 cm in diameter is as follows. If the solitary nature is confirmed on gadolinium enhanced MRI, patients receive two fractions of 10 Gy 1 or 2 days apart enclosing the region of enhancement plus a 2 mm margin within the 90% isodose. The additional use of whole brain irradiation is optional and currently not fully defined. Future studies should assess the dose/volume dependence and fractionation of SRT, although in such poor prognosis patients a single fraction or two fractions may be sufficient. The studies of the control of solitary brain metastases should also include randomization between localized treatment alone compared to local treatment plus whole brain irradiation.

Meningiomas

The conventional treatment of meningioma is surgical resection and, following complete excision, the recurrence rate is low. In patients with residual tumour after surgery the approximate recurrence rate is 40% at 5 years (Barbaro et al 1987, Salazar 1988, Taylor et al 1988). The addition of conventional fractionated external beam radiotherapy after incomplete tumour excision improves local control (Barbaro et al 1987, Salazar 1988, Glaholm et al 1990) but it is not clear if radiotherapy as a sole or adjuvant treatment is curative.

Stereotactic radiotherapy/radiosurgery has been introduced as an alternative adjuvant treatment in patients with incompletely excised tumours, those not accessible to surgical excision, as well as in the treatment of patients who are medically unfit for surgery. 17 patients with intracranial meningioma were treated with single fraction radiosurgery (Engenhart et al 1990). Of these, 13 had had previous surgery (six had residual disease and seven recurrent tumour) and four had unresectable tumours. They received 10–50 Gy (mean 29 Gy) in a single fraction by linear accelerator to field diameters ranging from 18 to 52 mm (mean 40 mm). Four patients died 1–23 months after radiosurgery. One patient had herniation associated with shunt occlusion at 1 month after treatment and one patient developed oedema and herniation at 4 months. These are likely to represent the complication of radiosurgery. Two other patients died of unrelated causes. The remaining 13 patients were alive without tumour progression at a median follow-up of 14 months.

The early experience of 50 patients with meningioma treated with gamma unit radiosurgery was reported from Pittsburgh (Kondziolka & Lunsford 1991). Patients were selected largely by meningioma size (<5 cm in diameter). The group was heterogenous, including 36 patients who had had previous surgery, two patients with unresectable disease, four previously irradiated and 16 apparently unbiopsied tumours. The actuarial 2 year control rate was 96% following doses of 10–25 Gy (mean 17 Gy). The results are difficult to evaluate. In an indolent disease such as meningioma it is difficult to accept 2 year progression-free survival of this heterogenous group of patients as proof of effectiveness of therapy.

The reported studies also demonstrate the difficulty of selecting the appropriate dose for single fraction treatment. Large doses were shown to cause morbidity and mortality (Engenhart et al 1990) and doses below the radiation tolerance of normal brain used in proximity to critical structures (Kondziolka et al 1991) are of uncertain effectiveness. It is possible that fractionated stereotactic radiotherapy may offer a better therapeutic window than single fraction treatment but there are no studies examining this issue.

Stereotactic radiotherapy has entered neurosurgical thinking as an effective treatment modality for meningiomas. There is insufficient evidence to support this view. Although there is a clear need for improvements in the treatment of incompletely excised meningiomas, it is debatable whether a single fraction of stereotactic radiotherapy/radiosurgery provides the most appropriate approach. In addition, tumours are rarely within the size range suitable for stereotactic radiotherapy. To evaluate the role of stereotactic radiotherapy it is necessary to define selection criteria and compare the results of conventional treatment, including fractionated radiotherapy, with SRT. The feasibility of SRT based on tumour size is not a sufficient reason for the use of this technique, particularly with single fraction treatment, and at present it cannot be considered as a proven alternative to surgery.

Following the failure of conventional treatment with surgery and radiotherapy, stereotactic radiotherapy remains a treatment option in lesions of an appropriate size, providing further excision is not possible. However, this approach needs full evaluation and the effectiveness of SRT in this situation is also not defined.

Acoustic neuromas

Acoustic neuromas are benign tumours with an indolent natural history. Untreated tumours may be observed over years and up to 40% remain unchanged in size. In approximately half the cases the tumours slowly enlarge, with a 1–2 mm increase in diameter per year (Bederson et al 1991). A small proportion of tumours rapidly increase in size and require urgent treatment but the majority may be safely observed with interval scans. Surgical resection is the primary treatment of acoustic neuroma and complete excision is curative. The procedure is not without surgical complications and almost invariably results in hearing loss and, frequently, facial weakness.

Radiosurgery was developed as a non-invasive alternative to surgery. 91 unilateral tumours were treated at the Karolinska Institute with the gamma knife. On CT, 49% became smaller, 42% were unchanged in size and 5% progressed at an unspecified time after therapy (Leksell 1987). Of 40 patients treated in Pittsburgh, 55% of tumours were smaller, 43% were unchanged and 2% progressed at 1 year (Flickinger et al 1991). There are no long term actuarial progression-free survival figures available for radiosurgery. Stereotactic radiotherapy is also not without complications. It produces hearing loss with more frequent deficit in larger tumours (Hirsch & Noren 1988).

Acoustic neuromas are indolent tumours. Left untreated they may remain unchanged for many years, particularly if small. It is therefore difficult to assess the efficacy of radiosurgery, particularly if patients are selected by tumour size alone. Radiosurgery may find a role in the treatment of acoustic neuromas. It may avoid the complications of surgery but is not without morbidity as it frequently causes a gradual hearing loss and the long term effectiveness is at present not fully defined.

Pituitary tumours

The current results of conservative surgery and radiotherapy in pituitary adenomas are excellent with a 90–95% 10 year and 85–90% 20 year tumour control rate (Flickinger et al 1989, Grigsby et al 1989). The 10 and 20 year progression-free survival of a cohort of 411 patients treated at The Royal Marsden Hospital was 94 and 88%, respectively (Brada et al 1992). The complications of conventional treatment include surgical morbidity and mortality and the late effects of irradiation. Radiation damage to the pituitary gland may cause late pituitary failure. Visual impairment due to radiation damage to the optic nerve and chiasma is less than 1% and is usually caused by incorrect technique or fractionation. Pituitary irradiation carries a risk of a second brain tumour, which is 1.3% at 10 years and 1.9% at 20 years (Brada et al 1992). This is a 10-fold increase in risk compared to the normal population.

It is difficult to see how stereotactic radiotherapy, particularly using unconventional fractionation, could improve such results. Unconventional fractionation may increase the toxicity to the optic pathway and the long term tumour control with large single doses is also not known. A reduction in the volume of normal brain irradiated may reduce the risk of second tumours, but a reduction of such a low risk event would be almost impossible to prove. Avoiding irradiation of the hypothalamus may reduce the incidence of pituitary failure. Although individual patients have been treated with stereotactic radiotherapy there are no studies available assessing the efficacy and toxicity of radiosurgery in non-secreting pituitary adenomas.

The results of conventional radiotherapy in acromegaly and pituitary Cushing's disease uncontrolled with surgery and medical treatment are not satisfactory. Although hormonal control can be achieved there is a considerable delay in the normalization of hormone levels (Feek et al 1984, Ciccarelli et al 1988). Focal irradiation has been practised in the form of proton beam therapy. 435 patients with acromegaly without suprasellar or parasellar extension were treated (Kliman et al 1987). Approximately 30% achieved remission (growth hormone <5 ng/ml) at 2 years and 50% at 5 years. The median fall in growth hormone was 40% in 1 year. Eight patients (1.7%) experienced partial visual impairment of whom two lost vision in both eyes. Two patients were reported to develop sarcoma. Although the reported rate of pituitary deficiency was lower than that for conventional therapy, it was not shown in actuarial terms and it is not clear if the risk increases with time. Although more patients reach normal growth hormone levels earlier than following conventional radiotherapy such results are dependent on pretreatment growth hormone levels and there is no published data demonstrating a faster decline in individual growth hormone level with proton treatment.

Patients with pituitary Cushing's disease have been treated with radiosurgery and protons, but it is difficult to prove that the results are superior to conventional treatment. 53 adults with Cushing's disease were treated with radiosurgery at The Karolinska Hospital (Degerblad et al 1986). Radiosurgery was delivered with the gamma unit to the centre of the pituitary using single doses of 70–100 Gy. Only 29 patients were followed and of these 14 (48%) achieved normalization of urinary cortisol levels after the first treatment. Following a second dose of radiosurgery, four of 11 patients (36%) achieved remission. Some patients had three or four treatments and a similar proportion reached remission. In total, 22 of 26 patients reached normal urine cortisol levels. The remission rate is similar to other techniques of irradiation and was not without toxicity. Of 22 patients in remission, 12 had pituitary insufficiency (Degerblad et al 1986).

Proton beam therapy was used to treat 145 patients with Cushing's disease to doses of 120–140 Gy (Kjellberg et al 1984). The actuarial remission rate (measured by diurnal cortisol and 24 hour urine-free cortisol) was 55% at 2 years and 80% at 5 years. Further surgery was required in 11 patients and the ophthalmological complication rate was low. Although the reported number of cases requiring hormone replacement was low this was not quoted in actuarial terms. One patient developed glioblastoma, suggesting that highly localized irradiation does not entirely avoid the risk of a second malignancy (see above). Overall, it is not clear if high dose proton beam therapy is superior to conventional treatment.

In summary, there is currently no justification for single fraction SRT/radiosurgery in the initial treatment of non-secreting pituitary adenomas. So far no clear benefit has been demonstrated for localized irradiation in the treatment of acromegaly or Cushing's disease. However, conventional methods, even though effective, are not ideal and SRT technology continues to evolve. It is likely that in the future the combination of high precision stereotactic localization, delivery, conformal therapy and fractionation will be utilized to treat pituitary adenomas with greater accuracy and potentially lower toxicity.

The treatment options in patients with recurrent pituitary adenomas are limited, particularly if surgery is considered hazardous. Stereotactic radiotherapy may be used in particular as a high precision technique which may avoid re-irradiating sensitive structures such as the optic pathway, although in many cases tumours lie in close proximity to the chiasma. The appropriate dose and fractionation for SRT of previously irradiated recurrent adenomas are not defined. Based on the experienced of proton therapy in previously irradiated patients the toxicity of SRT in this situation is likely to be considerable.

Other Tumours

Stereotactic radiotherapy has been used in other tumour types and the criteria has largely been the tumour size. Casentini et al (1990) reported the treatment of pineal tumours with single fraction SRT in addition to whole brain radiotherapy. Pineal germinomas are highly radiosensitive as well as chemosensitive, and localized treatment with SRT therefore will show responses. However, pineal germinomas are curable with conventional radiotherapy using relatively low dose fractionated treatment with a near 100% tumour control rate (Dearnaley et al 1990). They are also locally invasive and have a propensity for dissemination through the cerebrospinal fluid (CSF) (Brada and Rajan 1990). It is not clear what potential benefit single fraction SRT provides over conventional radiotherapy.

The future direction in the treatment of pineal germinoma is to reduce the radiotherapy dose and, if possible, substitute radiation, at least in part, with chemotherapy. This would avoid some of the late effects of cranial irradiation. Wide field craniospinal irradiation in patients at risk from CSF seeding is unlikely to be superseded by localized irradiation unless chemotherapeutic agents effectively enter the CSF space.

Cranial non-seminomatous germ cell tumours are incurable with conventional radiotherapy (Dearnaley et al 1990). As with teratomas of primary testicular origin there may be residual masses remaining after successful chemotherapy. SRT may have a role in controlling these masses as an alternative to potentially hazardous surgical excision.

Clivus tumours (chordoma/chondrosarcoma) are poorly controlled with conventional treatment, including surgery and conventional radiotherapy. Major advances in neurosurgery with skull base approaches have improved resection rates although tumour masses often remain; these may be amenable to treatment with SRT providing they are small and not invading the brain stem. The results of this treatment are not as yet reported, but skull base tumours have been treated using proton therapy, with results apparently superior to conventional treatment (Austin-Seymour et al 1989). However, patients may have been selected for proton therapy on the basis of tumour size, which is an independent prognostic factor for survival, and have received higher tumour doses (mean 69 cobalt Gy equivalent). It is not clear whether the results of proton beam therapy are the result of patient selection, higher radiation dose or more effective localized irradiation. In addition, there are many sensitive structures within the irradiated region and proton therapy has not been without toxicity.

Although the results of treatment in patients with medulloblastoma have improved, 30–40% of patients fail, and the majority do so at the primary site in the posterior fossa (Evans et al 1990, Jenkin et al 1990, Tait et al 1990). Conventional treatment includes surgery followed by craniospinal irradiation and a boost to the posterior fossa. A stereotactically guided localized boost of radiation away from sensitive structures in the brain stem may further improve the local control of incompletely excised tumours beyond that achieved with adjuvant chemotherapy. Such an approach is at present theoretical but medulloblastoma is a highly radiosensitive and frequently radiocurable tumour. A higher dose of irradiation may truly improve disease control and survival.

SRT may also be of value in patients with locally recurrent medulloblastoma who are rarely salvaged with other forms of therapy. Three patients treated with fractionated SRT at the Royal Marsden Hospital achieved local control but 2 subsequently recurred at adjacent or distant sites. The long term benefits of SRT and the potential toxicity are not defined.

Craniopharyngiomas have been treated with radiosurgery. They are indolent tumours and, following conservative surgery and conventional fractionated external beam radiotherapy, the 10 year progression-free survival is of the order of 70–80% with little morbidity. Craniopharyngiomas are frequently large and closely associated with sensitive structures such as the optic chiasma and hypothalamus. Large single fractions of radiosurgery, although potentially effective, may carry higher morbidity and should be employed with caution. In patients with good long term prognosis radiosurgery has little proven benefit over conventional irradiation and on present evidence its use is not encouraged.

CONCLUSION

Stereotactic external beam radiotherapy is a new and exciting technologically advanced form of radiotherapy. It offers superior dose distribution in the treatment of small lesions compared to conventional irradiation. Its relative simplicity is open to widespread use in many radiotherapy centres equipped with modern linear accelerators. The only proven role of SRT is in the treatment of small inoperable AVMs. They are relatively uncommon and the application of radiosurgery requires a very high precision technique, a high standard of quality control and extensive neurosurgical, neuroradiological and radiosurgical expertise. The treatment of AVMs should therefore be carried out only in specialized centres.

There is growing pressure to use stereotactic radiotherapy as a new and promising treatment for brain tumours. It is at present an unproven and entirely experimental mode of therapy with major limitations, particularly in terms of the size of tumours suitable for treatment.

Present and future application of SRT should not be guided simply by tumour size. The treatment is not without side-effects and despite its image as an advanced technology it should be applied only in situations where it is likely to result in better tumour control, survival and reduced toxicity in comparison with standard treatments. Although there is potential for benefit in a number of small tumours listed above, it cannot at present be recommended as the initial treatment of choice in any tumour. In addition, its use should be discouraged in the treatment of unbiopsed brain lesions and as the major form of treatment of pineal germinomas.

The technology of SRT is evolving. With advances in conformal therapy using dynamic multileaf collimators it may be possible to treat non-spherical volumes and larger lesions. The high precision tumour localization and treatment delivery will have a major impact on standard radiotherapy. It is likely that the relocatable techniques of immobilization and the methods of planning using a stereotactic system of coordinates will be introduced into conventional therapy. The separation of stereotactic and conventional external beam radiotherapy is likely to become a semantic point of the past.

REFERENCES

Austin-Seymour M, Munzenrider J, Goitein M et al 1989 Fractionated proton radiation therapy of chordoma and low-grade chondrosarcoma of the base of the skull. Journal of Neurosurgery 70: 13–17

Barbaro N M, Gutin P H, Wilson C B, Sheline G E, Boldrey E B, Wara W M 1987 Radiation therapy in the treatment of partially resected meningiomas. Neurosurgery 20(4): 525–528

Bederson J, von Ammon K, Wichmann W, Yasargil M 1991 Conservative treatment of patients with acoustic tumors. Neurosurgery 28: 646–651

Berg N O, Lindgren M 1963 Relation between field size and tolerance of rabbit's brain to roentgen irradiation (200 kV) via a slit-shaped field. Acta Radiologica 1: 147–168

Bernstein M, Laperriere N, Leung P, McKenzie S 1990 Interstitial brachytherapy for malignant brain tumours: preliminary results. Neurosurgery 26: 371–380

Bleehen N M, Stenning S P 1991 A Medical Research Council trial of two radiotherapy doses in the treatment of grades 3 and 4 astrocytoma. British Journal of Cancer 64: 769–774

Bova F J, Friedman W A 1991 Stereotactic angiography: an inadequate database for radiosurgery? International Journal of Radiation, Oncology, Biology, Physics 20(4): 891–895

Brada M 1989 Back to the future — radiotherapy in high grade gliomas. British Journal of Cancer 60: 1–4

Brada M, Rajan B 1990 Spinal seeding in cranial germinoma. British Journal of Cancer 61: 339–340

Brada M, Ford D, Ashley S et al 1992 Risk of second brain tumour following conservative surgery and radiotherapy of pituitary adenoma. British Medical Journal 304: 1343–1346

Bradshaw J D 1986 The stereotactic radiosurgery unit in Sheffield. Clinical Radiology 37(3): 277–279

Brenner D J, Martel M K, Hall E J 1991 Fractionated regimens for stereotactic radiotherapy of recurrent tumors in the brain. International Journal of Radiation, Oncology, Biology, Physics 21(3): 819–824

Burger P, Heinz E, Shibata T, Kleihues P 1988 Topographic anatomy and CT correlations in the untreated glioblastoma multiforme. Journal of Neurosurgery 68: 698

Casentini L, Colombo F, Pozza F, Benedetti A 1990 Combined radiosurgery and external radiotherapy of intracranial germinomas. Surgical Neurology 34: 79–86

Chang C H, Horton J, Schoenfeld D et al 1983 Comparison of postoperative radiotherapy and combined postoperative radiotherapy and chemotherapy in the multidisciplinary management of malignant gliomas. Cancer 52: 997–1007

Ciccarelli E, Corsello S, Plowman P, Besser G, Wass J 1988 Prolonged lowering of growth hormone after radiotherapy in acromegalic patients followed for over 15 years. Advances in Biosciences 69: 269–272

Coffey R J, Flickinger J C, Bissonette D J, Lunsford L D 1991 Radiosurgery for solitary brain metastases using the cobalt-60 gamma unit: methods and results in 24 patients. International Journal of Radiation, Oncology, Biology, Physics 20(6): 1287–1295

Colombo F, Benedetti A, Pozza F, Marchetti C, Chierego G 1989 Linear accelerator radiosurgery of cerebral arteriovenous malformations. Neurosurgery 24(6): 833–840

Daumas-Duport C, Scheithauer B W, Kelly P J 1987 A histologic and cytologic method for the spatial definition of gliomas. Mayo Clinic Proceedings 62: 435–449

Dearnaley D A, Hern R, Whittaker S, Bloom H 1990 Pineal and CNS germ cell tumours: Royal Marsden Hospital experience 1962–1987. International Journal of Radiation, Oncology, Biology, Physics 18: 773–781

Degerblad M, Rahn T, Bergstrand G, Thoren M 1986 Long-term results of stereotactic radiosurgery to the pituitary gland in Cushing's disease. Acta Endocrinologica (Copenhagen) 112(3): 310–314

Engenhart R, Kimmig B N, Hover K H et al 1990 Stereotactic single high dose radiation therapy of benign intracranial meningiomas. International Journal of Radiation Oncology, Biology, Physics 19(4): 1021–1026

Evans A, Jenkin D, Sposto R et al 1990 Results of a prospective randomised trial of radiation therapy with and without CCNU, vincristine and prednisone. Journal of Neurosurgery 72: 572–582

Feek C M, McLelland J, Seth J et al 1984 How effective is external pituitary irradiation for growth hormone-secreting pituitary tumours? Clinical Endocrinology 20: 401–408

Flickinger J C, Nelson P B, Martinez A J, Deutsch M, Taylor F 1989 Radiotherapy of nonfunctional adenomas of the pituitary gland. Cancer 63: 2409–2414

Flickinger J C, Maitz A, Kalend A, Lunsford L D, Wu A 1990 Treatment volume shaping with selective beam blocking using the Leksell gamma unit. International Journal of Radiation, Oncology, Biology, Physics 19(3): 783–789

Flickinger J C, Lunsford L D, Coffey R J et al 1991 Radiosurgery of acoustic neurinomas. Cancer 67(2): 345–353

Florell R C, Macdonald D R, Irish W D et al 1992 Selection bias, survival and brachytherapy for glioma. Journal of Neurosurgery 76: 179–183

Gill S S, Thomas D G, Warrington A P, Brada M 1991 Relocatable frame for stereotactic external beam radiotherapy. International Journal of Radiation, Oncology, Biology, Physics 20(3): 599–603

Glaholm J, Bloom H J G, Crow J H 1990 The role of radiotherapy in the management of intracranial meningiomas: The Royal Marsden Hospital experience with 186 patients. International Journal of Radiation, Oncology, Biology, Physics 18: 755–761

Graham J D, Warrington A P, Gill S S, Brada M 1991a A non-invasive relocatable stereotactic frame for fractionated radiotherapy and multiple imaging. Radiotherapy Oncology 21(1): 60–62

Graham J D, Nahum A E, Brada M 1991b A comparison of techniques for stereotactic radiotherapy by linear accelerator based on 3-dimentional dose distributions. Radiotherapy Oncology 22: 29–35

Grigsby P W, Simpson J R, Emami B N, Fineberg B B, Schwartz H G 1989 Prognostic factors and results of surgery and postoperative irradiation in the management of pituitary adenomas. International Journal of Radiation, Oncology, Biology, Physics 16: 1411–1417

Gutin P H, Prados M D, Phillips T L et al 1991 External irradiation followed by an interstitial high activity iodine-125 implant "boost" in the initial treatment of malignant gliomas: NCOG Study 6G82-2. International Journal of Radiation, Oncology, Biology, Physics 21(3): 601–606

Halperin E C, Bentel G, Heinz E R, Burger P C 1989 Radiation therapy treatment planning in supratentorial glioblastoma multiforme: an analysis based on post mortem topographic anatomy with CT correlations. International Journal of Radiation, Oncology, Biology, Physics 17: 1347–1350

Hariz M I, Henriksson R, Lofroth P O, Laitinen L V, Saterborg N E 1990 A non-invasive method for fractionated stereotactic irradiation of brain tumours with a linear accelerator. Radiotherapy Oncology 17(57): 57–72

Hirsch A, Noren G 1988 Audiological findings after stereotactic radiosurgery in acoustic neurinomas. Acta Otolaryngologica (Stockholm) 106(3–4): 244–251

Hochberg F, Pruitt A 1980 Assumptions in the radiotherapy of glioblastoma. Neurology 30: 907

Hopewell J W, Morris A D, Dixon B A 1987 The influence of field size on the late tolerance of rat spinal cord to single doses of X-rays. British Journal of Radiology 60(11): 1099–1108

Houdek P V, Schwade J G, Landy H, Serago C F, Pisciotta V 1990 Computer controlled stereotaxic radiotherapy. International Journal of Radiation, Oncology, Biology, Physics 19(suppl 1): 135 (abstract)

Jenkin D, Goddard K, Armstrong D et al 1990 Posterior fossa medulloblastoma in childhood: treatment results and a proposal for a new staging system. International Journal of Radiation, Oncology, Biology, Physics 19: 265–274

Jones D, Christopherson D, Haferman M D, Rieke J, Travaglini J, Vermeulen S 1990 Experience with a technique for fractionated radiosurgery. International Journal of Radiation, Oncology, Biology, Physics 19(suppl 1): 134

Kelly P J, Daumas-Duport C, Scheithauer B W, Kispert D B 1987 Stereotactic histologic correlations of computed tomography- and magnetic resonance imaging-defined abnormalities in patients with glial neoplasms. Mayo Clinic Proceedings 62: 450–459

Kjellberg R N 1979 Isoeffective dose parameters for brain necrosis in relation to proton radiosurgical dosimetry. In: Szigla G. (ed) Stereotactic cerebral irradiation. Elsevier, Amsterdam, pp 157–166

Kjellberg R N, Hanamura T, Davis K R, Lyons S L, Adams R D 1983 Bragg-peak proton-beam therapy for arteriovenous malformations of the brain. New England Journal of Medicine 309(5): 269–274

Kjellberg R, Kliman B, Swisher B, Butler W 1984 Proton beam therapy of Cushing's disease and Nelson's syndrome. In: Black P M (ed) Secretory tumours of the pituitary gland. Raven Press, New York, pp 295–307

Kliman B, Kjellberg R, Swisher B, Butler W 1987 Long-term effects of proton beam therapy for acromegaly. In: Robbins M (ed) Acromegaly: a century of scientific and clinical progress. Plenum Press, New York, pp 221–228

Kondziolka D, Lunsford L D 1991 Stereotactic radiosurgery for squamous cell carcinoma of the nasopharynx. Laryngoscope 101(5): 519–522

Kondziolka D, Lunsford L D, Coffey R J, Flickinger J C 1991 Stereotactic radiosurgery of meningiomas. Journal of Neurosurgery 74(4): 552–559

Laing R, Graham J, Warrington A, Brada M 1993 Efficacy and toxicity of fractionated stereotactic radiotherapy in the treatment of recurrent gliomas (phase I & II study). Radiotherapy and Oncology (in press)

Lampert P W, Davis R L 1964 Delayed effects of radiation on the human central nervous system. "Early" and "late" delayed reactions. Neurology 14: 912–917

Laws E, Taylor W, Clifton M, Okazaki H 1984 Neurosurgical management of low-grade astrocytoma of the cerebral hemispheres. Journal of Neurosurgery 61: 665–673

Leibel S, Gutin P, Wara W et al 1989 Survival and quality of life after interstitial implantation of removable high-activity iodine-125 sources for the treatment of patients with recurrent malignant gliomas. International Journal of Radiation, Oncology, Biology, Physics 17: 1129–1139

Leksell L 1951 The stereotaxic method and radiosurgery of the brain. Acta Chirurgica Scandinavica 102: 316–319

Leksell L 1983 Stereotactic radiosurgery. Journal of Neurology, Neurosurgery and Psychiatry 46(9): 797–803

Leksell D G 1987 Stereotactic radiosurgery — present status and future trends. Neurology Research 9: 60–68

Loeffler J, Alexander E III 1991 Stereotactic radiosurgery for malignant gliomas. Second International Neuro-oncology Conference, London

Loeffler J, Alexander E III, Wen P et al 1990a Results of stereotactic brachytherapy used in the initial management of patients with glioblastoma. Journal of the National Cancer Institute 82(24): 1918–1921

Loeffler J S, Kooy H M, Wen P Y et al 1990b The treatment of recurrent brain metastases with stereotactic radiosurgery. Journal of Clinical Oncology 8(4): 576–582

Lutz W, Winston K R, Maleki N 1988 A system for stereotactic radiosurgery with a linear accelerator. International Journal of Radiation, Oncology, Biology, Physics 14(2): 373–381

Marks L B, Spencer D P 1991 The influence of volume on the tolerance of the brain to radiosurgery. Journal of Neurosurgery 75: 177–180

Mundinger F, Braus D F, Krauss J K, Birg W 1991 Long-term outcome of 89 low-grade brain-stem gliomas after interstitial radiation therapy. Journal of Neurosurgery 75: 740–746

Nedzi L A, Kooy H, Alexander E III, Gelman R S, Loeffler J S 1991 Variables associated with the development of complications from radiosurgery of intracranial tumours. International Journal of Radiation, Oncology, Biology, Physics 21(3): 591–599

Ostertag C 1989 Stereotactic interstitial radiotherapy for brain tumours. Journal of Neurological Sciences 33: 83–89

Ostertag C, Warnke P 1991 Interstitial radiotherapy for brain tumours. British Journal of Neurosurgery 5: 421–436 (Second International Neuro-oncology Conference abstract)

Patchell R, Tibbs P, Walsh J et al 1990 A randomised trial of surgery in the treatment of single metastases to the brain. New England Journal of Medicine 322(8): 494–500

Peters T M, Clark J, Pike B, Drangova M, Olivier A 1987 Stereotactic surgical planning with magnetic resonance imaging, digital subtraction angiography and computed tomography. Applied Neurophysiology 50(1–6): 33–38

Phillips M H, Frankel K A, Lyman J T, Fabrikant J I, Levy R P 1990 Comparison of different radiation types and irradiation geometries in stereotactic radiosurgery. International Journal of Radiation, Oncology, Biology, Physics 18(1): 211–220

Pozza F, Colombo F, Chierego G et al 1989 Low-grade astrocytomas: treatment with unconventionally fractionated external beam stereotactic radiation therapy. Radiology 171(2): 565–569

Salazar O M 1988 Ensuring local control in meningiomas. International Journal of Radiation, Oncology, Biology, Physics 15: 501–504

Schad L R, Boesecke R, Schlegel W et al 1987 Three dimensional image correlation of CT, MR, and PET studies in radiotherapy treatment planning of brain tumors. Journal of Computer Assisted Tomography 11(6): 948–954

Serago C F, Lewin A A, Houdek P V et al 1991 Stereotactic target point verification of an X ray and CT localizer. International Journal of Radiation, Oncology, Biology, Physics 20(3): 517–523

Shapiro W R 1986 Therapy of adult malignant brain tumours: what have the clinical trials taught us? Seminars in Oncology 13: 38

Shaw E, Daumas-Duport C, Scheithauer B et al 1989 Radiation therapy in the management of low-grade supratentorial astrocytomas. Journal of Neurosurgery 70: 853–861

Sheline G E, Wara W M, Smith V 1980 Therapeutic irradiation and brain injury. International Journal of Radiation, Oncology, Biology, Physics 6: 1215–1228

Souhami L, Olivier A, Podgorsak E B, Pla M, Pike G B 1990 Radiosurgery of cerebral arteriovenous malformations with the dynamic stereotactic irradiation. International Journal of Radiation, Oncology, Biology, Physics 19(3): 775–782

Souhami L, Olivier A, Podgorsak E B, Villenmure J G, Pla M, Sadikot A F 1991 Fractionated stereotactic radiation therapy for intracranial tumors. Cancer 68: 2101–2108

Stenning S, Freedman L, Bleehen N 1987 An overview of published results from randomized studies of nitrosoureas in primary high grade malignant glioma. British Journal of Cancer 56: 89

Sturm V, Kober B, Höver K et al 1987 Stereotactic percutaneous single dose irradiation of brain metastases with a linear accelerator. International Journal of Radiation, Oncology, Biology, Physics 13: 279–282

Tait D, Thornton-Jones H, Bloom H, Lemerle J, Morris-Jones P 1990 Adjuvant chemotherapy for medulloblastoma: the first multi-centre control trial of the International Society of Paediatric Oncology (SIOP I). European Journal of Cancer 26(4): 464–469

Taylor W B J, Marcus R B J, Friedman W A, Ballinger W E J, Million R R 1988 The meningioma controversy: postoperative radiation therapy. International Journal of Radiation, Oncology, Biology, Physics 15: 299–304

Thomson E S 1990 Stereotactic multiple arc radiotherapy. PhD, University of London

Tsai J S, Buck B A, Svensson G K et al 1991 Quality assurance in stereotactic radiosurgery using a standard linear accelerator. International Journal of Radiation, Oncology, Biology, Physics 21(3): 737–748

van der Kogel A J 1987 Effect of volume and localization on rat spinal cord tolerance (abstract). In: Fielden J F F E M, Hendry J H, Scott D (eds) Proceedings of the 8th International Congress of Radiation Research. Taylor and Francis, London, p 352

Walker M D, Strike T A, Sheline G E 1979 An analysis of dose-effect relationship in the radiotherapy of malignant gliomas. International Journal of Radiation, Oncology, Biology, Physics 5: 1725

Wallner K E, Galicich J H, Krol G, Arbit E, Malkin M G 1989 Patterns of failure following treatment for glioblastoma multiforme and anaplastic astrocytoma. International Journal of Radiation, Oncology, Biology, Physics 16: 1405–1409

Wu A, Lindner G, Maitz A H, Kalend A M, Lunsford L D, Flickinger J C, Bloomer W D 1990 Physics of the gamma knife approach on convergent beams in stereotactic radiosurgery. International Journal of Radiation, Oncology, Biology, Physics 18: 941–949

11. Gamma knife radiosurgery for brain tumours

L. D. Lunsford D. Kondziolka

INTRODUCTION

During the last decade, advanced neuroimaging techniques such as computerized tomography (CT) and magnetic resonance imaging (MRI) were incorporated into the diagnostic neurosurgical armamentarium. Low risk graphic brain imaging, recently supplemented by neurophysiological evoked potential studies, has facilitated earlier recognition and precise definition of brain tumours. The widespread use of stereotactic surgery followed the pairing of stereotactic technology and imaging. Although stereotactic surgery had its origins in the 1950s and 1960s as a *therapeutic* modality (for functional neurosurgery), in the 1980s it attained general use as a *diagnostic* technique (CT guided stereotactic biopsy). In the 1990s therapeutic stereotactic surgery again will be used for many purposes, including cyst or abscess drainage, interstitial or intracavitary irradiation, guidance for microsurgical resection during craniotomy, functional neurosurgery and, especially, radiosurgery.

Stereotactic radiosurgery is the closed skull destruction of a precisely defined intracranial target using ionizing beams of radiation, delivered during a single treatment session. To precisely define the intracranial tumour for treatment, neuroimaging is used to visualize the normal and abnormal anatomy. Leksell initiated the radiosurgical technique in 1951 by coupling an orthovoltage X-ray tube to a stereotactic guiding device (Leksell 1951). For the next 25 years, the use of stereotactic radiosurgery was dependent upon whether the tumour could be defined with either angiography, encephalography or skull roentgenography. Although first used to create lesions in normal brain targets for functional neurosurgery, subsequently radiosurgery was used most often to treat mass lesions localized by angiography (e.g. arteriovenous malformations (AVMs) or by contrast cisternography (e.g. a tumour near the skull base) Leksell 1983). Imaging was unsatisfactory for the radiosurgical treatment of most intra-axial lesions. Stereotactic CT and MRI overcame these inadequacies by providing high resolution information on the shape, volume and location of brain tumours.

In this chapter, we discuss the indications for our techniques, and the results of treatment in 278 patients with benign and malignant brain tumours using gamma knife radiosurgery. During this initial 3 year experience, 268 patients with cerebral vascular malformations were also treated (Fig. 11.1) (Kondziolka et al 1990, Lunsford et al 1990a).

STEREOTACTIC RADIOSURGERY TECHNIQUE

General considerations

Either photons or charged particle irradiation can be used to provide focal single session destruction of an intracranial target using stereotactic guidance. Currently, two methods are available for the delivery of photon irradiation. The gamma unit consists of a permanent 18 000 kg shield surrounding a primary hemispheric array of 201 sources of cobalt-60 (Lunsford et al 1989). The central beam of radiation is fixed at an angle of 55° to

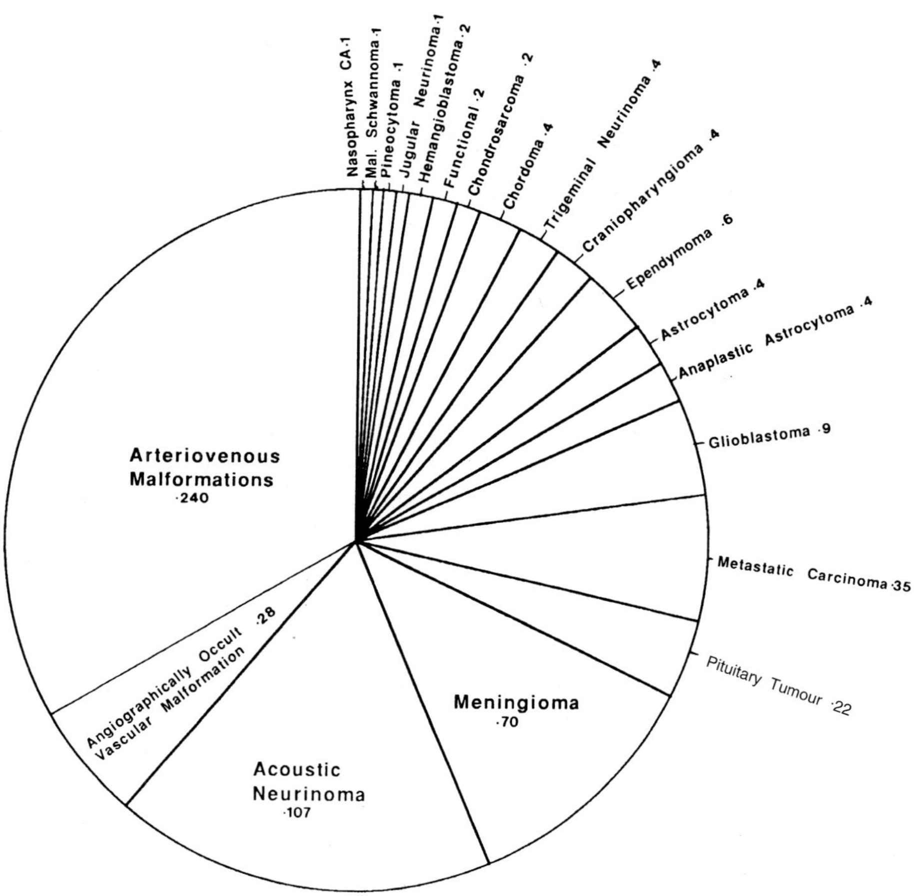

Fig. 11.1 Distribution of diagnoses in the first 546 patients treated with gamma knife radiosurgery at the University of Pittsburgh.

the horizontal plane, with the other beams arranged in an arc, all reaching a focal point 403 mm from the sources. A secondary collimator helmet with beam channel diameters of 4, 8, 14 or 18 mm is used to vary the volume of prescribed radiation. The stereotactic frame, firmly attached to the patient's head, is suspended within the secondary collimator helmet to ensure that the centre of the radiation volume (the target isocentre) is held at the focal point of the 201 cobalt sources. The second system for photon irradiation uses a modification of a standard linear accelerator (linac) (Colombo et al 1985, Hartmann et al 1985, Podgorsak et al 1988, Winston & Lutz 1988, Friedman & Bova 1989). A cyclotron is necessary to accelerate heavy charged particles towards an intracranial target with steep radiation fall-off. The Bragg peak of protons, helium ions or carbon ions can be used to provide focal radiation (Fabrikant et al 1984, Kjellberg & Abe 1988, Steinberg et al 1990). Because of the high initial cost and the need for a large physical plant, this technique is available at only a limited number of centres (Levy et al 1990).

At the University of Pittsburgh

At our institution, gamma knife radiosurgery in adult patients is performed under local anaesthesia supplemented with mild intravenous sedation. Children under the age of 14 years are treated under general endotracheal anaesthesia. After applying the stereotactic coordinate frame to the patient's head, the intracranial mass that will be treated is imaged by cerebral angiography,

CT or MRI. We use these images to determine the rectilinear (x, y and z) stereotactic coordinates of the irradiation target. For brain tumours, CT is most often used; MRI is performed to obtain coordinates for tumours poorly delineated by CT scans or coronal plane images of pituitary tumours. Along with the stereotactic coordinates of the target, determination of the γ angle (angle of beam incidence) and an estimation of the patient's head configuration are necessary to begin computer dose planning. Two or three dimensional multiplanar isodose plots are integrated with the intraoperative images. The goal of treatment dose planning is to enclose the lesion margin as closely as possible within the 50% isodose line or greater in order to maintain a steep fall-off of the radiation dose beyond the lesion margin (Fig. 11.2) (Wu et al 1990). After determination of the appropriate number of isocentres required for treatment, the tumour dose is selected jointly by the neurosurgeon and radiation oncologist.

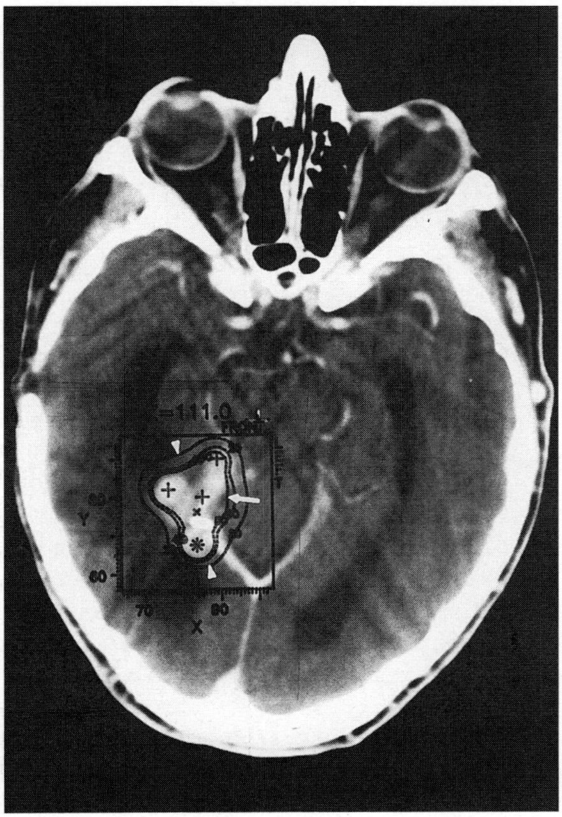

Fig. 11.2 Irregular isodose configuration constructed by combining multiple isocentres to treat a recurrent tentorial meningioma in a 72-year-old woman (contrast enhanced CT scan). The 50% isodose line at the tumour margin is identified by an arrow; the 20% line is identified by arrowheads.

Treatment planning can take as little as 20 minutes for simple tumours, but can extend to several hours for tumours of a complicated shape. The total treatment time within the gamma unit varies and is related to the dose and the strength of the cobalt sources. The entire procedure, from application to removal of the stereotactic frame, takes from 2 to 5 hours. We usually treat two patients per day. A therapeutic level of anticonvulsant medication is obtained in all patients with lobar or subcortical lesions. After radiosurgery, patients receive a single 40 mg dose of methylprednisolone, and those at risk from seizures also receive a single intravenous dose of phenobarbital (90 mg). Patients are discharged from the hospital the day after treatment.

Dose selection is one part of the 'art' of radiosurgery. The selection of the dose depends on the tumour pathology, location and size, as well as prior therapy. To help choose radiosurgical doses for our first patients with brain tumours, we used an integrated logistic formula, originally developed for the treatment of AVMs (Flickinger 1989). This formula predicts the dose likely to be associated with an approximate 3% risk of permanent delayed radiation-induced complications, a risk believed to be tolerable. Location of the tumour in a critical part of the brain (e.g. the cavernous sinus or adjacent to the brain stem) did not in itself lead to a reduction in the radiosurgical dose.

For parasellar or suprasellar tumours, the tumour margin must be at least 4 mm from the optic chiasma. We believe that the optic apparatus is especially radiosensitive and thus limits the dose received by the optic chiasma to 8 Gy. For example, if the dose to the optic chiasma must be 8 Gy or less (at the 20% isodose line), then the corresponding maximum tumour dose must be limited to 40 Gy.

We recommend that patients have follow-up clinical and imaging examinations at 3 and 6 months after radiosurgery and then at intervals of 6 months thereafter. Contrast enhanced MRI or CT scans are used to monitor tumour size and to detect possible complications.

RADIOSURGERY FOR BENIGN TUMOURS

Acoustic tumours

Microsurgical removal remains the standard treatment for healthy patients with unilateral acoustic nerve sheath tumours. However, alternatives to conventional surgery may be important to consider for patients who have tumours on the side of their only ear with hearing, for elderly patients or for those whose medical problems make microsurgery unacceptably dangerous. In such patients, stereotactic radiosurgery of small to moderately sized acoustic tumours offers an important treatment option.

The goal of radiosurgery in the treatment of acoustic tumours is to arrest growth, preserve cranial nerve function and prevent further neurological deficits. Whereas microsurgery enables tumour removal in many patients, only recently have attempts at preserving facial and even auditory function been possible. Furthermore, though microsurgical techniques have reduced the incidence of early postoperative meningitis, cerebrospinal fluid leakage, and stroke, such complications never occur after radiosurgery. In order to define the efficacy of radiosurgery in arresting tumour growth and maintaining cranial nerve function, we reviewed our experience in the radiosurgical treatment of 107 patients with acoustic tumours. Over a 3 year interval, more than 300 patients with newly diagnosed or recurrent acoustic tumours were referred to our centre for consideration of radiosurgery. We recommended radiosurgery when one or more of the following criteria existed: (1) the patient had significant concomitant medical illness; (2) the patient was elderly; (3) the tumour was recurrent after microsurgery; (4) the tumour was on the side of the patient's only ear with hearing; (5) the patient had bilateral acoustic tumours with at least unilateral hearing preservation; (6) the patient refused surgical removal. Young, healthy patients were advised that microsurgery was the current standard treatment. All patients accepted for treatment underwent preradiosurgical high resolution CT or MRI scans, audiometry, brain stem evoked response testing, and facial electromyography.

The 107 treated patients varied in age from 14 to 83 years (mean 55 years). 15 patients (14%) had bilateral tumours in the setting of neurofibromatosis (type II). Microsurgery had been performed at least once in 25 patients (23%); six patients had had 'gross total removal' and 19 'subtotal resections'. Clinical symptoms included hearing loss (95%), imbalance or ataxia (63%), tinnitus (36%), facial weakness (24%) and facial sensory loss (27%).

In virtually all patients, the irregular shape of the tumours required the use of multiple isocentres of irradiation (range 2–7). At least one isocentre was placed in the extracanalicular portion of the tumour and one was placed in the intracanalicular portion. Tumour volumes varied from 225 to 28 000 mm^3 (mean 6110 mm^3). To maintain a sharp fall-off in the specified radiation dose, the 50% or greater isodose line was used to encircle the tumour margin in 93% of patients (Fig. 11.3). The mean dose delivered to the centre of the tumour was 34.6 Gy (range 24.3–50 Gy); the dose to the tumour margin varied from 13.6 Gy to 20 Gy (mean 17.8 Gy).

Tumour response

Serial imaging studies in 86 patients showed that loss of central tumour contrast enhancement (compatible with central necrosis) often occurred between 6 and 12 months after treatment (Fig. 11.4). In the total series (including patients with less than 1 year follow-up), 57% showed no further tumour growth, 42% showed tumour reduction; only one patient had delayed tumour growth. Of 40 patients who had a minimum of 1 year follow-up, central necrosis was seen in 25 (63%) and some degree of tumour shrinkage in 22 (55%) (Fig. 11.5). It is important to note that tumour shrinkage was not often dramatic, usually amounting to a reduction of a few millimetres in the average tumour diameter. Peritumoural

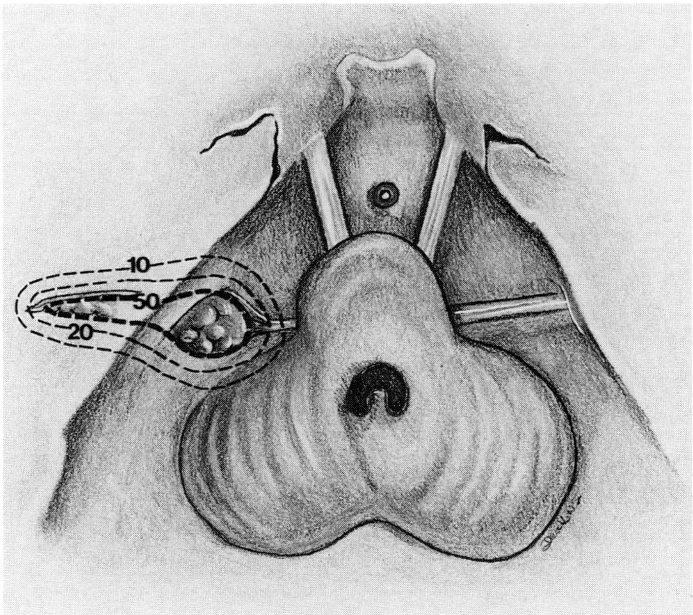

a

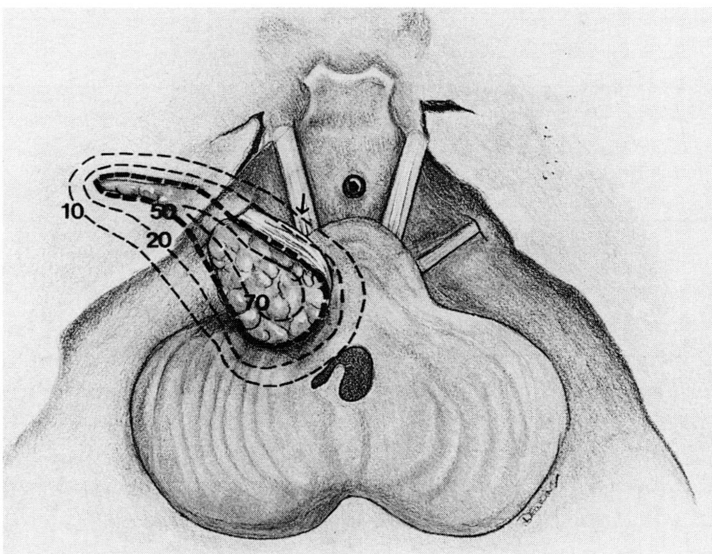

b

Fig. 11.3 Isodose plans to treat **a** a small and **b** a large acoustic neurinoma. Multiple isocentres of irradiation are used to cover both the intracanalicular and extracanalicular portions of the tumour margin within the 50% isodose line. In the large tumour, radiation (at a low isodose) reaches the trigeminal nerve (arrow).

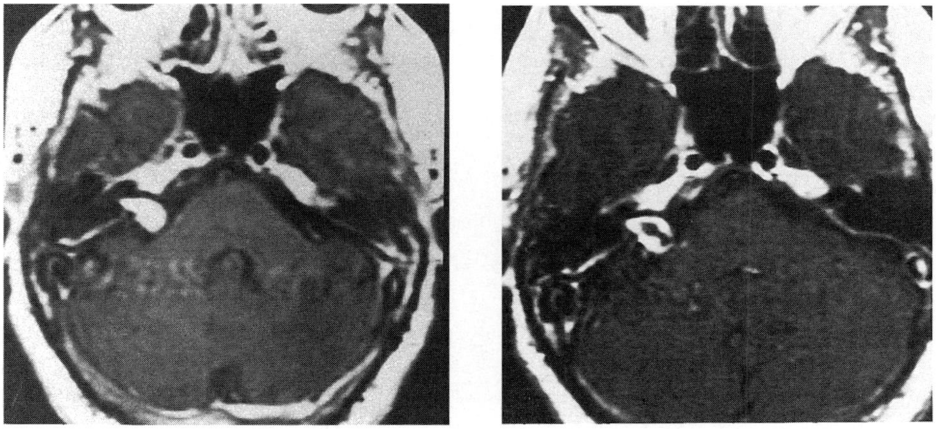

a b

Fig. 11.4 MRI scans (T_1 spin-echo with gadopentetic acid Gd-DTPA) of an acoustic neurinoma. **a** Before radiosurgery. **b** Although the tumour had not changed in size 6 months after radiosurgery, there was loss of central contrast enhancement.

(cerebellar or cerebellar peduncle) imaging changes (compatible with radiation induced oedema) were observed in two patients, as represented by either increased signal changes on T_2 weighted MRI or low attenuation changes on CT images.

The radiobiological effect by which radiosurgery arrests tumour growth is probably related to direct tumour cytotoxicity followed by delayed vascular obliteration (Thompson et al 1990). Relatively high rates of central tumour necrosis and delayed shrinkage indicate that the effect of radiosurgery on benign tumours is considerable (Linskey et al 1990). In contrast, tumour necrosis is an uncommon finding after conventional fractionated external beam radiation therapy. We believe that total necrosis of the entire tumour is not necessary to control tumour

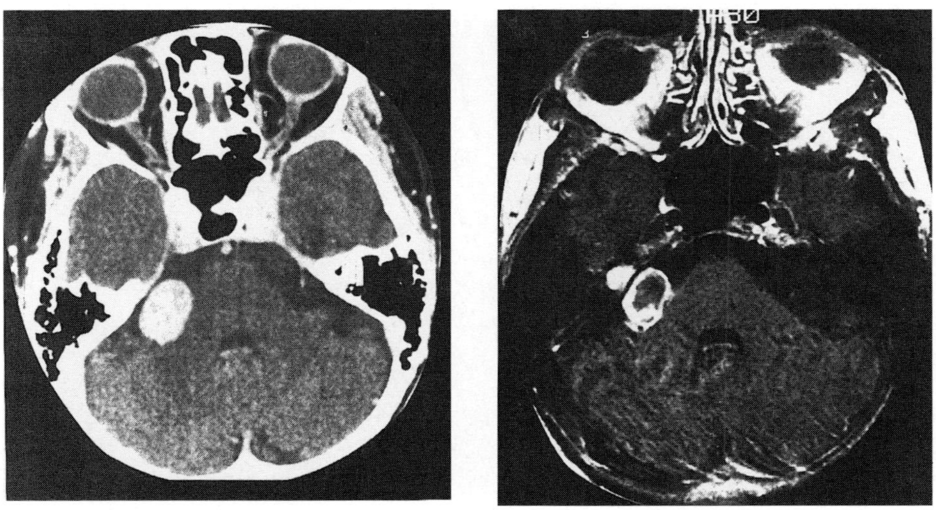

a b

Fig. 11.5 Axial images of a large acoustic tumour in a 73-year-old woman. **a** Before radiosurgery (CT scan with contrast). **b** 1 year after radiosurgery; the contrast enhanced MRI scan shows marked loss of central contrast enhancement, indicating tumour necrosis.

progression. The radiobiological mechanisms for prolonged growth inhibition remain to be understood.

Cranial nerve preservation

Audiometric findings were evaluable in 68 patients using the Gardner–Robertson classification system (Gardner & Robertson 1988). In 15 patients who had useful hearing preoperatively (22%; Gardner–Robertson class I or II), the actuarial 1 year rate of useful hearing preservation was 46%. Hearing improved significantly in only two patients, from class III to class I in one of them, and from class III to class II in the second. Loss of hearing was significantly associated with average tumour diameter ($p = 0.04$). No new hearing loss developed after radiosurgery in any of seven patients with an average tumour diameter less than 10 mm. Interestingly, we found no significant relationship between the treatment dose or the marginal tumour isodose and the subsequent development of hearing loss (Kondziolka et al 1990).

Using the House–Brackmann scale (House & Brackmann 1985) we evaluated facial nerve function in the first 85 patients treated. A new facial paresis developed during follow-up in 14 of 65 patients, with normal function preoperatively. The median time of facial neuropathy onset was 6 months after radiosurgery. By the end of our current follow-up period, only two patients had new permanent facial palsies; both were caused by a loss of facial nerve continuity after these patients underwent delayed microsurgery at other institutions. The actuarial risk of developing a previously undetected facial neuropathy (House–Brackmann grades II–VI) was 33% at 1 and 2 years. We evaluated seven patients 1–10 months after their postradiosurgical facial neuropathy began to improve and found that function had returned to pretreatment levels in four patients. The median time from the beginning of improvement in facial function to complete recovery was 8 months. Hirsch and Noren reported 'recovery' in all patients who had delayed onset of facial weakness after stereotactic radiosurgery (Noren et al 1983, Hirsch & Noren 1988). In our own series, additional follow-up will be necessary to confirm whether satisfactory recovery of facial neuropathy occurs in all patients. No new facial neuropathy developed after radiosurgery in any of the seven patients whose average tumour diameter was less than 10 mm. No significant relationship could be detected between the treatment dose or isodose and the subsequent development of facial neuropathy.

Incomplete neuropathy of the trigeminal nerve resulted in 12 of 42 patients who had normal preoperative facial sensation. The median onset of sensory loss was 7 months after treatment. The actuarial risk of developing a new trigeminal neuropathy was 37% at both 1 and 2 years. Trigeminal neuropathy began to improve 1–17 months after onset, and at 17 months the projected improvement rate was 100%. As with seventh and eighth nerve deficits, fifth nerve deficits did not develop in patients whose tumour diameter was less than 10 mm and did not correlate with dose or isodose.

The incidence of facial or trigeminal neuropathy in our series was higher than that reported by Hirsch and Noren. This discrepancy in part may be related to our treatment of tumours substantially larger than previously treated at the Stockholm gamma unit. At the end of our first year's experience, we reduced our minimum marginal tumour dose from 20 Gy to a dose usually varying between 16 and 18 Gy in an attempt to reduce complications. To date, we have found no relationship between the dose delivered and the risk of a new cranial neuropathy. Lowering the treatment dose neither decreased the risk of developing delayed cranial neuropathies nor changed the tumour control rate. Additional clinical and radiobiological data is necessary to assess the lowest effective and maximally tolerable doses.

Patients with neurofibromatosis type II continue to present a special challenge. Our current policy with such patients who have bilateral acoustic tumours is the following: (1) staged microsurgical resection is recommended if both tumours are large and hearing is absent; (2) if hearing is functional, both microsurgery and radiosurgery are withheld until hearing deteriorates. Radiosurgery can be offered as a treatment alternative if the

tumour is small (< 25–30 mm in greatest diameter).

Radiosurgery has proved to be a safe and effective treatment alternative for carefully selected patients with acoustic tumours. Its attractive features include the absence of major perioperative risks, the rapid return of patients to their preoperative level of function, a 30–70% reduction in the cost of the procedure as compared to microsurgery, a high tumour growth control rate, and an acceptable rate of delayed complications, most of which are reversible.

Meningiomas

Meningiomas are potentially ideal tumours for stereotactic radiosurgery. They are usually well demarcated and rarely invade brain; thus, the steep radiation fall-off achieved by radiosurgery can be directed at the tumour margin. Meningiomas are easily visible on MRI or CT scans used for targeting and dose planning, and now can be recognized even when small (< 30 mm in diameter). They are usually slow growing, allowing time for the radiation induced obliterative effect to develop. Because their blood supply arises from the dura (which can be included within an optimal isodose) the tumour blood supply can be obliterated. Whereas open microsurgical resection of some skull base meningiomas can carry a high risk for the development of new neurological deficits, radiosurgery can reduce these risks. Finally, radiosurgery under local anaesthesia eliminates the surgical and anaesthetic risks associated with craniotomy, which is especially important for elderly or medically infirm patients (Kondziolka et al 1990).

Despite these potential advantages, for *most* patients surgical removal is the ideal goal. Long term disease free survival can be achieved after surgical resection of the tumour and its dural base (Simpson 1957, Adegbite et al 1983). Although most meningiomas can be resected with low morbidity and mortality, the morbidity rate after resection of basal meningiomas continues to be high (Mayberg and Symon 1986, Guidetti et al 1988, Samii et al 1989, Sekhar et al 1989). During the CT era, mortality after meningioma surgery (in any brain location) in elderly patients has varied from 8 to 23% (Papo 1983, Djindjian et al 1988, Awad et al 1989). Despite advances in microsurgical techniques, tumour recurrence after surgery can be a problem. After documented tumour recurrence, some surgeons advocate clinical observation and serial imaging studies, reserving repeat surgery for when tumour growth becomes symptomatic. Others advocate fractionated external beam radiation therapy, while recognizing that its role remains controversial (Wara et al 1975, Carella et al 1982, Petty et al 1985, Barbaro et al 1987, Taylor et al 1988). Stereotactic radiosurgery can be offered as a primary or adjuvant treatment for selected high risk meningioma patients.

We used radiosurgery to treat 70 patients with meningiomas (50 women, 20 men, aged 14–82 years) during our first 3 years' experience. Patients were accepted for treatment only if the lesion was less than 35 mm in average diameter. Radiosurgery was not recommended if the tumour was amenable to open surgical resection with acceptable risk or was within 4 mm of the optic chiasma (Kondziolka et al 1991). As a result, no convexity meningiomas were treated with radiosurgery. Contrast enhanced CT or MRI revealed a well demarcated dural based or intraventricular tumour in all patients; 87% of patients had basal meningiomas, and 69% had undergone at least one prior surgical procedure.

The radiation dose was selected on the basis of tumour location and volume. The presence of adjacent major intracranial vessels, cranial nerves or brain stem structures usually restricted the peripheral treatment dose to 18 Gy or less. We limited the dose received by the optic nerve and chiasma to 8 Gy or less (Fig. 11.6), which correspondingly limited the dose to the tumour margin. All patients received what was anticipated to be a therapeutic radiation dose. Dose per volume estimates were based on the integrated logistic formula as described above. The radiosurgical dose thus calculated was reduced further if the patient had received prior external beam radiation therapy ($n = 4$).

Multiple isocentres of irradiation were necessary in 58 patients to create irregular isodose configurations that closely corresponded to the

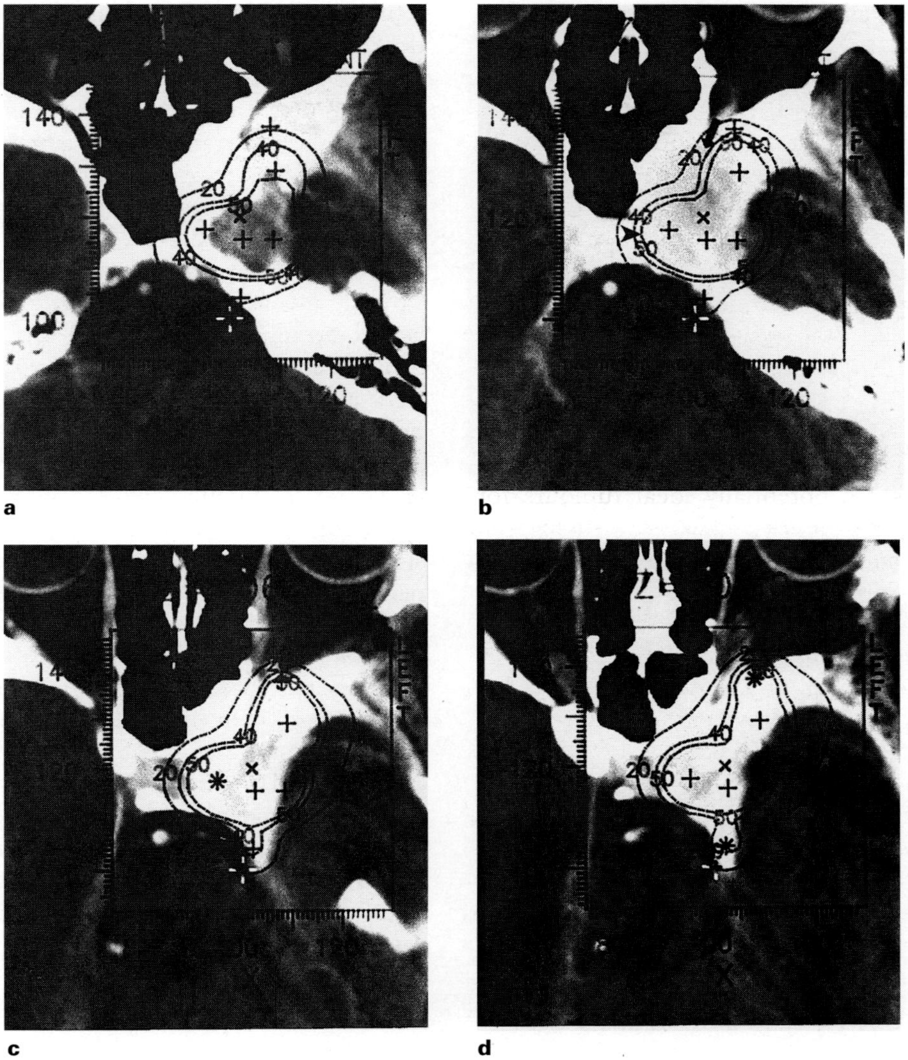

Fig. 11.6 Consecutive 3 mm thick axial contrast enhanced CT images showing the isodose plan for a left cavernous sinus meningioma. A dose of 16 Gy was delivered to the 50% isodose line (arrowhead) using six isocentres of irradiation. The optic nerve was contained within the 20% isodose line (arrow) and received a dose of 6.4 Gy (see **b**).

tumour volumes (Flickinger et al 1990a). An irregular tumour contour was almost the rule if a previous resection had been performed. Dose plans were especially difficult to devise for cavernous sinus or parasellar tumours because of their tendency to extend into multiple intracranial and extracranial compartments; however, multiple isocentres succeeded in providing satisfactory isodose configurations for these. The presence of major vessels (e.g. the internal carotid or anterior cerebral arteries) within the tumour did not cause us to limit the radiosurgical dose below an anticipated therapeutic level.

The radiosurgical treatment of basal meningiomas (or any basal lesion) currently has its inferior limit at the foramen magnum. The stereotactic frame must be applied as low as possible on the head to place the target near the

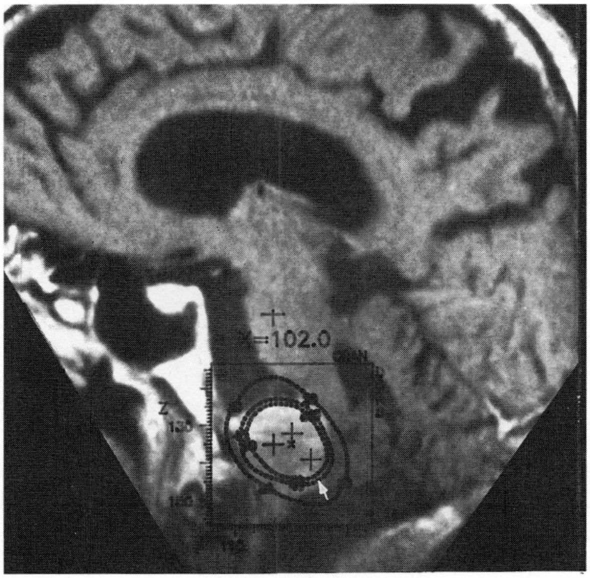

Fig. 11.7 Sagittal MRI scan (T_1 spin-echo with Gd-DTPA) of a large recurrent foramen magnum meningioma in an 82-year-old man. This tumour was treated with 14 Gy to the 40% isodose line using three isocentres of irradiation delivered with the 18 mm collimator.

centre of the collimator helmet (Kondziolka & Lunsford 1991). Although this posed only minor technical problems for patients with anterior foramen magnum meningiomas (Fig. 11.7), we were unable to treat patients with tumour extension into the upper cervical spinal canal.

We evaluated CT or MRI scans performed 4–34 months after treatment in the first 61 patients. The actuarial 2 year tumour control rate was 96%. Among 25 patients who had imaging studies 12–34 months after treatment, tumours appeared smaller in 13 (52%) (Fig. 11.8). Loss of central contrast enhancement (an imaging finding we believe consistent with intratumoural necrosis) was noted in nine patients and was related to the occurrence of subsequent tumour shrinkage ($p <$ than 0.001). In nine patients, we saw no change in tumour size; and in two patients tumour had grown outside the radiosurgical treatment volume. Large size and lack of well demarcated borders (resulting in suboptimal treatment) was responsible for treatment failure in two patients who had delayed tumour growth. One of these patients had a malignant torcular meningioma treated by radiosurgery after three operations and conventional radiation therapy.

Clinical evaluation 12–34 months after treatment in 30 patients found that 22 remained clinically stable and five improved. Of the 40 patients examined 3–12 months after treatment, 36 were in a stable condition and two were improved. Two patients died in the course of follow-up. The first was a 64-year-old woman who

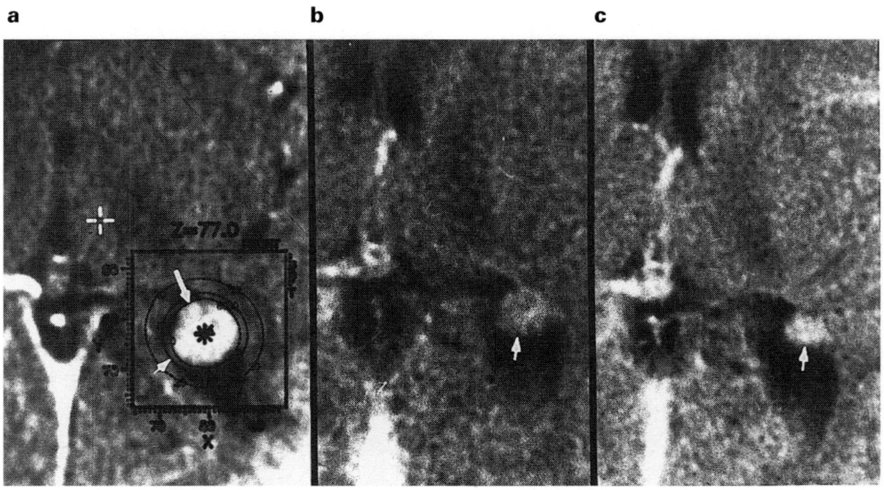

Fig. 11.8 Serial contrast enhanced CT images in a 14-year-old boy with an intraventricular meningioma, recurrent after two craniotomies. **a** At radiosurgery the 13 mm tumour was treated with 25 Gy to the 80% isodose margin (large arrow); the 50% line is identified by the small arrow. **b** 4 months after treatment the tumour measured 10 mm in diameter. **c** By 9 months after radiosurgery the diameter had further decreased to 8 mm.

had growth from a cavernous sinus tumour 1 year after radiosurgery; she suffered a seizure and died of respiratory complications. The second patient was a 71-year-old man who died of unrelated glomerulonephritis 6 months after radiosurgery of a posterior clinoid region meningioma.

No immediate postoperative complications or perioperative seizures occurred. Temporary new neurological deficits were seen in three patients who had petrous apex meningiomas.

Contralateral weakness occurred in two of them (both at 12 months after treatment), and the other developed a third nerve palsy 3.5 months after treatment. All three were given a brief course of oral corticosteroid therapy and subsequently improved. Although the pathological nature of these complications is not known, we speculate that radiation induced axonal swelling, demyelination or small vessel infarction, alone or in combination, may have played significant roles.

In contrast to our experience with acoustic tumours, where approximately 30% of patients had a new transient postoperative facial or trigeminal neuropathy, we detected no new neuropathy or worsening of any pre-existing cranial neuropathy in 59 of 61 patients (97%) with basal meningiomas. None of the 24 patients with cavernous sinus tumours acquired a new cranial neuropathy after treatment. The reasons for this are as yet unclear, although we suspect that motor cranial nerves are more tolerant than sensory cranial nerves, which in turn are more tolerant than special sensory nerves.

Further follow-up is necessary to evaluate the benefits of radiosurgery in long-term control of meningiomas. To date, encouraging results have been seen in carefully selected patients with small meningiomas in high risk locations.

Pituitary adenomas

The use of pharmacological agents, surgery, radiation or a combination of these is required for successful management of pituitary tumours (Baskin et al 1982, Boggan et al 1983). We consider radiosurgery to be an adjuvant treatment for pituitary adenomas recurrent or residual after surgical resection and a primary treatment for patients whose advanced age or medical condition militates against surgery. In contrast to the treatment of acoustic tumours and meningiomas, conventional fractionated radiation therapy has proven valuable in the treatment of pituitary tumours (Eastman et al 1979, Flickinger et al 1989). The total fractionated dose is limited by the amount of radiation that can be delivered safely to critical structures such as the adjacent optic nerves and hypothalamus.

The initial radiosurgical efforts in the treatment of pituitary tumours began in the 1950s with the use of charged particles. Linfoot & Lawrence (1985) reported on 781 patients who received charged particle single fraction irradiation to the pituitary gland. Kjellberg and coworkers subsequently described the Bragg peak stereotactic proton irradiation of 1125 pituitary adenomas (Kjellberg & Abe 1988). Their series included patients with acromegaly, Cushing's disease, Nelson's syndrome, prolactinoma, thyrotrophin secreting adenomas and non-functioning adenomas. In most of the patients with acromegaly, they found that clinical features and elevated growth hormone levels began to abate 3–6 months after treatment. However, normalization of growth hormone levels occurred slowly; at 2 years 28% of patients had attained levels less than 5 ng/ml, and at 5 years 75% of patients had reached this level. Of the patients with Cushing's disease, 55% had no adrenocortical production of hormone 2 years after treatment. This rate improved to 80% at 5 years and 90% at 20 years. They noted a 10% rate of delayed hypopituitarism and a 13% incidence of delayed visual field disturbances.

The results of gamma knife radiosurgery at the Karolinska Institute in Stockholm have been reported for patients with Cushing's disease (Degerblad et al 1986, Rahn & Thoren 1988). Normalization of urinary cortisol levels was seen in more than 75% of patients within the first 3 years after treatment. In most of these patients, multiple radiosurgical procedures were required to achieve eventual disease control. Pituitary insufficiency developed in 55% of patients.

At the University of Pittsburgh, we performed radiosurgery in 22 patients with pituitary adenomas. Transsphenoidal or transcranial tumour resection had been performed previously in 20 patients. Nine of the 13 patients with microadenomas underwent follow-up imaging studies (mean time 17 months). Tumour sizes were smaller in four patients, no tumour growth was seen in three patients, and two had tumour growth. Of the nine patients with macroadenomas, eight had imaging follow-up (mean time 18 months). Five had smaller tumours, and three had no change.

Hormonal hypersecretion was present in 14 patients (eight with acromegaly and six with Cushing's disease). No patient had a prolactinoma. Evaluation of growth hormone levels in four acromegalic patients showed that levels had fallen to 2 ng/ml in one patient, to 7 ng/ml in another and from 150 to a range of 30–100 ng/ml in the third; levels in the fourth patient remained unchanged at the last follow-up. The other four patients with acromegaly were treated too recently to have been studied. In five patients with Cushing's disease, three had continued elevation of cortisol levels and two had normalization with clinical improvement (mean follow-up 14 months). Because of persistent cortisol hypersecretion, surgical resection was repeated 14 months after radiosurgery in one patient, and at 27 months in another. Eight patients with non-secreting pituitary tumours developed pituitary insufficiency during follow-up, extending to 32 months. The maximum doses used in all patients with pituitary tumours ranged from 28 to 60 Gy, the mean being 40 Gy.

Early radiosurgical efforts at other centres in treating pituitary adenomas were directed towards ablation of the sellar contents. In this era of high resolution imaging, we believe that the tumour alone, if possible, should be identified and treated. Proper selection of radiosurgical candidates with pituitary tumours depends on such imaging studies. First, the tumour must be distinct from the gland, a feature best demonstrated by contrast enhanced coronal MRI. Coronal images also provide important information on the relationship of the tumour to the optic nerves and chiasma; treatment is prohibited if the tumour–chiasma distance is less than 5 mm (Fig. 11.9). Selective radiation beam blocking permits the lower isodoses to be moved away from the optic

a b

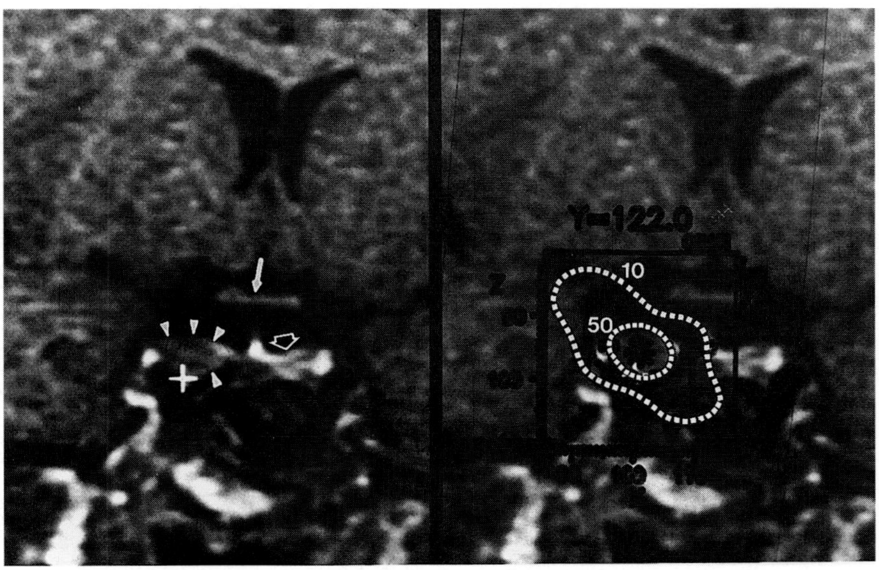

Fig. 11.9 Treatment planning for a pituitary microadenoma. Coronal contrast enhanced MRI scans show **a** the tumour (arrowheads) and **b** the isodose configuration for radiosurgery using one isocentre of irradiation with the 8 mm collimator. Selective beams were blocked to move the lower isodose lines (10% line, identified) away from the optic chiasma (white arrow) and pituitary gland (open arrow).

apparatus (Flickinger et al 1990b). Lateral tumour invasion of the cavernous sinus is not a contraindication to radiosurgery.

The availability of successful medical treatment has virtually eliminated the use of radiosurgery for prolactinomas. The role of radiosurgery is more important in Cushing's disease, because the rate of hormonal relapse can be high after microsurgery (Friedman et al 1989). We are currently considering multiple radiosurgical treatments in patients with Cushing's disease who have persistent cortisol hypersecretion 12–24 months after radiosurgery. Taking greater advantage of modern imaging tools, we hope ultimately to control hormonal hypersecretion and to avoid the high incidence of delayed pituitary insufficiency reported by Rahn and colleagues (Rahn & Thoren 1988). Radiosurgery seems best reserved for the adjuvant treatment of residual or recurrent pituitary tumours after failed microsurgery or as a primary treatment for small tumours in elderly or medically infirm patients.

Other benign tumours

We have also used radiosurgery to treat patients with other types of benign intracranial tumours. The solid portion of a craniopharyngioma was treated in three patients who had recurrent tumours after resection or fractionated radiotherapy. One patient underwent two separate radiosurgical procedures for recurrent craniopharyngiomas in different locations. Her residual tumour in the posterior third ventricle regressed 1 year after treatment (Fig. 11.10). A separate regrowth in the sella subsequently was treated and was slightly smaller 10 months later.

Two patients with haemangioblastomas (cerebellar hemisphere and foramen magnum) and four patients with trigeminal nerve sheath tumours were treated. We also treated one patient with a pineocytoma and another with a nerve sheath tumour of the jugular foramen. The value of radiosurgery for treating pineal region tumours was emphasized initially by Backlund et al (1974). Astrocytomas will be discussed in the next section under the heading of 'Glial tumours'.

RADIOSURGERY FOR MALIGNANT TUMOURS

Solitary brain metastases

Because radiosurgery had proved valuable for the treatment of circumscribed benign brain

a b

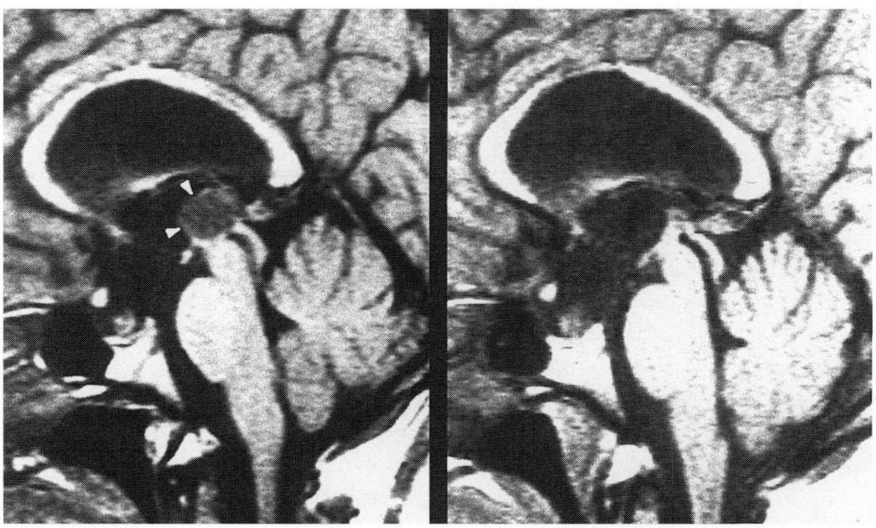

Fig. 11.10 Sagittal MRI scans (T_1 spin-echo with Gd-DTPA) **a** before and **b** 12 months after radiosurgery of a residual posterior third ventricular craniopharyngioma (arrowheads) in an 11-year-old girl.

tumours, we anticipated that small solitary brain metastases (that appear to be well circumscribed on CT or MRI scans) might also respond favourably. Based on the hypothesis that stereotactic radiosurgery could replace the benefit provided by surgical resection for solitary brain metastases, we began a phase I/II trial of 'boost radiosurgery' in 1987 (Lunsford et al 1990a). For this purpose, radiosurgery is used to enhance, not replace, fractionated radiotherapy. Due to the possibility of microscopic metastases in other brain locations not revealed by neuroimaging studies and the risk of local tumour infiltration beyond the contrast enhanced imaging margin, fractionated whole brain irradiation remains necessary (Coffey et al 1991).

Modern neuroimaging techniques enable the earlier detection of metastatic brain tumours, including those diagnosed as part of tumour staging examinations in asymptomatic patients. However, despite earlier diagnosis and a variety of treatment options, results have not improved significantly (Black 1979, Madajewicz et al 1984, Mandell et al 1986). The median survival in patients with untreated metastatic brain cancer is approximately 1 month. The best treatment results to date were demonstrated by a recent randomized study that compared surgical excision plus radiotherapy with radiotherapy alone; this study found increased survival and improved quality of life with the combined treatment (Patchell et al 1990). However, with almost all types of metastatic tumours, median survival remains under 1 year.

We have used stereotactic radiosurgery to treat selected small (< 3 cm), solitary metastatic tumours. Our goal was to equal the rate of tumour control provided by surgical excision. Radiosurgery would then obviate the need for craniotomy, reduce the length and cost of hospitalization, and lessen the potential morbidity associated with surgical resection (Sturm et al 1987, Lindquist 1989). The first 35 such patients we treated had the following primary tumours: malignant melanoma (n = 13), non-small cell lung carcinoma (n = 7), renal cell carcinoma (n = 5), breast carcinoma (n = 3), colorectal carcinoma (n = 1), choriocarcinoma (n = 1), oropharyngeal carcinoma (n = 1), lymphoma (n = 1) and adenocarcinoma of unknown origin (n = 3). 34 patients received 16–20 Gy to the tumour margin as a radiosurgical 'boost' to 30–43 Gy whole brain fractionated radiotherapy. One patient refused conventional radiotherapy and was treated with radiosurgery alone.

The majority of patients improved clinically after radiosurgery, usually in association with CT or MRI evidence of a reduction in the amount of cerebral oedema surrounding the tumour (Fig. 11.11). Patient demise was related uniformly to systemic disease progression or to the development of distant brain metastases. Two patients developed growth of the treated tumour and had surgical resection; these patients were alive at 4 and 12 months after radiosurgery. For the entire series, the mean survival after metastatic brain tumour diagnosis was 9.2 months (after utilization of combined treatments). Mean survival after radiosurgery was 6.2 months, at which time 15 patients were still living. Analysis by histological type found that mean survival after diagnosis of metastasis was longest in the seven patients with lung carcinoma (12 months; range 1–30 months); the five patients with renal cell carcinoma had a mean survival of 9.3 months (range 0.25–18 months); and the 13 patients with metastatic melanoma 8.2 months (range 3–20 months).

Post-treatment imaging studies performed 6 months or more after treatment were evaluable in 19 patients. A reduction in tumour size was demonstrated in 13 (68%) of these patients, three of whose tumours had disappeared completely (Fig. 11.12). The other six patients had no change in tumour size. One patient had a haemorrhage into a tumour cyst 6 months after treatment and required craniotomy.

Loeffler and coworkers (1990) reported results in 18 patients with 21 recurrent brain metastases treated by linac radiosurgery. All patients had previously received conventional radiotherapy to total doses of 30 - 49 Gy. Local tumour control was achieved within the prescribed radiation field in every patient, but two tumours recurred at the treatment margin. As in our series, most patients showed evidence of clinical improvement, often accompanied by a reduction in the amount of surrounding cerebral oedema. Engenhart reported

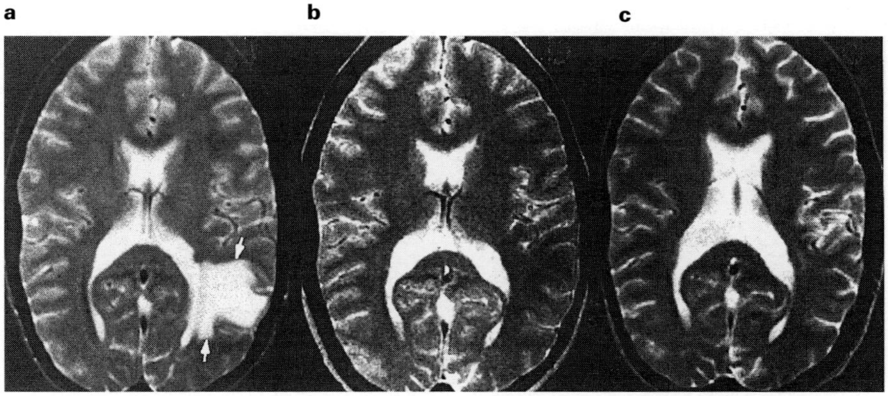

Fig. 11.11 Serial MRI scans (T_2 spin-echo) of a metastatic melanoma in the left parietal lobe **a** before, **b** 4 months after and **c** 7 months after radiosurgery. The peritumoural oedema (arrows) before treatment resolved after radiosurgery.

the Heidelberg experience with linac radiosurgery in 37 patients (Engenhart et al 1989). Symptomatic improvement was seen in 84% of patients after treatment. Although median survival in this series was only 5 months, their report covered a mean follow-up of only 6.8 months. 28 patients died of systemic disease, and two died from progression of the treated tumour. This may have been because only nine patients in their series received external beam radiotherapy in addition to radiosurgery.

Radiosurgery offers two attractive features for the treatment of solitary brain metastases. First, because stereotactic technique is used, the problem of locating subcortical or deep, small tumours during craniotomy is avoided. Second, radiosurgery offers potential treatment to patients with tumours in locations associated with a high risk of neurological deficit after conventional surgery (Coffey et al 1991). It is unlikely that the three brain stem tumours in our series would have been amenable to conventional resection.

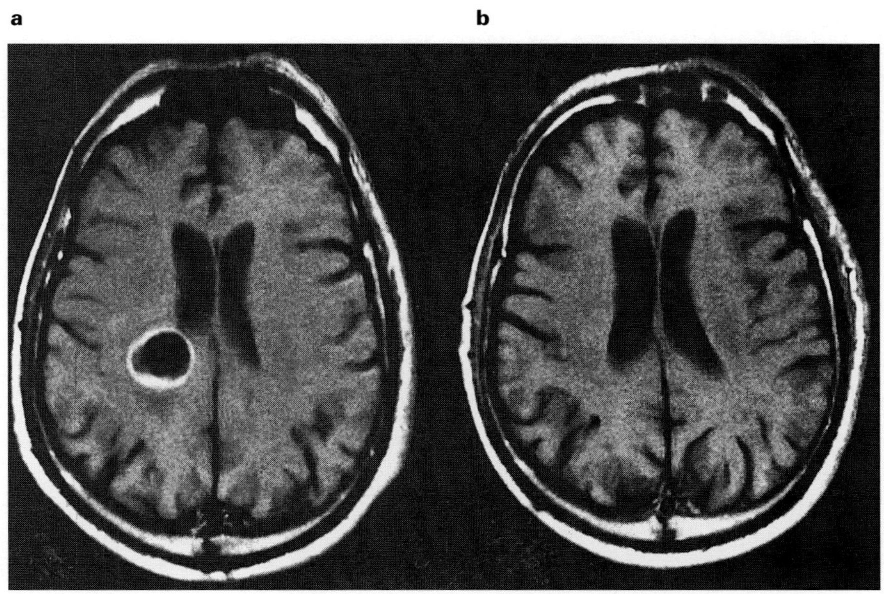

Fig. 11.12 Contrast enhanced CT images at **a** the time of and **b** 8 months after radiosurgery illustrate disappearance of the tumour in a 75-year-old man with metastatic adenocarcinoma of unknown origin.

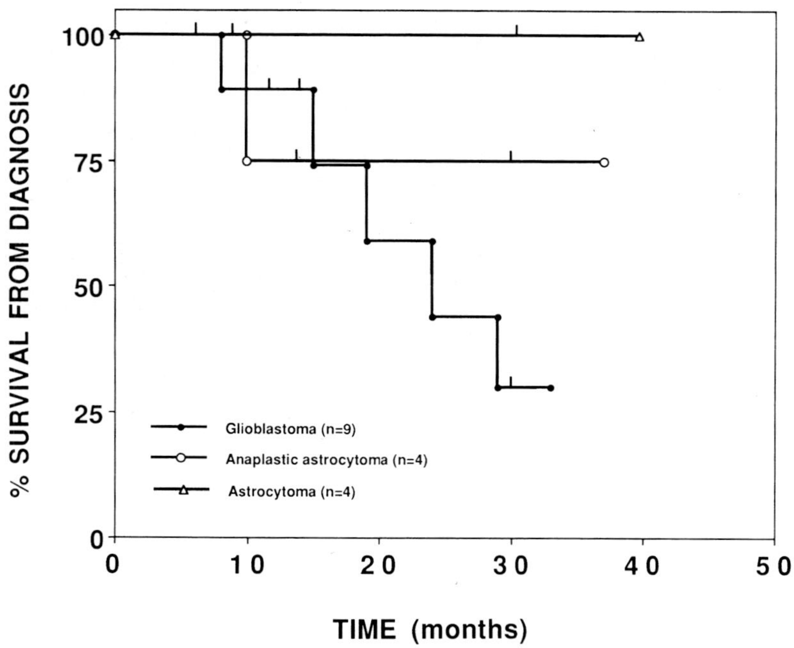

Fig. 11.13 Kaplan–Meier plots of survival after diagnosis for 17 patients with glioblastoma multiforme, anaplastic astrocytoma or astrocytoma treated by radiosurgery. Vertical bars indicate patients still alive.

We believe that radiosurgery offers satisfactory local control for patients with small solitary brain metastases. For patients with systemic disease and solitary metastases greater than 3 cm in diameter, surgical resection followed by whole brain radiotherapy still represents the best treatment option.

Glial tumours

Both primary and secondary malignant brain tumours are characterized by their tendency for local invasion and infiltration beyond imaging defined margins. It is this uncontrolled local growth that eventually leads to demise of the patient (Hochbert & Pruitt 1980, Bashir et al 1988). In an attempt to control local growth, interstitial brachytherapy has been used to deliver a radiation boost to selected, well circumscribed supratentorial malignant gliomas less than 5 cm in diameter (Gutin et al 1984, Lunsford et al 1985, Leibel et al 1989, Bernstein et al 1990). We have used radiosurgery as an alternative treatment to boost the fractionated radiation dose delivered to biopsy proven gliomas less than 3 cm in diameter.

Brachytherapy differs from radiosurgery by delivering a greater radiation dose over a longer period (usually 4–5 days) and can be used for larger tumour volumes. Brachytherapy also treats malignant cells in different phases of the cell cycle. Brachytherapy is less sensitive to definition of the brain adjacent to the tumour margin, because the radiation fall-off is less steep than in radiosurgery. Failure after glial neoplasm radiosurgery is related in part to an inability to clearly define the actual tumour margin and to the size most glial tumours reach before detection. Patients are currently accepted for radiosurgery if the tumour measures less than 3 cm in diameter and the margins appear well circumscribed on both CT and MRI (Fig. 11.13).

From December 1990, we have used radiosurgery as an adjuvant to fractionated external beam radiation therapy in 10 patients with biopsy proven glioblastoma. One patient had also received brachytherapy. The mean age of patients was 48 years (range 6–59 years). All

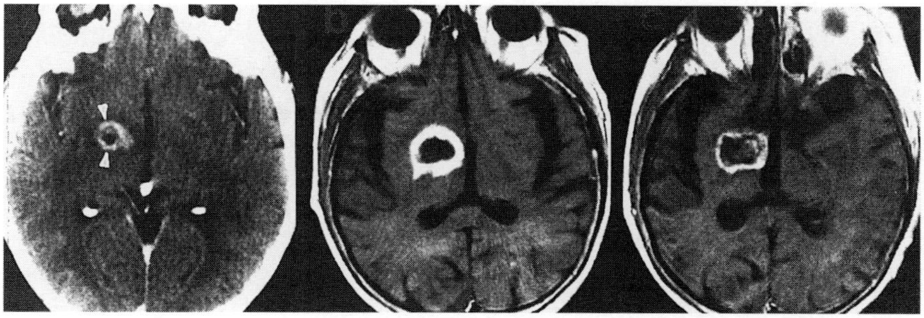

Fig. 11.14 Serial contrast enhanced CT images in a 55-year-old woman with biopsy-proven glioblastoma multiforme adjacent to the third ventricle; **a** the tumour was small and appeared well circumscribed (arrowheads) at the time of treatment. The patient remained stable **b** 7 and **c** 22 months after radiosurgery, despite apparent local progression of the mass.

tumours were supratentorial (two frontal, two temporoparietal, one frontoparietal, two parietal, one temporal, one in the basal ganglia and one thalamic). The mean dose delivered to the tumour margin was 15.7 Gy (range 12.5–20 Gy). During follow-up ranging from 3 to 22 months (mean 10 months), no imaging or clinical evidence of cerebral radiation injury was seen. Radiosurgery was used an average of 10 months after diagnosis (range 3–23 months). The mean survival after initial diagnosis was 20.3 months; four patients were still alive 11, 14, 30 and 33 months after diagnosis (Fig. 11.14).

Five patients with anaplastic astrocytoma also were treated with radiosurgery after first receiving external beam fractionated radiation. Radiosurgery in this group was performed an average of 8 months after diagnosis (range 3–15 months). One patient died 10 months after diagnosis. Three other patients (with follow-up longer than 2

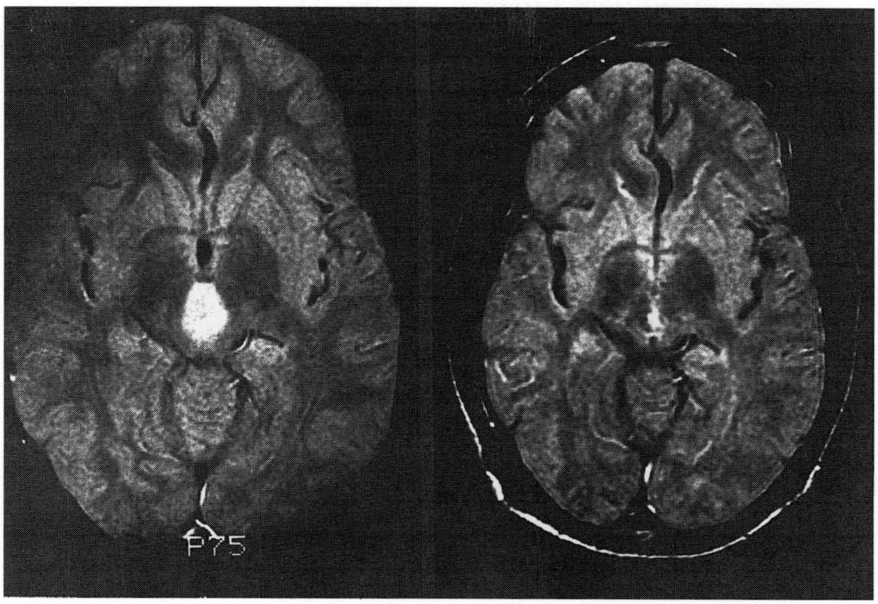

Fig. 11.15 Serial MRI scans (T_2 spin-echo) **a** before and **b** 2 years after radiosurgical treatment of an anaplastic astrocytoma of the dorsal midbrain–pineal region in a 14-year-old boy.

months) were alive at 14, 30 and 37 months after diagnosis. In one of these, a tumour in the posterior third ventricle virtually disappeared on both CT and MRI studies, performed 12 months after radiosurgery, and clinical symptoms also were in complete remission (Fig. 11.15).

Radiosurgery was used as an alternative, rather than an adjunct, to fractionated irradiation in four patients with biopsy proven non–malignant astrocytomas. Two of these patients had lesions within the midbrain. A mean dose of 17 Gy was delivered to the tumour margin (15–20 Gy). One patient with a midbrain tumour had imaging evidence of radiation induced blood–brain barrier breakdown in the region surrounding the tumour 3 months after radiosurgery (Fig. 11.16). Marked loss of central contrast enhancement within the neoplasm suggested tumour necrosis. Progression of symptoms and associated hydrocephalus required cerebrospinal fluid diversion and prolonged corticosteroid therapy. All four patients were alive an average of 22 months after diagnosis (range 7–40 months).

We used radiosurgery as a boost to prior external beam radiation therapy to treat six recurrent ependymomas (in five patients), a mean of 60 months after initial diagnosis. Four of the tumours were intraventricular and two were located at the cerebellopontine angle. Four tumours were in children (the mean age of patients with ependymomas was 21 years). During follow-up, two patients died, both with malignant ependymomas. At the time of writing, the mean length of survival after diagnosis for this series was 75 months (range 26–131 months).

Chordomas and chondrosarcomas

Tumour recurrence and progression of clinical symptoms is the rule following conventional multimodality treatment of chordomas and chondrosarcomas of the skull base. In an effort to improve results, more aggressive microsurgical skull base approaches and a variety of irradiation techniques have been advocated (Suit et al 1982,

a **b**

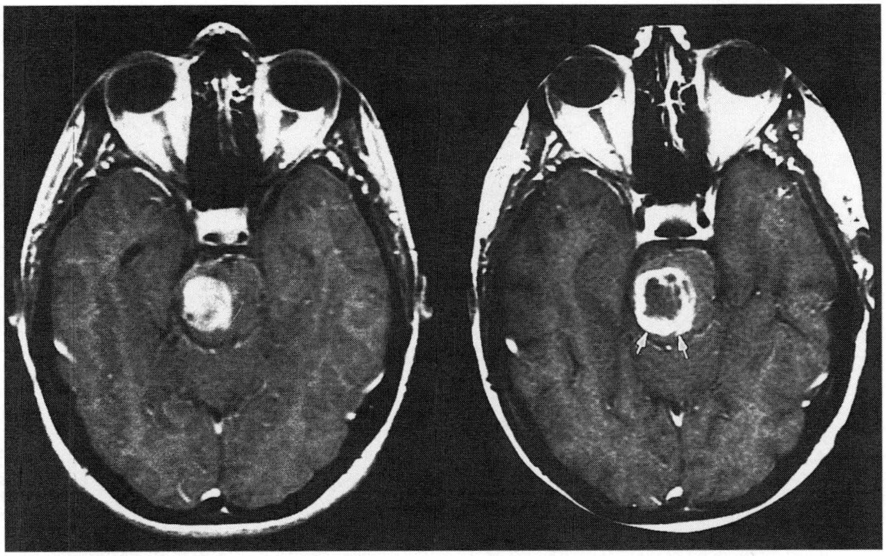

Fig. 11.16 Serial MRI scans (T_1 spin-echo with Gd-DTPA) **a** before and **b** 6 months after radiosurgery of a midbrain pilocytic astrocytoma in a 35-year-old woman. Ataxia and nystagmus developed in this patient 3 months after treatment. The post-treatment scans showed evidence of central tumour necrosis and contrast enhancement within the adjacent brain stem (arrows).

Cummings et al 1983, Raffel et al 1985, Sen et al 1989, Cocke et al 1990). Although these tumours are considered radioresistant, some centres have reported benefit from high dose fractionated radiotherapy (Pearlman & Friedman 1970), brachytherapy (Gutin et al 1987) and fractionated heavy charged particle irradiation (Saunders et al 1985, Austin-Seymour et al 1989). However, the use of these techniques has been limited by tissue intolerance to high fractionated doses, by the technical difficulties associated with isotope implantation, and by the delivery of radiation to adjacent critical brain structures. To examine the role of radiosurgery in the treatment of these refractory cranial base tumours, we treated four patients with chordoma and two with chondrosarcoma. Five of these patients underwent radiosurgery as adjuvant treatment after microsurgery (1–3 resections). No patient received fractionated external beam radiotherapy. During follow-up (mean 21 months, range 8–36 months), pretreatment neurological deficits (abducens nerve palsies) improved in three patients, while the other three patients remained in a stable neurological condition. Serial imaging studies showed that two patients had smaller tumours and four patients had no growth of the treated tumour volume (Fig. 11.17 and 11.18).

The failure of radiosurgery to provide long-term tumour control was demonstrated in two patients. One patient underwent treatment of a seemingly well circumscribed chordoma that recurred after radical skull base surgery. Although the treated nodule decreased in size 8 months after radiosurgery, there was remote growth of tumour outside the radiosurgical treatment volume. Another patient developed a metastatic parietal lobe chondrosarcoma 19 months after radiosurgery of a primary cavernous sinus–middle fossa tumour residual from microsurgery. This patient remained stable at 36 months after radiosurgery.

Because the radiation dose can be delivered in

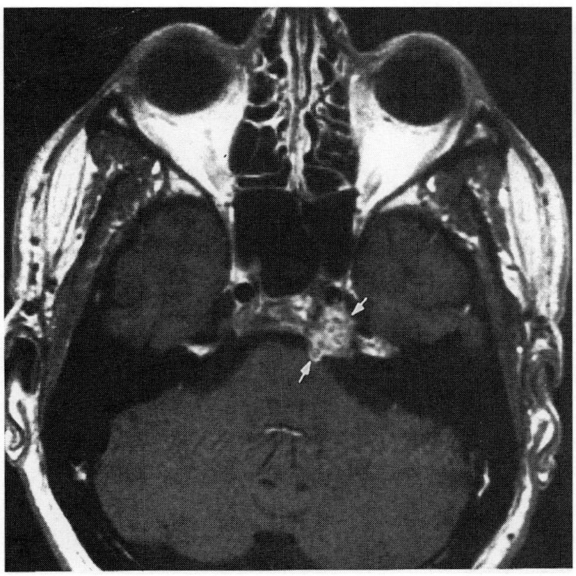

a

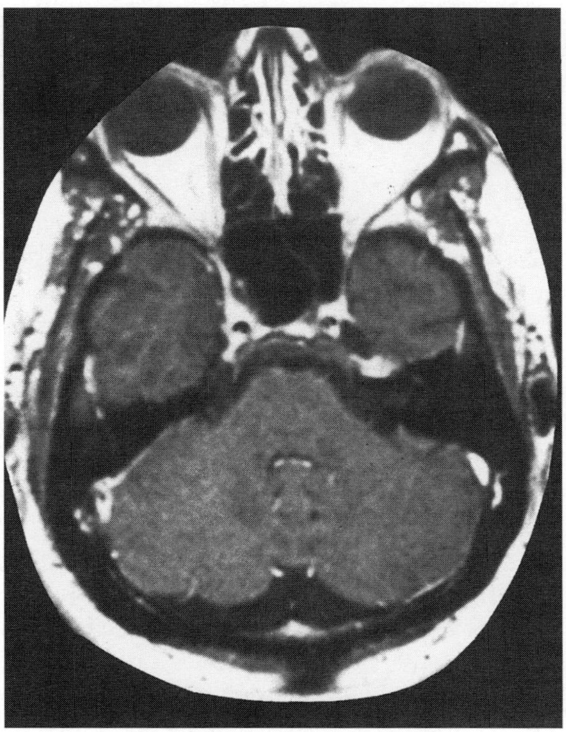

b

Fig. 11.17 Serial contrast enhanced MRI scans showing **a** a recurrent petroclival chordoma (arrows) and **b** disappearance of tumour 9 months after treatment with 20 Gy to the tumour margin.

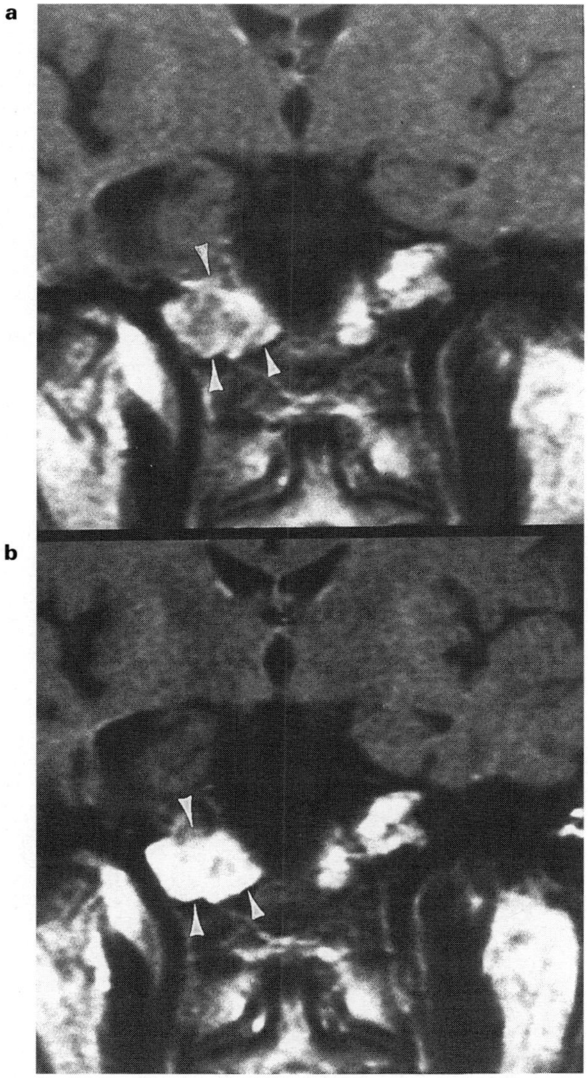

Fig. 11.18 Serial coronal MRI scans with contrast show **a** a residual cavernous sinus chondrosarcoma (arrowheads) and **b** no change in the size of the tumour (arrowheads) 16 months after radiosurgery. A dose of 20 Gy was delivered to the tumour margin with two isocentres of irradiation using the 18 mm collimator.

a single treatment session and can spare surrounding critical vascular, cerebral and cranial nerve structures, stereotactic radiosurgery has potential advantages over fractionated irradiation techniques for treating skull base chordomas and chondrosarcomas. We hope that this multi-avenue approach (skull base microsurgery, fractionated irradiation, radiosurgery or some combination of these) will lengthen survival and reduce patient morbidity.

Other malignant tumours

We used radiosurgery to treat a recurrent poorly differentiated squamous cell carcinoma of the nasopharynx after the patient had undergone biopsy, fractionated radiotherapy, interstitial irradiation and chemotherapy (Kondziolka & Lunsford 1991). Stereotactic MRI was used to identify this extracranial tumour for treatment. The patient remained in a stable condition without imaging defined tumour growth 11 months after treatment, but another biopsy found focal tumour cells. An additional patient had a malignant metastatic schwannoma of the cerebellopontine angle treated with radiosurgery. Although radiosurgery currently is limited to tumours anatomically above the level of the foramen magnum, some extracranial midline lesions could potentially be treated.

FUTURE EFFORTS

Imaging advances

As each new imaging technique has been developed, it has been incorporated into stereotactic radiosurgery for lesion targeting. In general, cerebral angiography is mandatory for treatment of AVMs, and CT scans are required for the treatment of tumours. We recently compared the accuracy of target determination by stereotactic MRI to that by stereotactic CT. In 25 consecutive patients for whom stereotactic MRI target localization was indicated, we also obtained stereotactic CT scans for comparison. The MRI studies were performed either on a 1.5 or a 0.5 T unit. In all patients, coordinates in both axial and coronal planes were virtually identical on both CT and MRI (differences were usually 2 mm or less in two dimensions). Fiducial measurements on the stereotactic frame were always accurate to within 1 mm when calculated using the software measure-distance function. We are confident in the use of stereotactic MRI alone for target selection and now use it as the sole imaging procedure for lesions that are poorly visualized with CT (e.g. pituitary tumours).

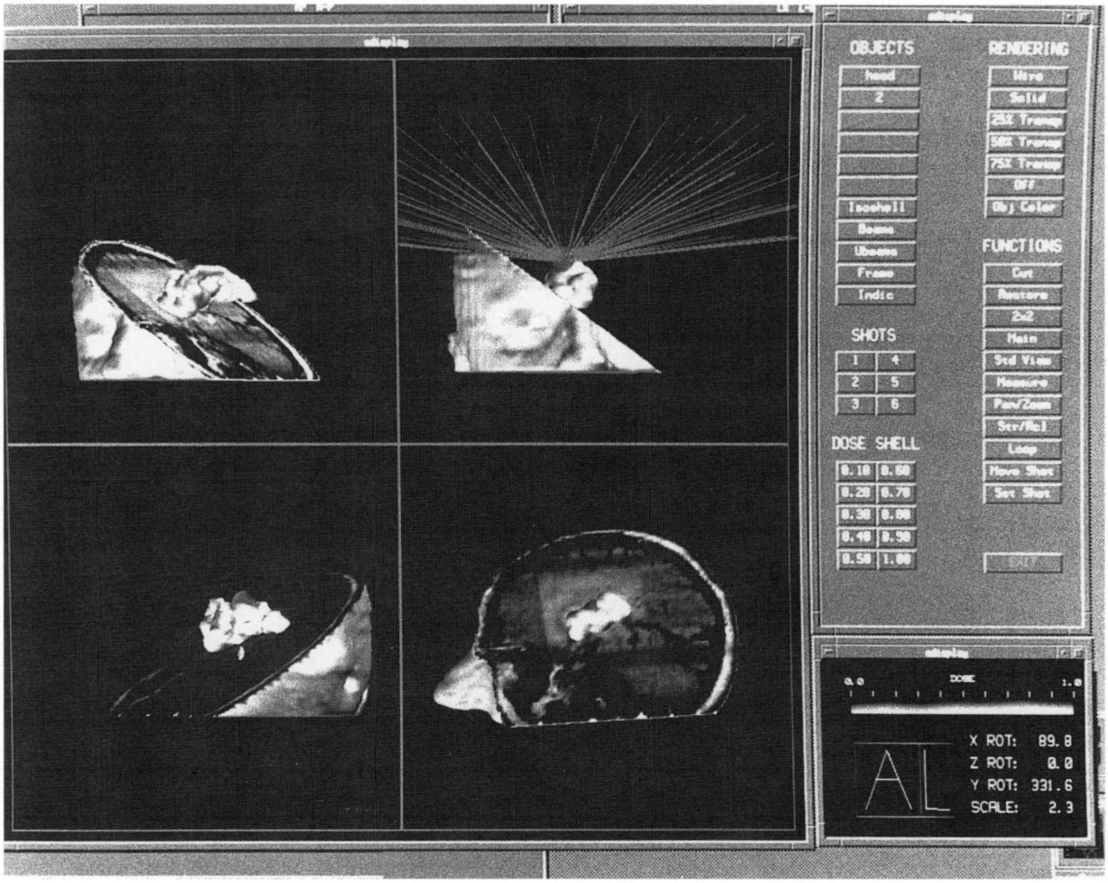

Fig. 11.19 Three dimensional gamma knife radiation dose planning (Leksell GammaPlan works-in-progress; courtesy of Elekta Instruments, Inc., Atlanta, Georgia, USA).

Computerized graphics for three dimensional reconstruction of brain tumours and surrounding critical brain structures will be an important development in radiosurgical planning techniques. The ability to confine the effective treatment isodose to the tumour margin in three dimensions (rather than sequential two dimensional slices) will facilitate faster and more accurate dose planning (Fig. 11.19).

Radiobiological research

We have developed a rat glioma model to study the effects of radiosurgery in vivo. The implantation of C6 glioma cells into the frontal lobe of the rat, produces a rapidly growing, uniform tumour mass leading to demise of the animal approximately 30 days after implantation (San-Galli et al 1989). Currently, we are studying the effects of different radiosurgical tumour doses using this model. This study will improve our ability to determine therapeutic doses and increase our knowledge of the pathological effects of single session tumour irradiation. A second study will examine the dose and temporal effects of radiosurgery in a human acoustic neurilemmoma xenograft grown in nude mice. We are also now examining the effects of different radiosurgical doses on the normal ventrolateral pons in the primate, by analysing neuroimaging studies, cerebral blood flow, brain stem evoked potentials, the myelin basic protein level in cerebrospinal fluid, neurobehavioural status and neuropathological findings (Lunsford et al 1990b). Such investigations, designed to augment our knowledge of the basic radiobiological substrate of radiosurgery, should ultimately improve treatment. Proper patient selection, high resolution imaging lesion definition, and dose volume analyses will enhance the use of radiosurgery. We suspect that, in the future, specific tumour radiation sensitizers and selective brain protectors will further advance this rapidly emerging field.

ACKNOWLEDGEMENTS

The authors would like to thank Dr John C. Flickinger, Dr Robert J. Coffey and the staff of the Specialized Neurosurgical Center at the University of Pittsburgh for their dedicated assistance in this project, and Helene Marion for editorial support.

REFERENCES

Adegbite A B, Khan M I, Paine K W E, Tan L K 1983 The recurrence of intracranial meningiomas after surgical treatment. Journal of Neurosurgery 58: 51–56

Austin-Seymour M, Munzenrider J, Goitein M et al 1989 Fractionated proton radiation therapy of chordoma and low-grade chondrosarcoma of the base of the skull. Journal of Neurosurgery 70: 13–17

Awad I A, Kalfas I, Hahn J F 1989 Intracranial meningiomas in the aged: Surgical outcome in the era of computed tomography. Neurosurgery 24: 557–560

Backlund E O, Rahn T, Sarby B 1974 Treatment of pinealomas by stereotaxic radiation surgery. Acta Radiologica, Therapy, Physics, Biology 13: 368–376

Barbaro N M, Gutin P M, Wilson C B 1987 Radiation therapy in the treatment of partially resected meningiomas. Neurosurgery 20: 525–528

Bashir R, Hochberg F, Oot R 1988 Regrowth patterns of glioblastoma multiforme related to planning of interstitial brachytherapy radiation fields. Neurosurgery 23: 27–30

Baskin D S, Boggan J E, Wilson C B 1982 Transsphenoidal microsurgical removal of growth hormone-secreting pituitary tumors: a review of 137 cases. Journal of Neurosurgery 56: 634–641

Bernstein M, Laperriere N, Leung P, McKenzie S 1990 Interstitial brachytherapy for malignant brain tumours: preliminary results. Neurosurgery 26: 371–380

Black P 1979 Brain metastasis: current status and recommended guidelines for management. Neurosurgery 5: 617–631

Boggan J E, Tyrrell J B, Wilson C B 1983 Transsphenoidal microsurgical management of Cushing's disease: report of 100 cases. Journal of Neurosurgery 59: 195–200

Carella R J, Ransohoff J, Newall J 1982 Role of radiation therapy in the management of meningioma. Neurosurgery 10: 332–339

Cocke E W, Robertson J H, Robertson J T, Crook J P 1990 The extended maxillotomy and subtotal maxillectomy for excision of skull base tumours. Archives of Otolaryngology, Head and Neck Surgery 116: 92–104

Coffey R J, Flickinger J C, Bissonette D J, Lunsford L D 1991 Radiosurgery for brain metastases using the cobalt-60 gamma unit: methods and results in 24 patients. International Journal of Radiation, Oncology, Biology, Physics 20: 1287–1295

Colombo F, Benedetti A, Pozza F et al 1985 External stereotactic irradiation by linear accelerator. Neurosurgery 16: 154–160

Cummings B J, Hodson D I, Bush R S 1983 Chordoma: the results of megavoltage radiation therapy. International Journal of Radiation, Oncology, Biology, Physics 9: 633–642

Degerblad M, Rahn T, Bergstrand G, Thoren M 1986 Long term results of stereotactic radiosurgery to the pituitary gland in Cushing's disease. Acta Endocrinologica 112: 310–314

Djindjian M, Caron J P, Athayde A A 1988 Intracranial meningiomas in the elderly (over 70 years old): a retrospective study of 30 cases. Acta Neurochirurgica (Wien) 90: 121–123

Eastman R C, Gorden P, Roth J 1979 Conventional supervoltage irradiation is an effective treatment for acromegaly. Journal of Clinical Endocrinology and Metabolism 48: 931–940

Engenhart R, Kimmig B, Sturm V 1989 Stereotactically guided convergent beam irradiation of solitary brain metastases and cerebral arteriovenous malformations. In: Dyck P, Bouzaglou A (eds) Brachytherapy of brain tumours and related stereotactic treatment. Hanley and Belfus, Philadelphia, pp 119–132

Fabrikant J I, Lyman J T, Hosobuchi Y 1984 Stereotactic heavy-ion Bragg peak radiosurgery for intra-cranial vascular disorders: method for treatment of deep arteriovenous malformations. British Journal of Radiology 57: 479–490

Flickinger J C 1989 The integrated logistic formula and prediction of complications from radiosurgery. International Journal of Radiation, Oncology, Biology, Physics 17: 879–885

Flickinger J C, Nelson P B, Martinez A J, Taylor F H, Deutsch M, Robinson A G 1989 Radiotherapy of nonfunctional adenomas of the pituitary gland: results with long-term follow-up. Cancer 63: 2409–2414

Flickinger J C, Lunsford L D, Wu A, Maitz A H, Kalend A 1990a Treatment planning for gamma knife radiosurgery with multiple isocenters. International Journal of Radiation, Oncology, Biology, Physics 18: 1495–1501

Flickinger J C, Maitz A H, Kalend A, Lunsford L D, Wu A 1990b Treatment volume shaping with selective beam blocking using the Leksell gamma unit. International Journal of Radiation, Oncology, Biology, Physics 19: 783–789

Friedman R B, Oldfield E H, Nieman L K et al 1989 Repeat transsphenoidal surgery for Cushing's disease. Journal of Neurosurgery 71: 520–527

Friedman W A, Bova F J 1989 The University of Florida radiosurgery system. Surgical Neurology 32: 334–342

Gardner G, Robertson J H 1988 Hearing preservation in unilateral acoustic neuroma surgery. Annals of Otolaryngology, Rhinology and Laryngology 97: 55–56

Guidetti B, Ciapetta P, Domenicucci M 1988 Tentorial meningiomas: Surgical experience with 61 cases and long-term results. Journal of Neurosurgery 69: 183–187

Gutin P H, Phillips T L, Wara W M et al 1984 Brachytherapy of recurrent malignant brain tumours with removable high-activity iodine-125 sources. Journal of Neurosurgery 60: 61–68

Gutin P H, Leibel S A, Hosobuchi Y et al 1987 Brachytherapy of recurrent tumours of the skull base and spine with iodine-125 sources. Neurosurgery 20: 938–945

Hartmann G H, Schlegel W, Sturm V 1985 Cerebral radiation surgery using moving field irradiation at a linear accelerator facility. International Journal of Radiation, Oncology, Biology, Physics 11: 1185–1192

Hirsch A, Noren G 1988 Audiological findings after stereotactic radiosurgery in acoustic neurinomas. Acta Otolaryngologica (Stockholm) 106: 244–251

Hochberg F H, Pruitt A 1980 Assumptions in the radiotherapy of glioblastoma. Neurology 30: 907–911

House W F, Brackmann D E 1985 Facial nerve grading system. Otolaryngology, Head and Neck Surgery 93: 184–193

Kjellberg R N, Abe M 1988 Stereotactic Bragg peak proton beam therapy. In: Lunsford LD (ed) Modern stereotactic neurosurgery. Martinus Nijhoff, Boston, pp 463–470

Kondziolka D, Lunsford L D 1991 Stereotactic radiosurgery for squamous cell carcinoma of the nasopharynx. Laryngoscope 101: 519–522

Kondziolka D, Lunsford L D, Coffey R J, Flickinger J C 1990 Cranial nerve preservation after radiosurgery for acoustic neurinoma. Surgical Forum 41: 508–510

Kondziolka D, Lunsford L D, Coffey R J, Flickinger J C 1991 Stereotactic radiosurgery of meningiomas. Journal of Neurosurgery 74: 552–559

Leibel S A, Gutin P H, Wara W M et al 1989 Survival and quality of life after interstitial implantation of removable high-activity iodine-125 sources for the treatment of patients with recurrent malignant gliomas. International Journal of Radiation, Oncology, Biology, Physics 17: 1129–1139

Leksell L 1951 The stereotaxic method and radiosurgery of the brain. Acta Chirurgica Scandinavica 102: 316–319

Leksell L 1983 Stereotactic radiosurgery. Journal of Neurology, Neurosurgery and Psychiatry 46: 797–803

Levy R P, Fabrikant J I, Frankel K A, Phillips M H, Lyman J T 1990 Charged-particle radiosurgery of the brain. Clinics of North America 1(4): 955–990

Lindquist C 1989 Gamma knife surgery for recurrent solitary metastasis of a cerebral hypernephroma: case report. Neurosurgery 25: 802–804

Linfoot J A, Lawrence J H 1985 Treatment of functioning pituitary tumours. In: Wilkins R H, Rengachary S S (eds) Neurosurgery. McGraw-Hill, Toronto, pp 1119–1126

Linskey M E, Lunsford L D, Flickinger J C 1990 Radiosurgery for acoustic neurinomas: early experience. Neurosurgery 26: 736–745

Loeffler J S, Kooy H M, Wen P Y et al 1990 The treatment of recurrent brain metastases with stereotactic radiosurgery. Journal of Clinical Oncology 8: 576–582

Lunsford L D, Deutsch M, Yoder V 1985 Stereotactic interstitial brachytherapy — current concepts and concerns in twenty patients. Applied Neurophysiology 48: 117–120

Lunsford L D, Flickinger J C, Lindner G, Maitz A H 1989 Stereotactic radiosurgery of the brain using the first United States 201 source cobalt-60 gamma knife. Neurosurgery 24: 152–159

Lunsford L D, Flickinger J, Coffey R J 1990a Stereotactic gamma knife radiosurgery: initial North American experience in 207 patients. Archives of Neurology 47: 169–175

Lunsford L D, Altschuler E, Flickinger J C, Wu A, Martinez A J 1990b In vivo biological effects of stereotactic radiosurgery: a primate model. Neurosurgery 27: 373–382

Madajewicz S, Karakousis C, West C R, Caracandas J, Avellanosa A 1984 Malignant melanoma brain metastases. Review of Roswell Park Memorial Institute experience. Cancer 53: 2550–2552

Mandell L, Hilaris B, Sullivan M et al 1986 The treatment of single brain metastasis from non-oat cell lung carcinoma. Surgery and radiation versus radiation therapy alone. Cancer 58: 641–649

Mayberg M R, Symon L 1986 Meningiomas of the clivus and apical petrous bone. Report of 35 cases. Journal of Neurosurgery 65: 160–167

Noren G, Arndt J, Hindmarsh J 1983 Stereotactic radiosurgery in cases of acoustic neurinomas: further experiences. Neurosurgery 13: 12–22

Papo I 1983 Intracranial meningiomas in the elderly in the CT scan era. Acta Neurochirurgica (Wien) 67: 195–204

Patchell R A, Tibbs P A, Walsh J W et al 1990 A randomized trial of surgery in the treatment of single metastases to the brain. New England Journal of Medicine 322: 494–500

Pearlman A W, Friedman M 1970 Radical radiation therapy of chordoma. American Journal of Roentgenology 108: 333–341

Petty A M, Kun L E, Meyer G A 1985 Radiation therapy for incompletely resected meningiomas. Journal of Neurosurgery 62: 502–507

Podgorsak E B, Olivier A, Pla M, Lefebvre P Y, Hazel J 1988 Dynamic stereotactic radiosurgery. International Journal of Radiation, Oncology, Biology, Physics 13: 1553–1557

Raffel C, Wright D C, Gutin P H, Wilson C B 1985 Cranial chordomas: clinical presentation and results of operative and radiation therapy in 26 patients. Neurosurgery 17: 703–710

Rahn T, Thoren M 1988 Radiosurgery in pituitary adenomas. Advances in the Biosciences 69: 451–453

Samii M, Ammirati M, Mahran A, Bini W, Sepehrnia A 1989 Surgery of petroclival meningiomas: report of 24 cases. Neurosurgery 24: 12–17

San-Galli F, Vrignaud P, Robert J, Coindre J M, Cohadon F 1989 Assessment of the experimental model of transplanted C6 glioblastoma in wistar rats. Journal of Neuro-Oncology 7: 299–304

Saunders W M, Chen G T Y, Austin-Seymour M et al 1985 Precision, high-dose radiotherapy. II. Helium ion treatment of tumours adjacent to critical central nervous system structures. International Journal of Radiation, Oncology, Biology, Physics 11: 1339–1347

Sekhar L N, Sen C N, Jho H D, Janecka I P 1989 Surgical treatment of intracavernous neoplasms: a four year experience. Neurosurgery 24: 18–30

Sen C N, Sekhar L N, Schramm V L, Janecka I P 1989 Chordoma and chondrosarcoma of the cranial base: an 8-year experience. Neurosurgery 25: 931–941

Simpson D 1957 The recurrence of intracranial meningiomas

after surgical treatment. Journal of Neurology, Neurosurgery, Psychiatry 20: 22–39
Steinberg G K, Fabrikant J I, Marks M P et al 1990 Stereotactic heavy-charged-particle Bragg-peak radiation for intracranial arteriovenous malformations. New England Journal of Medicine 323: 96–101
Sturm V, Kober B, Hover K H et al 1987 Stereotactic percutaneous single dose irradiation of brain metastases with a linear accelerator. International Journal of Radiation, Oncology, Biology, Physics 13: 279–282
Suit H D, Goitein M, Munzenrider J et al 1982 Definitive radiation therapy for chordoma and chondrosarcoma of base of skull and cervical spine. Journal of Neurosurgery 56: 377–385
Taylor B W, Marcus R B, Friedman W A, Ballinger W E, Million R R 1988 The meningioma controversy: postoperative radiation therapy. International Journal of Radiation, Oncology, Biology, Physics 15: 299–304
Thompson B G, Coffey R J, Flickinger J C, Lunsford L D 1990 Stereotactic radiosurgery of small intracranial tumors: neuropathological correlation in three patients. Surgical Neurology 33: 96–104
Wara W M, Sheline G E, Newman M 1975 Radiation therapy of meningiomas. American Journal of Roentgenology 123: 453–458
Winston K R, Lutz W 1988 Linear accelerator as a neurosurgical tool for stereotactic radiosurgery. Neurosurgery 22: 454–464
Wu A, Lindner G, Maitz A M et al 1990 Physics of gamma knife approach on convergent beams in stereotactic radiosurgery. International Journal of Radiation, Oncology, Biology, Physics 18: 941–949

12. The mathematics of stereotactic localization

L. Lemieux   C. J. Henri   R. Wootton   D. L. Collins   T. M. Peters

PART 1
AN INTRODUCTION

L. Lemieux   C. J. Henri

Stereotaxis refers to the localization of structures within the body (from the Greek: stereos, solid; taxis, arrangement). In medicine, and neurosurgery in particular, stereotaxis has two distinct meanings: first, the localization of structures based on the analysis of image data and the ability to reach surgically those structures precisely by surgical means using a stereotactic frame; second,the localization of structures relative to an anatomically defined coordinate system, enabling the accurate comparison of image data from various modalities.

In the following we will be interested in the analysis of image data acquired in conjunction with a stereotactic frame. However, anatomically defined coordinate systems also make it possible to relate the image data to some physically based coordinate system. Of particular practical interest here is the comparison of data obtained from various modalities and/or anatomical atlases. When interpreting functional image data, such as positron emission tomography (PET), the analysis is often facilitated by displaying it in relation to anatomical data, such as magnetic resonance imaging (MRI). Although less precision might be tolerated here than in surgical applications, the problem to be solved is the same in each case: to find a common coordinate system within which to relate each data set. We will call this coordinate system the stereotactic coordinate system.

In surgical applications we also must be able to relate the positions of anatomical structures to those of the surgical instruments. A stereotactic frame is a rigid structure that is attached to the skull and serves the dual purpose of defining a three dimensional (3D) coordinate system for target localization and providing a physical support for the surgical instruments. The patient's skull, therefore, is the reference upon which the frame coordinate system is based. This may not be considered ideal in the sense that neurosurgery is mostly concerned with the brain, which is not rigidly connected to the skull.

Stereotactic localization refers to the process of determining the position relative to the 3D coordinate system of a point in the image data. The principle at the basis of stereotactic localization is the calculation of mathematical transformations which map image coordinates (2D) on to stereotactic frame coordinates (3D), and vice versa, for each type of image data. While these transformations exist for tomographic images, the situation is different for radiographic projections (e.g. standard X-ray or angiography). In this case, only the frame-to-image transformation is available. The inverse mapping requires two or more distinct projections (e.g. anteroposterior and lateral, or stereoscopic pair) in which a point must be identified unambiguously. The following chapter describes how the above transformations are determined from points on the stereotactic frame (called 'fiducials' or 'fiducial markers') which appear in each acquired image.

Modern stereotactic frames are compatible with several imaging modalities, such as computerized tomography (CT), MRI, X-ray, digital subtraction angiography (DSA) and PET. This allows features in each type of data to be related accurately. A necessary prerequisite is that the stereotactic frame must remain fixed in position with respect to the skull when imaged in each modality. Then the frame coordinates of a particular anatomical point as determined in any data set will be the same.

We proceed in the following two parts to discuss the mathematical methods at the basis of the display and analysis of image data acquired under stereotactic conditions. The first part addresses stereotactic localization based on tomographic data, while the second part covers stereotactic localization for radiographic projections. While the distinction between the two is logical, it also conveniently reflects the personal expertize of the authors.

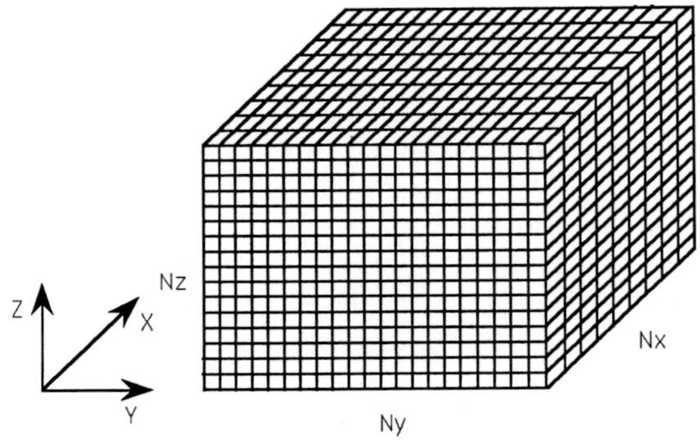

Fig. 12.1 Tomographic volume data set and voxel coordinates. Slices are parallel to the *XY* plane, *Z* is the slice number.

PART 2

THE MATHEMATICS OF STEREOTACTIC TOMOGRAPHIC IMAGE DISPLAY AND ANALYSIS

L. Lemieux R. Wootton

INTRODUCTION

The aim is to present here, in a unified form, a review of the mathematics necessary for the display and analysis of stereotactically acquired tomographic volume data sets based on the use of stereotactic frames. Although this part is primarily concerned with the mathematics of stereotactic image display and analysis, a number of issues relating to the accuracy of localization will be discussed*. Since our experience is mainly with the Brown–Roberts–Wells (BRW) stereotactic frame (Brown 1979a, b) our discussion will be directly relevant to the analysis of data acquired with this device. The methods presented here stem from what may be called the *algebraic* approach to stereotactic localization, as first described by Brown et al (1980).

Tomographic image data consists of rectangular arrays of pixels, which can be represented as a volume consisting of voxels (see Fig. 12.1). When acquired under stereotactic conditions it is possible to calculate the coordinates of any voxel relative to the coordinate system of the stereotactic frame. A slice transformation matrix (STM) may be calculated for each slice. This is a one-to-one mapping between image and frame coordinates. This is made possible by the use of the stereotactic localizer, the geometry of which effectively enables the determination of the position, orientation and size of each tomographic cut (Fig. 12.2). Stereotactic localization based on the STMs is perfectly satisfactory if it is only necessary to examine the data slice by slice, as the appropriate coordinate transformation is used for each slice. In this situation the STMs are independent and the slices are effectively mathematically 'unconnected'.

If the volume as a whole is going to be manipulated then one may use a single coordinate transformation, called the volume transformation matrix (VTM). The VTM maps voxel coordinates on to frame coordinates. The application of the VTM is possible only if the data set satisfies certain conditions, the most critical being that the slices are exactly parallel. This volume transformation maps voxel space (3D) on to frame coordinate space. The modalities of the calculation of this transformation will be described.

We will also discuss the resampling of the volume along a specified plane ('slice reconstruction') and the implications for localization. As will be shown, the reconstruction process can be described in terms of coordinate transformations, facilitating the calculation of frame coordinates from reconstructed voxel coordinates.

* Note that this is only one aspect of the accuracy of stereotactic surgical procedures (Galloway & Maciunas 1990).

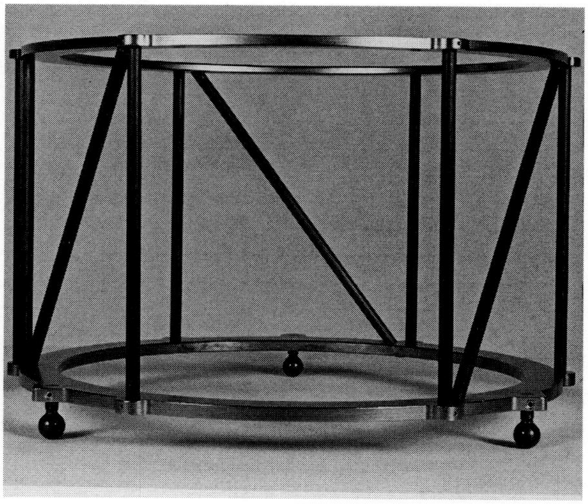

a

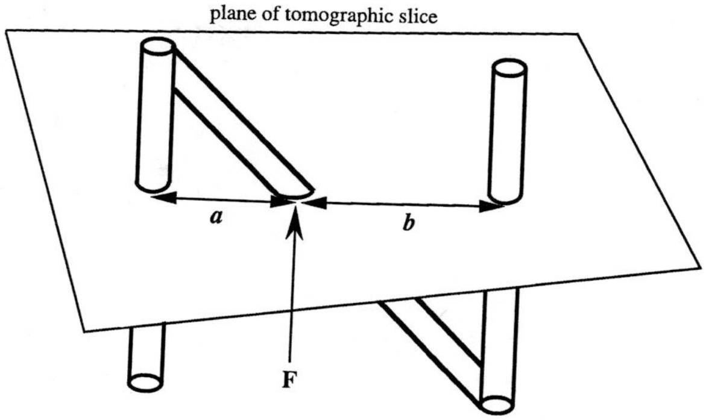

b

Fig. 12.2 **a** BRW tomographic stereotactic localizer, **b** Geometric principle of the localizer: the height in the frame coordinate system of fiducial ***F*** is given by the ratio $b/(a+b)$ measured in the image.

4-vector representation

Assuming that the volume data sets consist of parallel slices, then all data manipulations and coordinate transformations described here (i.e. slice and volume transformations) may be expressed in terms of the rigid body coordinate transformations translation and rotation, plus scaling and skew (also called shearing) (see Gonzalez & Wintz 1987, Rogers & Adams 1990)*. For non-parallel slices, this still applies to each individual slice (apart from skew), but not for the volume data set as a whole.

The coordinates of a point in 3D space, $\boldsymbol{x}$,

$$\mathbf{x} = \begin{pmatrix} x \\ y \\ z \end{pmatrix} \qquad (1)$$

can be expressed as a 4-vector, $\underline{\boldsymbol{X}}$, (represented as an underlined character) of the form:

$$\boldsymbol{X} = \begin{pmatrix} X \\ Y \\ Z \\ 1 \end{pmatrix}. \qquad (2)$$

The fourth dimension allows the inclusion of translation in a 4×4 square matrix formalism.

For stereotatic localization we seek the transformation matrix **F**, which maps coordinates in one system ($\underline{\boldsymbol{X}}$) on to another system ($\underline{\boldsymbol{X}}'$):

$$\underline{\boldsymbol{X}}' = \mathbf{F}\underline{\boldsymbol{X}} \qquad (3)$$

$$\underline{\boldsymbol{X}} = \mathbf{F}^{-1}\underline{\boldsymbol{X}}' \qquad (4)$$

Since **F** must include rotation, translation, scaling and skew transformations it has the form

$$\mathbf{F} = \begin{pmatrix} F_{11} & F_{12} & F_{13} & F_{14} \\ F_{21} & F_{22} & F_{23} & F_{24} \\ F_{31} & F_{32} & F_{33} & F_{34} \\ 0 & 0 & 0 & 1 \end{pmatrix} \qquad (5)$$

The upper right 3×1 submatrix of **F** produces translation. The upper left 3×3 submatrix of **F** produces a linear transformation consisting of rotation, scaling and skew. Note that the unit basis vectors are mapped from a coordinate system to another system via the 3×3 submatrix.

APPLICATION TO STEREOTACTIC IMAGES

When the geometric relationship between two coordinate systems is known in terms of successive rotations, translation and scaling, the matrix **F** can be calculated as the product of the

* Skew transformations may be involved if the scanner gantry is not perpendicular to the scanning axis.

appropriate rotation, translation and scaling matrices in the correct order (Gonzalez & Wintz 1987). As explained later, stereotactic localizers are designed to allow the precise determination of this geometric relationship (i.e. the position, orientation and dimensions of the tomographic slices). Certain stereotactic frame designs favour a geometrical approach to stereotactic localization (Galloway & Maciunas 1990). For example, the angles determining the orientation of a given slice may be calculated explicitly. These angles are then used in the transformation between pixel and frame coordinates.

The approach we present is rather based on algebraic methods to calculate the matrix which best maps two sets of points: the coordinates in both image and frame coordinate systems of a number of points. These points are commonly referred to as *fiducials*. The advantage of this approach is the possibility of using more points than required by geometric considerations alone, therefore reducing the error due to uncertainty in fiducial localization ('noise'). An *over-determined* set of equations is obtained and a solution may be obtained which minimizes some norm. The geometric part of the method consists of the calculation of the frame coordinates of the fiducials based on their position within each slice (Brown 1979a, Weaver et al 1990).

Image acquisition under stereotactic conditions

A stereotactic localizer is used during the acquisition of tomographic images. The geometry of the localizer varies between the various makes of frames currently available, and may vary for different modalities (e.g. CT, MRI and PET) (Galloway & Maciunas 1990). However, the general principle is that the geometry is such that the position and orientation of the plane corresponding to a tomographic slice relative to the stereotactic frame's coordinate system can be calculated by analysing information contained in that slice. In the case of the BRW stereotactic frame, the CT localizer comprises nine rods, six running perpendicular to the base ring and three positioned obliquely (see Fig. 12.2). This configuration allows the determination of the three points, the minimum necessary to define the plane corresponding to the slice, at which a given slice intersects the oblique rods by analysing the relative positions of the nine points in the slice. The OBT (Olivier et al 1985) device comprises 12 such rods, therefore allowing the calculation of four points. Other systems (e.g. Leksell (Leksell & Jernberg 1980) rely on the fact that the slices are perpendicular to the longitudinal axis.

Slice transformation matrix

We now come to the problem of finding the coordinate transformation between voxel space and real space. Let us start by restricting ourselves to a single slice, and follow the development by Brown et al (1980). We are seeking the frame transformation matrix, **F**, which maps pixel coordinates, $\underline{\boldsymbol{x}}$, onto frame coordinates, $\underline{\boldsymbol{X}}$,

$$\underline{\boldsymbol{X}} = \mathbf{F}\underline{\boldsymbol{x}}. \qquad (6)$$

The relationship between the slice coordinate system and that of the stereotactic frame is illustrated in Figure 12.3. In equation (6) the pixel coordinates are expressed as a 4-vector. However, since we are restricted to a plane in voxel space we can eliminate the z=0. This

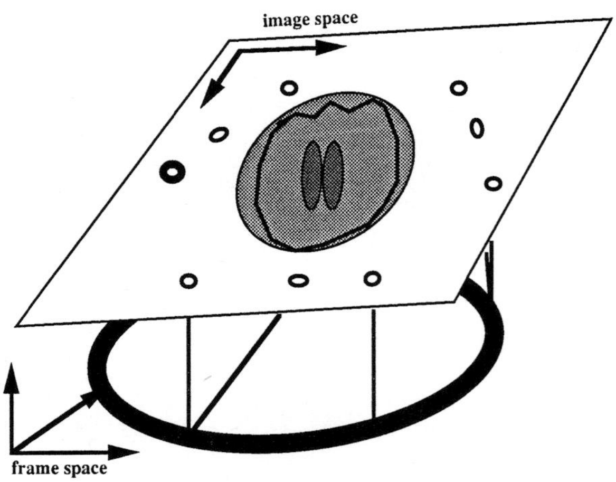

Fig. 12.3 Relationship between the image coordinate system and the stereotactic frame coordinate system. The nine hollow circles and ellipsoids represent the intersection between the image plane and the rods of the localizer. The calculation of the transformation between image and frame coordinates is based on the determination of their coordinates in both systems.

enables us to remove the third column as well as the fourth row in **F**. We therefore obtain **F** as a reduced 3×3 transformation matrix:

$$\begin{pmatrix} X \\ Y \\ Z \end{pmatrix} = \mathbf{F} \begin{pmatrix} x \\ y \\ 1 \end{pmatrix} \quad (7)$$

F can be calculated from a minimum of three non-colinear fiducials, the coordinates of which are determined in the image and frame coordinate systems. Taking the case of three fiducials, matrices **A** and **B** are constructed from the known coordinates of the points expressed as 3-vectors, pixel coordinates $\boldsymbol{x}_i = (x_i, y_i, 1)^T$ and frame coordinates $\boldsymbol{X}_i = (\boldsymbol{X}_i, \boldsymbol{Y}_i, \mathbf{Z}_i)^T$:

$$\mathbf{A} = (\boldsymbol{x}_1\ \boldsymbol{x}_2\ \boldsymbol{x}_3), \quad (8)$$

$$\mathbf{B} = (\boldsymbol{X}_1\ \boldsymbol{X}_2\ \boldsymbol{X}_3). \quad (9)$$

From equation (6) we then have

$$\mathbf{B} = \mathbf{FA} \quad (10)$$

and, therefore,

$$\mathbf{F} = \mathbf{BA}^{-1}. \quad (11)$$

B is non-singular if the points have been properly selected. Note that the inverse transformation, $\mathbf{F}^{-1}$ (frame coordinates to slice coordinates), is only valid for points in the plane of the slice (see the Appendix).

The above solution is an exact geometric one and effectively corresponds to the determination of the equation of the plane through the three selected points. The transformation **F** is therefore subject to the error of localization of the fiducials. This effect may be reduced by making use of more than the minimum three points⋆. If the number of fiducials, **N**, is greater than three then the matrices **A** and **B** are 3×N, and the equation system is overdetermined; in general, no exact solution exists.

A least squares solution, i.e. which minimizes the norm

$$\|\mathbf{B}\text{-}\mathbf{FA}\| \quad (12)$$

is given by

$$\mathbf{F} = \mathbf{BA}^T(\mathbf{AA}^T)^{-1}, \quad (13)$$

provided $\mathbf{AA}^T$ is non-singular.

A better (more robust) solution is obtained by using singular value decomposition (SVD) (Noble & Daniel 1977, Press et al 1988). SVD effectively takes care of the possible redundancies in the selected fiducials (e.g. three colinear points) and automatically gives the least squares solution. We rewrite equation (10) such that the elements of **F** form a vector, $\boldsymbol{f}'$:

$$\mathbf{A}'\boldsymbol{f}' = \mathbf{B}', \quad (14)$$

where $\boldsymbol{f}'$ is the 9-vector

$$\boldsymbol{f}' = \begin{pmatrix} F_{11} \\ F_{12} \\ F_{13} \\ F_{21} \\ F_{22} \\ F_{23} \\ F_{31} \\ F_{32} \\ F_{33} \end{pmatrix} \quad (15)$$

where **A**' is the 3N×9 matrix of pixel coordinates,

$$\mathbf{A}' = \begin{pmatrix} x_1 & y_1 & 1 & 0 & 0 & 0 & 0 & 0 & 0 \\ 0 & 0 & 0 & x_1 & y_1 & 1 & 0 & 0 & 0 \\ 0 & 0 & 0 & 0 & 0 & 0 & x_1 & y_1 & 1 \\ x_2 & y_2 & 1 & 0 & 0 & 0 & 0 & 0 & 0 \\ 0 & 0 & 0 & x_2 & y_2 & 1 & 0 & 0 & 0 \\ 0 & 0 & 0 & 0 & 0 & 0 & x_2 & y_2 & 1 \\ \cdots \\ \cdots \\ \cdots \\ x_N & y_N & 1 & 0 & 0 & 0 & 0 & 0 & 0 \\ 0 & 0 & 0 & x_N & y_N & 1 & 0 & 0 & 0 \\ 0 & 0 & 0 & 0 & 0 & 0 & x_N & y_N & 1 \end{pmatrix} \quad (16)$$

and **B**' is the 3N vector of frame coordinates,

$$\mathbf{B}' = \begin{pmatrix} X_1 \\ Y_1 \\ Z_1 \\ X_2 \\ Y_2 \\ Z_2 \\ \cdot \\ \cdot \\ \cdot \\ X_N \\ Y_N \\ Z_N \end{pmatrix} \quad (17)$$

⋆ Indeed, as noted by Galloway & Maciunas (1990), nine such points are available for the BRW localizer.

A least squares solution is then given by

$$f' = (A')^{-} B' \qquad (18)$$

where $(\mathbf{A}')^{-}$ is the generalized inverse of $\mathbf{A}'$ as given by SVD. The desired matrix **F** is then built from the elements of f' according to the definition of equation (15).

Volume transformation matrix

For certain applications it is necessary to have a single coordinate transformation between the tomographic volume (voxel coordinates) and the frame coordinate system. For example, it is not convenient to use the STMs to map a point of known frame coordinates on to a volume data set. On the other hand, it is useful to manipulate the tomographic volume as a whole, for example when the volume is matched stereotactically to data from another modality, as described later.

It is possible to define a single global transformation, contained in a 4×4 matrix, for the whole volume. In order to be able to do this the slices must be parallel, equally spaced and aligned. In other words the slices must be such that the volume they form can be mapped on to frame coordinates via a rigid body transformation (translation and rotation), scaling and skew. If one of the slices has been shifted then a global transformation matrix derived from points in the other slices will not be accurate for that slice. If the slices are not equidistant or not parallel then the global transformation matrix will not allow the Z voxel axis (which a priori is the slice number) to be properly mapped onto frame coordinates.

If the data satisfy the above geometric conditions, then it is a simple generalization of the concepts of the preceding section to calculate the VTM, F. Therefore, instead of having a different 3×3 matrix for each slice, a single 4×4 matrix is used throughout the volume with the voxel coordinates being composed of the in-slice pixel coordinates, x and y, and the slice number, z*.

* In the case of unevenly spaced parallel slices, one can map the Z voxel axis on to an axis Z' such that the slices have a z' corresponding to the relative separation. In order to do this one must know their separation in real-world units (millimetres).

A minimum of four fiducial points is now needed in order to define the transformation. One can then write the equation corresponding to equation (10) for the whole volume as a product of 4×4 matrices:

$$\mathbf{B} = \mathrm{F}\mathbf{A}, \qquad (19)$$

where

$$\mathbf{A} = (\underline{\boldsymbol{x}}_1\ \underline{\boldsymbol{x}}_2\ \underline{\boldsymbol{x}}_3\ \underline{\boldsymbol{x}}_4) \qquad (20)$$

and

$$\mathbf{B} = (\underline{\boldsymbol{X}}_1\ \underline{\boldsymbol{X}}_2\ \underline{\boldsymbol{X}}_3\ \underline{\boldsymbol{X}}_4) \qquad (21)$$

Again,

$$\mathrm{F} = \mathbf{B}\mathbf{A}^{-1}, \qquad (22)$$

The four points necessary to calculate the transformation matrix must not lie on a plane, which in turn means that no three points should be colinear. If so, **A** would then be singular since it would be possible to put it in a form having a row of zeros through the elementary row/column operations. Geometrically, three points are necessary to determine the position, orientation and size of the slices; the fourth point is necessary to obtain the scaling along the axis perpendicular to the slice plane. A straightforward choice is therefore to select three points in one slice and a fourth one in a different slice.

In order to obtain a better estimate of F in the least squares sense, one must use more fiducials than the minimum of four. This is due to the error in localizing the fiducials in the images. Using all available points (i.e. three in each slice) will give a matrix F which is more accurate for the whole volume. Again, SVD may be used to calculate the best matrix F in a least squares sense. **A** is rewritten as a $3N \times 12$ matrix similar to A' (equation (16)) with an extra z_i entry in each row. The 12 non-trivial elements of F are put into a 12-vector and **B** is put into a $3N$ vector identical to **B**' in equation (17).

The use of a VTM instead of the STMs can introduce a degradation of the accuracy of localization. The amount of inaccuracy is dependent on the degree of misalignment of the slices. This inaccuracy can be measured by calculating the difference between the calculated frame coordinates of a number of selected voxels using the STMs and the VTM:

$$\boldsymbol{Dx} = | \mathbf{F}\boldsymbol{x} - \mathbf{F}\underline{\boldsymbol{x}} | . \qquad (23)$$

The geometric inconsistencies can be reduced

by fixing the frame to the scanner table in order to limit patient movement. However, it may be possible to 'correct' this problem, as discussed in a further section.

IMAGE ANALYSIS AND STEREOTACTIC LOCALIZATION

Volume resampling

Volume resampling (also called *reconstruction*) is the process by which a new data set is obtained by resampling the volume of data along a different plane. An example is the reconstruction of sagittal slices from an axial data set. One can also imagine two stereotactic data sets of different modalities (MRI and CT, for example) where a fraction of the two sets overlaps in real space but the slices of which might not coincide. If one wants to do a direct comparison of the two sets of images slice by slice, then one must be able to reconstruct one of the sets such that the slices in both coincide. We will discuss how this can be done based on the concept of coordinate transformation.

The method we describe is based on the fact that resampling is simply a coordinate transformation, where the value of the resampled voxel at coordinates $\underline{\boldsymbol{x}}'$, $\mathbf{I}'(\underline{\boldsymbol{x}}')$ is equal to that of the voxel at $\underline{\boldsymbol{x}}$, $\mathbf{I}(\underline{\boldsymbol{x}})$,

$$\mathbf{I}'(\underline{\boldsymbol{x}}') = \mathbf{I}(\underline{\boldsymbol{x}}), \tag{24}$$

where

$$\underline{\boldsymbol{x}} = \mathbf{M}\underline{\boldsymbol{x}}'. \tag{25}$$

$\mathbf{M}$ is the 4×4 transformation matrix which maps resampled voxel coordinates on to original voxel coordinates. The *reconstruction matrix*, $\mathbf{M}$, represents the geometric relationship between the original data and the reconstructed image (data set). Since $\mathbf{I}(\ )$ and $\mathbf{I}'(\ )$ are discrete functions, this is strictly true only if $\underline{\boldsymbol{x}}$ falls precisely on a voxel. Equation (24) therefore represents the nearest neighbour case, where $\underline{\boldsymbol{x}}$ is rounded to the nearest voxel in the original data. If an interpolating algorithm is used, the value $\mathbf{I}(\ )$ can be calculated for any $\underline{\boldsymbol{x}}$.

The problem of resampling is the calculation of the mapping $\mathbf{M}$. From a computational point of view it is not efficient to calculate the product (25) at each resampled voxel. Instead, we use a stepping process between neighbouring voxels in a row-by-row and slice-by-slice fashion. This is described in the section entitled 'The stepping process'.

Stereotactic reconstruction

Imagine that we have two tomographic data sets, for example CT and MRI, which span approximately the same physical volume, but with different orientations and slice spacing, as illustrated in Figure 12.4. We want to resample one of the two data sets according to the sampling in the other, called the *master* side. In order to resample a data set V_2 according to the slice orientation of data set V_1 one has to calculate the matrix $\mathbf{M}_{12}$ which maps the voxels in V_1 on to V_2. If the two data sets have been acquired in a stereotactically consistent fashion, then the frame transformation matrices F_2 and F_1 both relate the voxels in V_1 and V_2 to the same coordinate system. The voxel coordinates in V_1, $\underline{\boldsymbol{x}}'$, are first mapped to the frame and then mapped on to V_2:

$$\boldsymbol{x} = F_2^{-1}\,(F_1\,\underline{\boldsymbol{x}}'). \tag{26}$$

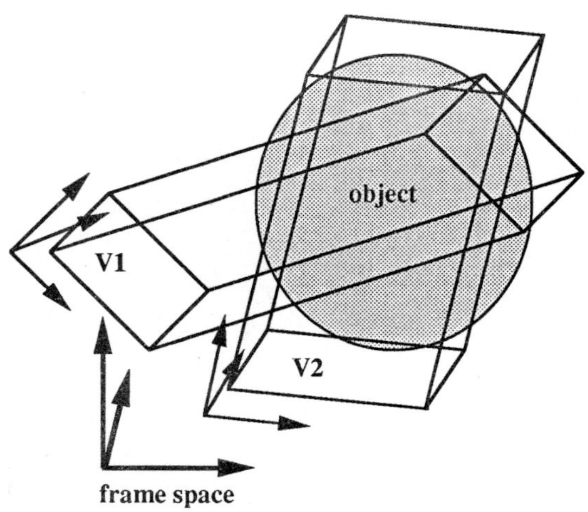

Fig. 12.4 Representation of two volume data sets which overlap in frame space. For example, CT and MRI data sets acquired along planes at different orientation. The accurate comparison of anatomical features in the two sets is possible if the frame remains fixed relative to the skull.

The desired matrix **M** is therefore given by the product

$$\mathbf{M}_{12} = F_2^{-1} F_1. \quad (27)$$

Stereotactic slice reconstruction

To increase the accuracy, instead of resampling V_2 according to V_1 one may also resample V_2 according to a single slice in V_1, using the STM **F**, of equation (6) instead of F_1. In order to calculate $\mathbf{M}_{12}$, **F** must be augmented to a 4×4 form, F_{1S}, in the following way*:

$$F_{1s} = \begin{pmatrix} F_{11} & F_{12} & 0 & F_{13} \\ F_{21} & F_{22} & 0 & F_{23} \\ F_{31} & F_{32} & 1 & F_{33} \\ 0 & 0 & 0 & 1 \end{pmatrix}. \quad (28)$$

M is given by the product (see Fig. 12.5)

$$\mathbf{M}_{12} = F_2^{-1} F_{1s}. \quad (29)$$

Obviously the resampling process then has to be limited to a single slice.

An example of stereotactic reconstruction is given in Figure 12.6. The data sets were acquired with different patients, and therefore are not anatomically consistent. Nonetheless, the result serves to illustrate the principle, as the fiducials appear at the same position in both images.

The stepping process

As explained before, the resampling of a tomographic volume data set requires the calculation of the transformed coordinates of the resampled voxels on to the original volume according to equation (25). Instead, we make use of the fact that the voxels are on a regular array. On a given row the coordinates of the current resampled voxel, x'_i, are given by the 3-vector sum of the coordinates of the preceding voxel and the unit vector along the row axis, $(\boldsymbol{u}')'$:

$$\boldsymbol{x}'_i = \boldsymbol{x}'_{i-1} + (\mathbf{u}_{x'})'. \quad (30)$$

The $(\boldsymbol{u}_x')'$ step is mapped on to the original coordinate system via the 3×3 submatrix† of **M**, *M*:

$$\boldsymbol{u}_x' = \mathbf{M}(\boldsymbol{u}_{x'})'. \quad (31)$$

* Since there is no information on the mapping of the Z_1 axis, the contents of the third column can be set arbitrarily.

† By the scaling and rotation submatrix we mean the top left 3×3 submatrix. No translation is needed since $\boldsymbol{u}'$ is a free vector.

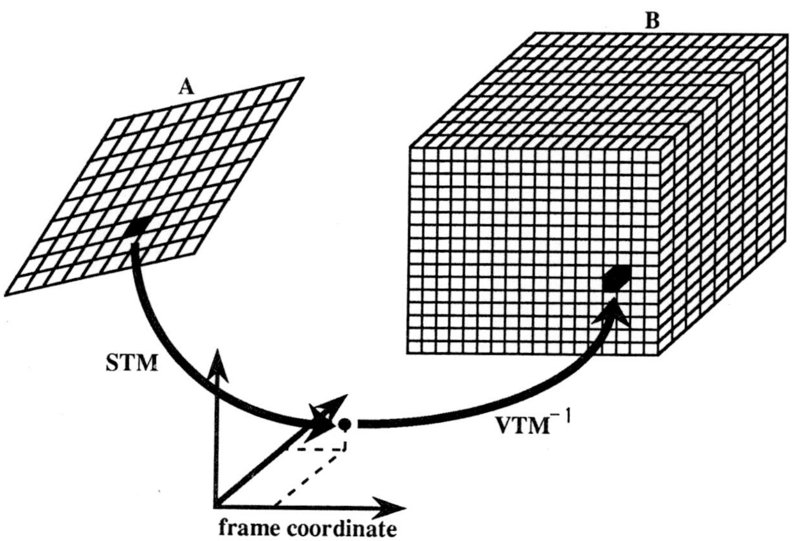

Fig. 12.5 Illustration of the principle of stereotactic reconstruction for a single slice. The mapping of the pixels in a slice in data set *A* on to the voxels in a set *B* via the STM of *A* and the inverse of the VTM of *B*.

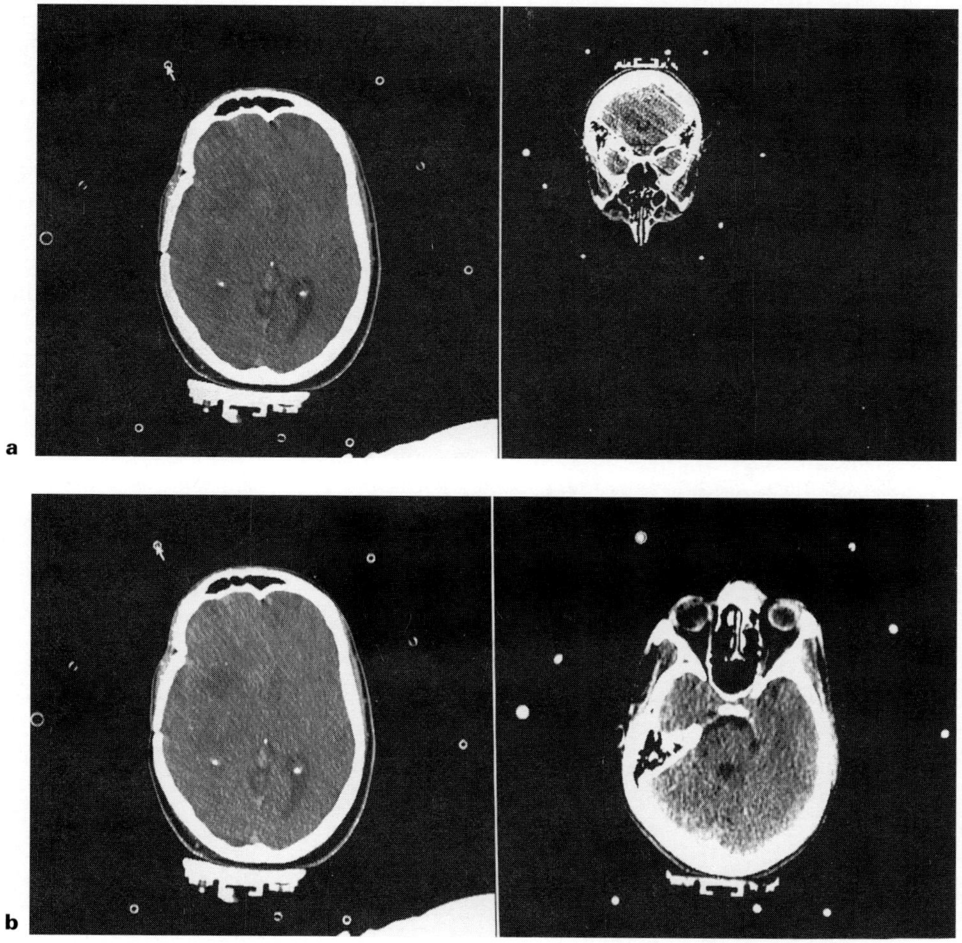

Fig. 12.6 Example of stereotactic reconstruction. In order to illustrate the principle two CT data sets were used. **a** Original data: the data set on the left consists of 12 512x512 slices with a separation of 4 mm; the set on the right consists of 15 320x320 slices with a separation of 5 mm. **b** The image on the right was obtained by resampling the right hand side set according to the plane defined by the slice on the left. The coordinates of the nine fiducials in both images agree to within one pixel. (Scans are from different patients, see text.)

M is called the *step matrix*. It consists of the three 3-vectors $\boldsymbol{u}$ corresponding to the displacements along the X', Y' and Z' axes. Once the values for $\boldsymbol{u}_{x'}$ have been calculated using equation (31) the stepping process can be expressed in the original data set. We then have

$$\boldsymbol{x}_i = \boldsymbol{x}_{i\text{-}1} + \boldsymbol{u}_x'. \quad (32)$$

This equation, along with similar equations in y and z, is therefore used to calculate the coordinates of the resampled voxels in equation (25). The process is started at the origin of the resampled data set, $(0\ 0\ 0\ 1)^{\mathrm{T}}$. The coordinates in the original data set are given by

$$\underline{\boldsymbol{x}}_0 = \mathbf{M}\begin{pmatrix}0\\0\\0\\1\end{pmatrix}, \quad (33)$$

which is called the *starting vector*. At the end of each row in the resampled data one has to step by $\boldsymbol{u}_{Y'}$ in the Y direction, then by $\boldsymbol{u}_{z'}$ in the Z direction to move up one slice. Therefore, each step involves only three additions, instead of nine multiplications and three additions as in equation (25).

The stepping process described above can be seen as a general tool for image reconstruction, as it is used to calculate the coordinates of successive resampling points. It can be used to step along arbitrary planes with arbitrary step sizes, with original voxels of arbitrary size and with any interpolating algorithm.

Calculation of frame coordinates from reconstructed data

The calculation of the frame coordinates of the resampled voxels follows the same lines as the resampling process. The point of interest in the resampled image, $\underline{\boldsymbol{x}}'$, is mapped on to original data set voxel coordinates, $\underline{\boldsymbol{x}}$, via the reconstruction matrix **M** as in equation (25). The VTM F (or STM **F**) for the original data set is then used to map this point on to frame coordinates (see Fig. 12.7). Therefore,

$$\underline{\boldsymbol{X}} = \mathrm{F}(\mathbf{M}\underline{\boldsymbol{x}}'). \qquad (34)$$

In order to be accurate the mapping from resampled to original data depends upon whether the resampling algorithm used is based on nearest neighbour or more sophisticated interpolation (i.e. trilinear interpolation, see Parker et al 1983). Equation (34) is a general equation where the VTM is used because it applies to all voxel space. However, it is effectively accurate only if the resampled value corresponds to the exact position specified by the mapping **M**, which is the case for trilinear interpolation.

In the case of nearest neighbour resampling the displayed value is that of the voxel nearest to the one specified by **M**. Therefore, it is necessary to use a different mapping for the calculation of the coordinates: from resampled voxel coordinates to nearest original voxel coordinates, then to the frame coordinate system using the STM of the original data:

$$\underline{\boldsymbol{X}} = \mathbf{F}_z \mathrm{nint}(\mathbf{M}\underline{\boldsymbol{x}}), \qquad (35)$$

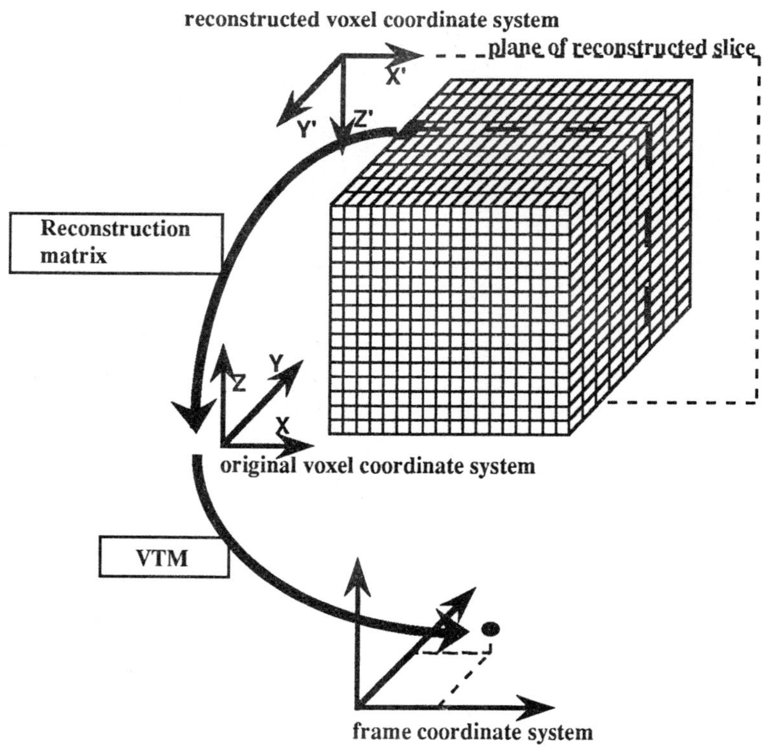

Fig. 12.7 Calculation of frame coordinates from reconstructed data. The reconstruction matrix maps reconstructed voxels(or pixels) on to original voxel coordinates. As explained in the text, this depends on the interpolating algorithm. The VTM is then used to calculate the frame coordinates.

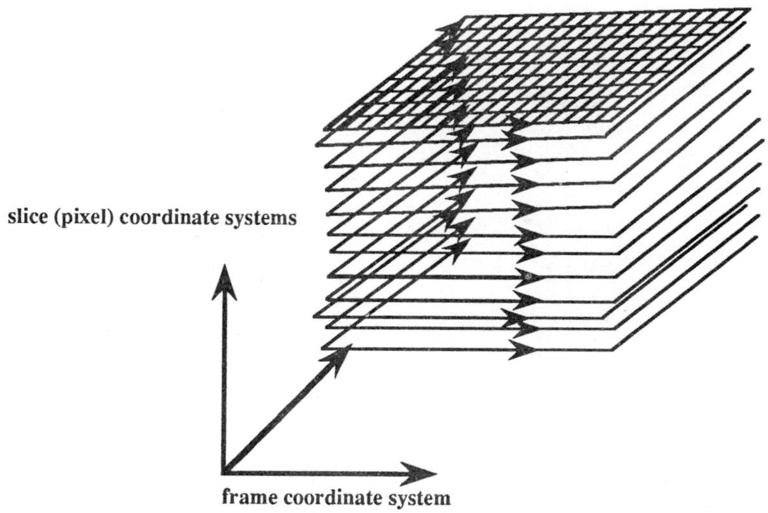

Fig. 12.8 Representation of misalignment of data set in frame space due to patient movement. Assuming that the positional information in each individual slice is coherent, it is possible to reconstruct a data set consisting of cubic voxels by interpolating along a cubic array.

where 'nint' represents the nearest integer. $\mathbf{F}_z$ is the STM for slice z, the Z component of nint($\mathbf{M}\underline{\boldsymbol{x}}$):

$$z = \text{nint}(\mathbf{M}\,\underline{\boldsymbol{x}})_z. \tag{36}$$

For stereotactic reconstruction, **M** is given by equation (27). For nearest neighbour resampling, substituting equation (27) in equation (35):

$$\underline{\boldsymbol{X}} = \mathbf{F}_{2z}\text{nint}[(\mathrm{F}_2^{-1}\,\mathrm{F}_1)\underline{\boldsymbol{x}}], \tag{37}$$

where $\mathbf{F}_{2z}$ is the STM of slice z(the Z component of nint[(F_2^{-1} F_1)$\underline{\boldsymbol{x}}$]). In the case of trilinear interpolation the resampled value is calculated at the position specified by the frame coordinates of the resampled voxel. Indeed, substituting F_2 for F and using equation (27), equation (34) becomes

$$\underline{\boldsymbol{X}} = \mathrm{F}_1\underline{\boldsymbol{x}}. \tag{38}$$

Therefore, the coordinates of the resampled voxels are the same as those of the master data set (V_1).

Correction of geometric inconsistencies and cubic voxels

As discussed previously, the accuracy of localization based on the VTM depends on inconsistencies in the geometry of acquisition of the data. Expressed in frame coordinates (using the individual STMs) the data can be described as a set of randomly distributed data points. More precisely, the voxels are regularly arranged within the slices*, but these may have irregular orientation and position (see Fig. 12.8). In other words, the voxels are not 'cubic'. As discussed in (Pelizzari et al 1989, Henri et al 1991), it is often advantageous to have a data set consisting of cubic voxels. Let us briefly discuss a possible solution to this problem based on the VTM†.

The first step in obtaining cubic voxels is the resampling of the data along a regular grid. As discussed previously, the VTM can account for rotations, translation, scaling and skew. Therefore, by using the VTM as a stepping matrix to resample the data set one can obtain voxels forming a volume which in general has the shape of a skewed rectangular box. In this instance the data consists of voxel values and voxel frame coordinates calculated using the

* We are not considering the issue of geometric distortion in MRI (see Schad et al 1987).

† The best results are likely to be obtained with the best data. Therefore, rigid fixation of the frame to the scanner couch will ensure that the slices are parallel.

appropriate STM. There are a number of algorithms for the interpolation of arbitrarily distributed data points (Sheppard 1968, Hayes & Halliday 1974). Some involve the determination of a number of nearest neighbours for each sampling point. In our case, the determination of the nearest neighbours may be facilitated by the fact that the data points lie on a nearly regular grid, and therefore can be referenced by integer indexing.

If the data were acquired with the scanner gantry not perpendicular to the scanning axis, then the resampled voxel coordinate axes are skewed relative to the frame coordinate axes, as illustrated in Figure 12.9. Therefore, if necessary, a skew correction may be applied (Collins & Henry 1991) and supplementary slices generated in order to obtain cubic voxels.

CONCLUSION

We have presented a review of mathematical methods useful for the analysis of tomographic image data acquired under stereotactic conditions. The stereotactic frame allows the determination of transformations which map pixel coordinates on to the stereotactic frame coordinate system. We have also shown how, under certain conditions, this can be extended to the whole volume data set, although possibly at the cost of accuracy loss. This leads to a unified formalism for the manipulation and display of tomographic images based entirely on coordinate transformations.

It is important to note that the determination of the VTM does not have to rely on stereotactic fiducials. In particular the determination of anatomically based coordinate systems allows the accurate comparison of data from various modalities and from different scanning sessions (Pelizzari et al 1989, Hill & Hawkes 1991). However, the determination of anatomically based coordinate systems relies on the identification of points or features *throughout* the image data, contrary to the stereotactic frame, which defines the coordinate system within each slice. This may limit the accuracy of localization as geometric inconsistencies in the data may not be recovered. Furthermore, in a surgical context there remains the problem of determining the position of the surgical tools relative to the coordinate system. Depending on the level of accuracy available through such techniques, they may one day also provide the basis for a non-invasive alternative to the stereotactic frame.

APPENDIX

Calculation of a 4x4 STM for the projection of points across slices

We have seen that the 3 x 3 STM maps a 2D space (the image space) on to 3D space (the frame

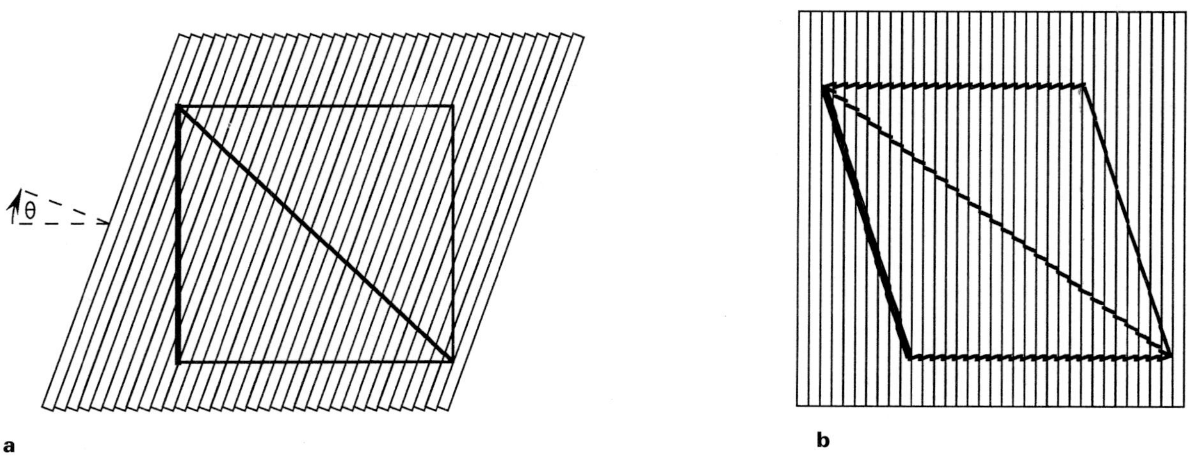

Fig. 12.9 Skew effect due to scanner gantry tilt relative to the the scanning axis. The skew angle, θ, is given by the angle between the *Z* (slice number) voxel axis and the voxel axis in the plane of skew (i.e. plane of the drawing in this example) expressed in the frame coordinate system.

space). The STM contains no information on the 'third dimension' of the image. This has the effect that points in frame space which are not in the plane of the slice are not mapped on to the image in a geometrically consistent way. However, by defining a third axis relative to the plane, we can correct this. In particular, we may take this axis to be perpendicular to the plane of the slice. Then, a point outside the plane of the slice will be mapped to the point on the plane nearest to it.

We know that the coordinates of at least four points, and not all coplanar, are needed to calculate the VTM which maps two 3D spaces. For a single tomographic slice, no non-coplanar point is available. However, such a point may be 'created' by taking the normal to the plane, therefore expanding the image space from 2D to 3D. As before, we take the (minimum) three points in the plane and assign them to the **z** = 0 plane,

$$\begin{pmatrix} x_1 \\ y_1 \\ 0 \\ 1 \end{pmatrix}, \begin{pmatrix} x_2 \\ y_2 \\ 0 \\ 1 \end{pmatrix}, \begin{pmatrix} x_3 \\ y_3 \\ 0 \\ 1 \end{pmatrix} \tag{A1}$$

in the expanded image coordinate system. In frame space,

$$\begin{pmatrix} X_1 \\ Y_1 \\ Z_1 \\ 1 \end{pmatrix} \begin{pmatrix} X_2 \\ Y_2 \\ Z_2 \\ 1 \end{pmatrix} \begin{pmatrix} X_3 \\ Y_3 \\ Z_3 \\ 1 \end{pmatrix}. \tag{A2}$$

The fourth point may be given coordinates

$$\begin{pmatrix} x_1 \\ y_1 \\ 1 \\ 1 \end{pmatrix} \tag{A3}$$

in the expanded image coordinate system, and

$$\begin{pmatrix} X_1+N_x \\ Y_1+N_y \\ Z_1+N_z \\ 1 \end{pmatrix} \tag{A4}$$

in frame space, where N is the normalized vector product of the two difference vectors $(\boldsymbol{X}_2 - \boldsymbol{X}_1)$ and $(\boldsymbol{X}_3 - \boldsymbol{X}_1)$. A new 4×4 STM can then be calculated by matrix inversion or by SVD.

The inclusion of the perpendicular axis insures that a point outside the plane of the slice will be mapped on to the image at the point on the slice nearest to it*. Note that the Z axis of the expanded image coordinate system contains direction information but lacks a proper scale and sign.

REFERENCES

Brown R A 1979a A stereotactic head frame for use with CT body scanners. Investigative Radiology 14: 300–304

Brown R A 1979b A computerized tomography–computer graphics approach to stereotaxic localization. Journal of Neurosurgery 50: 715–720

Brown R A, Roberts T S, Osborne A G 1980 Stereotaxic frame and computer software for CT-directed neurosurgical localization. Investigative Radiology 15(4): 308–312

Collins D L, Henri C J 1991 Personal communication

Galloway R L, Maciunas R J, 1990 Stereotactic neurosurgery. Clinical Reviews in Biomedical Engineering 18(3): 181–205

Gonzalez R C, Wintz P 1987 Digital image processing, 2nd ed., Addison-Wesley, Reading

Hayes J G, Halliday J 1974 The least-squares fitting of cubic spline surfaces to general data sets. Journal of the Institute of Mathematics and its Applications 14: 89–103

Henri C J, Collins D L, Peters T M 1991 Multimodality image integration for stereotactic surgical planning. Medical Physics 18(2): 167–177

Hill D L G, Hawkes D J 1991 3D Synergistic imaging as an aid to image interpretation and surgical planning. Presented at the Imaging Techniques for Medicine Colloquium, The Institution of Electrical Engineers, London, 18 April

Leksell L, Jernberg B 1980 Stereotaxis and tomography — a technical note. Acta Neurochirurgica 52: 1–7

Noble B, Daniel J W 1977 Applied linear algebra, 2nd ed, Prentice-Hall, Englewood Cliffs

Olivier A, Peters T, Bertrand G 1985 Stereotactic system and apparatus for use with MRI, CT, and DSA. Applied Neurophysiology 48: 94–96

Parker J A, Kenyon R V, Troxel D E 1983 Comparison of interpolating methods for image resampling. IEEE Transactions on Medical Imaging 2(1): 31–39

Pelizzari C A, Chen G T Y, Spelbring D R, Weichslebaum R R, Chen C T 1989 Accurate three-dimensional registration of CT, PET, and/or MR images of the brain. Journal of Computer Assisted Tomography 13(1): 20–26

Press W H, Flannery B P, Teukolsky S A, Vetterling W T 1988 Numerical recipes in C — the art of scientific computing, Cambridge University Press, Cambridge

Rogers D F, Adams J A 1990 Mathematical elements for computer graphics, 2nd edn. McGraw-Hill, New York

Schad L, Lott S, Schmitt F, Sturm V, Lorenz W J 1987 Correction of spatial distorsion in MR imaging: a prerequisite for accurate stereotaxy. Journal of Computer Assisted Tomography 11(3): 499–505

Shepard D 1968 A two-dimensional interpolation function

* Recall that the distance between a point and a plane is minimum along the perpendicular to the plane which includes the point.

for irregularly-spaced data. Proceedings of the 23rd National Conference ACM, Brandon/Systems Press, Princeton, pp 517–523

Weaver K, Smith V, Lewis J D, Lulu B, Barnett C M, Leibel S A, Gutin P, Larson D, Phillips T 1990 A CT-based computerized treatment planning system for I-125 stereotactic brain implants. International Journal of Radiation, Oncology, Biology, Physics 18: 445–454

PART 3 THE MATHEMATICS OF STEREOTACTIC LOCALIZATION AND MULTIMODALITY IMAGE MATCHING BASED ON PROJECTION RADIOGRAPHY

C. J. Henri D. L. Collins T. M. Peters

INTRODUCTION

Before the advent of tomographic imaging modalities, stereotactic neurosurgery was most commonly planned using projection radiographic techniques. Although these methods have been largely supplanted by CT and MRI, certain radiographic procedures, like angiography, are still performed. Because tomographic and radiographic images represent inherently different views of an object, the mathematics required to localize targets in each case also differ. For a tomographic image, there is a transformation matrix that allows us to determine the frame coordinates of a target given its position in the image (see previous part). Furthermore, the reverse transformation of coordinates may be accomplished via the inverse of this matrix, thus enabling us to switch freely between the coordinate systems of the image and stereotactic frame.

For a radiographic image, however, the situation is less straightforward. Here a single point in the image is the superposition of every point that lies along a ray emanating from the focal spot. This 'many-to-one' mapping does not allow us to determine the 3D frame coordinates of a point based on its position in an image. However, the reverse transformation is easily accomplished, enabling us to plot the position of a target if its coordinates have been determined previously or are known a priori.

In order to derive the frame coordinates of a target using radiographic images, two or more distinct projections are required. The target is subsequently identified in each image then, together with a description of the imaging geometries, a *triangulation* is performed to obtain the desired 3D frame coordinates.

In the following discussion, these procedures are described mathematically using a matrix formulation similar to the one used to describe target localization in tomographic images (see Part 2 of this chapter). We include a brief description of stereoscopic techniques in order to illustrate several aspects of the discussion to follow. In a later section, we address the issue of correlating observations among tomographic and radiographic data sets. Here we describe a method for combining the two for visualization purposes.

STEREOTACTIC TARGET LOCALIZATION USING PROJECTION RADIOGRAPHY

Image–frame coordinate transformations

A fundamental difference between tomographic and radiographic imaging modalities is that the former yield *orthographic* cross-sectional views of the object while the latter are *perspective* projections through the object's entire volume. The transformations we seek, therefore, must take into account the differential magnification inherent in a given projection. This is accomplished conveniently using a homogeneous coordinate representation. The discussion presented here follows the principles outlined by Sutherland (1974). (This reference provides an excellent description of the underlying mathematics and geometrical considerations involved.)

We represent the coordinates of a 3D point as a four-component vector $(\alpha x, \alpha y, \alpha z, \alpha)$, where α is the homogeneous scaling factor and (x, y, z) are the 3D coordinates of a given point. These coordinates are transformed into those of a different 3D coordinate system via a 4×4 homogeneous transformation matrix. The 16 elements of this matrix account for rotation, scaling, translation and perspective between the two coordinate systems, thus completely describing the transformations between them. The problem here, however, requires only a transformation from 3D frame coordinates to 2D image coordinates.

In this case, we may delete the third column of the 4 × 4 matrix since the image plane is at a fixed distance, z, from the focal spot (X-ray source). When we multiply the four-component vector, $(x, y, z, 1)$, by the remaining 4 × 3 matrix, we obtain a three-component vector, as follows:

$$(\gamma u \ \gamma v \ \gamma)=(x \ y \ z \ 1)\begin{bmatrix} m_{11} & m_{12} & m_{13} \\ m_{21} & m_{22} & m_{23} \\ m_{31} & m_{32} & m_{33} \\ m_{41} & m_{42} & m_{43} \end{bmatrix} \qquad (1)$$

Here u and v are image coordinates specified in pixels, and γ is an arbitrary scaling factor. The coordinates u and v are obtained by dividing the first two terms of the three-component vector by the third term, γ. The problem remains to determine the 12 elements of the 4 × 3 matrix.

This is accomplished in a manner similar to the approach used for tomographic image data; specifically, by using the fiducial markers appearing in each image. The fiducial markers serve as points whose 3D frame coordinates are known and whose corresponding positions in the image may be determined. In the case of radiography, the fiducials are usually small radiopaque pellets on the frame that are easily identified in each image. For algebraic consistency reasons, it is important that these points avoid certain 'degenerate' configurations*. In practice, eight fiducials are usually employed; each located at the corner of a cube surrounding the patient's head. In order to see how these points facilitate target localization, we perform the matrix multiplication in equation (1) to obtain three equations. After substituting the homogeneous coordinate, γ, into the first two and simplifying, we have the following two equations:

$$(m_{11}-m_{13}u)x+(m_{21}-m_{23}u)y+(m_{31}-m_{33}u)z+(m_{41}-m_{43}u)=0 \qquad (2)$$

and

$$(m_{12}-m_{13}v)x+(m_{22}-m_{23}v)y-(m_{32}-m_{33}v)z-(m_{42}-m_{43}v)=0. \qquad (3)$$

We see that for any point having real-world (i.e. frame) coordinates (x, y, z) and image coordinates (u, v), two equations are available in terms of the 12 m_{ij}. Six such points provide 12 equations; enough to solve for the elements of the transformation matrix.

Since each of the eight fiducial markers yields a pair of equations from equations (2) and (3), we have a total of 16 equations in the 12 m_{ij} unknowns. These equations may be written compactly as follows:

$$\mathbf{A}\boldsymbol{x} = 0, \qquad (4)$$

where $\mathbf{A}$ is a 16 x 12 matrix comprising (known) elements determined from the image and frame coordinates of each fiducial, and $\boldsymbol{x}$ is a vector comprising the 12 (unknown) elements of the desired 4 × 3 matrix.

Since equation (4) is homogeneous, it contains an arbitrary scale factor which allows us to set m_{43} in the vector $\boldsymbol{x}$ equal to 1. This allows us to rewrite equation (4) as

$$\mathbf{A}\chi = \boldsymbol{b}, \qquad (5)$$

where $\mathbf{A}$ is now a (known) 16 x 11 matrix; χ is a vector comprising 11 (unknown) elements, and $\boldsymbol{b}$ is a (known) 16 element vector resulting from having set m_{43} equal to 1 in equation (4). This over-determined system of equations may be solved using the technique described earlier (see Part 2). The 4 × 3 transformation matrix may then be used to determine where a given point, specified in frame coordinates, appears in the radiographic image. The following section addresses the issue of deriving the frame coordinates for a point given its position in two or more images acquired from different viewpoints.

3D target localization via triangulation

For a given projection and associated transformation matrix along with the image coordinates of a desired target, we are able to rewrite equations (2) and (3), respectively, as

$$a_2x+b_2y+c_2z+d_2= 0 \qquad (6)$$

and

$$a_3x+b_3y+c_3z+d_3=0, \qquad (7)$$

* No more than four points may be coplanar (Adams 1981).

where *a*, *b*, *c* and *d* correspond to the terms in parentheses in equations (2) and (3).

These equations represent geometrical planes whose intersection defines a line between the focal spot and image plane on which the target point must lie. Given a second projection with its transformation matrix and the image coordinates of the desired target point, we obtain a second pair of equations from equations (6) and (7). This yields a total of four equations in the three unknowns (x, y and z), which can then be solved in the same fashion as equation (5), above.

This process, referred to as 'triangulation', can be thought of as finding the coordinates of the point where the two rays between each image plane and focal spot intersect. It is important to note, however, that with uncertainties in the measured image coordinates the rays may no longer intersect. This means that the solution to the above system of equations is rarely exact and represents only the best solution in the least squares sense. The need for a robust (i.e. numerically stable) algorithm such as SVD is now understood. While any two images may be used for triangulation purposes, the difference in imaging geometries influences the accuracy of the results. As we will see below, this is an important consideration when deriving coordinates from images acquired stereoscopically.

STEREOSCOPY IN STEREOTACTIC NEUROSURGERY PLANNING

As we have seen above, stereotactic target localization using radiographic images requires the use of two or more projections acquired from different viewpoints. In this section we describe the use of stereoscopic imaging techniques in planning stereotactic procedures, and we comment on how the imaging geometries affect the localization results.

Stereoscopic image acquisition, visualization and analysis

Stereotactic procedures, by definition, require that targets be identified and measurements be performed in three dimensions. When using radiographic techniques, this is most commonly achieved using images acquired from orthogonal viewpoints; specifically, using lateral and antero-posterior projections. Since each image is inherently 2D, this method requires that the neurosurgeon draw upon his or her experience to assess the 3D spatial relationships between relevant structures in each of the two views. Difficulties arise, however, when there is some ambiguity in identifying the target, or when it is obscured in either of the images by overlying structures. Measurement accuracy can be affected and it may be difficult to obtain an appreciation of the target's position in relation to important anatomical landmarks. For this reason, a stereoscopic approach has some advantages over standard biplane methods.

Aside from the imaging geometries, the primary difference between the two techniques lies in how the data are analysed, i.e. how the observer infers 3D information from the images. Unlike a biplane approach in which the target is identified in each image independently of the other, a stereoscopic approach employs each image simultaneously and relies upon the observer to 'fuse' the images (via stereopsis) to perceive the object in three dimensions. The observers may, therefore, view the imaged structure directly without having to infer spatial relationships from separate projections. Although a target may still be obscured by overlying objects, the neurosurgeon often obtains valuable insights from his or her appreciation of the 3D structure that help to resolve further ambiguities (Worthington et al 1985). Fig. 12.10 illustrates an example of a stereoscopic digital subtraction angiogram.

Image acquisition, visualization and analysis

Stereoscopic image acquisition techniques vary and usually depend upon the intended application of the data. A number of authors have described mathematically the relationship between the shape of the perceived object and the image acquisition and viewing geometries (Jarre & Teschendorf 1933, Manilla 1956, Saunders 1968, DuMond 1932, Henri & Peters 1990). Their conclusions may be summarized as follows: *unless the acquisition geometry precisely*

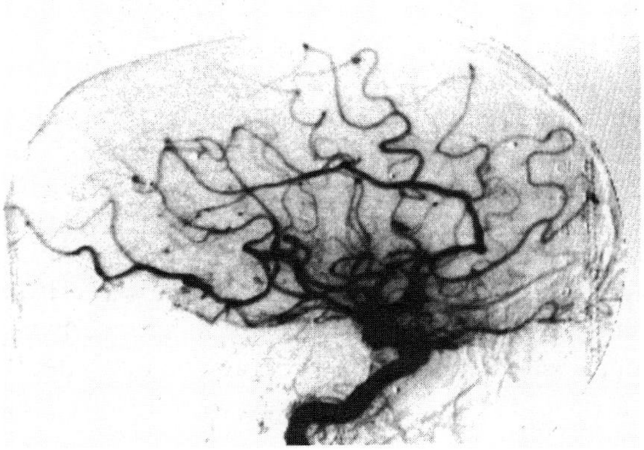

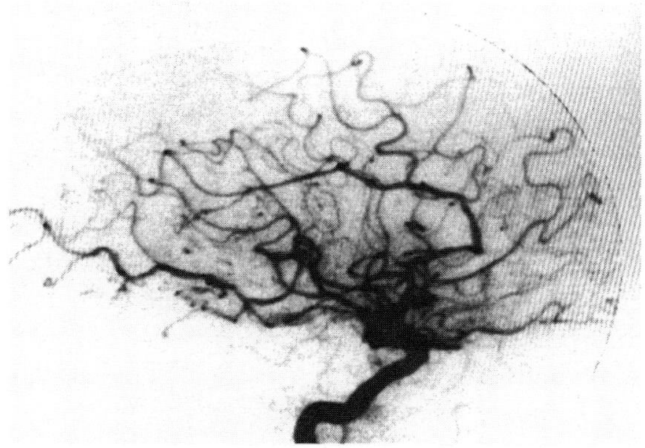

Fig. 12.10 A stereoscopic digital subtraction angiogram. A lateral view of the internal carotid arterial tree is shown here. The images are arranged for cross-eyed viewing (i.e. the stereo-pair may be fused by crossing one's eyes to the point where a third image appears between the given two. A 3D effect is achieved when this image is brought into focus).

matches the viewing geometry, the perceived structure will be distorted in shape and/or size when compared to its true form. We note that such idealized conditions are difficult to attain in practice and, in fact, are seldom sought. In most applications, the distortions are easily tolerated or simply do not affect the outcome of the given analysis. For this reason, there is a relatively wide range of 'acceptable' geometries that may be employed to acquire stereoscopic projections.

In practice, either of two acquisition techniques is commonly used (see Fig. 12.11). The first employs a lateral shift of the focal spot (or, alternatively, the patient) in a direction approximately parallel to the image plane (Sen et al 1983, Vogelsang & Dietz 1983, Hodges et al 1990). The second acquisition method employs a rotation of the imaging apparatus around the patient (Saunders 1968, Henri & Peters 1990).

In the past, a large number of stereoscopic viewing techniques and apparatus have been described, including simple cross-eyed viewing methods and stereoscopes using mirrors, lenses or a combination of both. Although these techniques are suitable for viewing purposes (i.e. qualitative analyses), they are difficult to use in

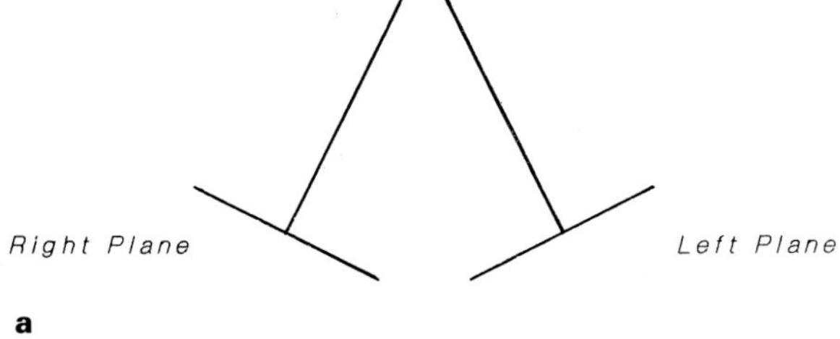

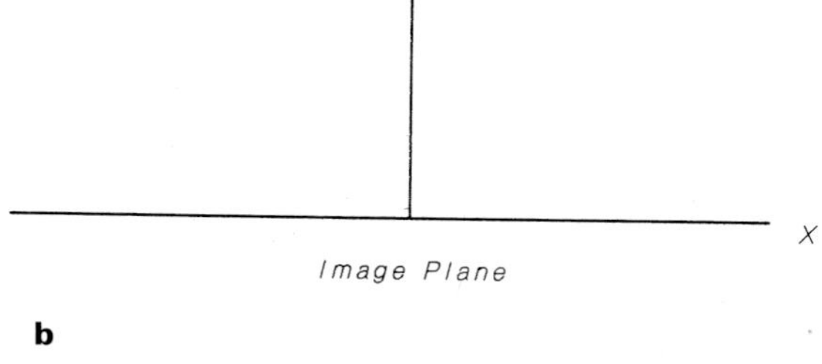

Fig. 12.11 Stereoscopic image acquisition geometries. Images are usually acquired using either **a** a rotation of the imaging apparatus around the object, or **b** by employing a lateral shift between the two centres of projection.

quantitative applications since there is no natural way to interact with the perceived structure. However, with new technologies for displaying digitized stereoscopic images, this is less of a problem. Several such systems have been described in the literature (Roese & Turner 1976, Lipton & Meyer 1984, Sand 1984, Haven 1987). The stereoscopic image is viewed on a high performance video monitor that displays right eye and left eye images alternately at a rate usually above 60 frames per second. The display of each image is synchronized with a 'polarizing shutter' in front of the monitor, allowing each image to be viewed through appropriately polarized glasses. A variation on this technique is to incorporate a shutter mechanism within the glasses themselves (Roese & Turner 1976).

Interaction with the perceived 3D object is achieved via computer graphics. A cursor drawn at the appropriate positions in each image appears as a single 3D cursor within the perceived object when viewed stereoscopically. By allowing the cursor to be manoeuvred in some fashion, it may then be used to identify targets, etc. Henri et al (1990) describe the operation of such a cursor using a conventional three-button mouse. 3D lines may be drawn and manipulated the same way, and are particularly useful for simulating the path for a biopsy needle or depth electrode.

MULTIMODALITY IMAGE MATCHING

In this section we describe a method to combine projection and tomographic image data to obtain a composite 3D view of the imaged structures. The aim here is to provide the surgeon with a method of visualizing the spatial relationships between complementary image data without having to derive such information from separate analyses. When the data are from CT and DSA, for instance, he may wish to understand how the vascular tree is oriented with respect to a target that is visible in only the CT data. While this information can be derived from a detailed analysis of the two data sets using the techniques discussed earlier, the approach described here is more convenient and better able to aid the surgeon in forming a 3D impression of the relevant anatomical structures.

The two types of data are combined by superimposing the projection image (DSA) on to a volume rendered image of CT or MRI data. In principle, the resulting composite image of anatomy and vasculature may then be used for surgical planning by treating it as an ordinary projection image and applying the analysis techniques described earlier.

The matching technique described here assumes that the rendered images are generated using orthographic projections (Pixar 1987, Drebin et al 1988). (Alternative ray tracing methods are more computationally intensive.) As a result, the tomographic volume must first be reshaped and oriented to yield a perspective view that matches the DSA projection. This will allow the two to be superimposed accurately in the sense that anatomical and vascular structures are correctly oriented with respect to each other in the final image.

In the following sections, we describe the mathematics involved in processing the tomographic data to obtain the desired view when rendered. We build upon the coordinate transformation methods described earlier and establish an improved understanding of the differences between those used for both tomographic and projection image data.

Methods

Having established the transformations between image and stereotactic frame coordinate systems (for CT, MRI and DSA), we begin by decomposing the DSA associated matrix into its components. The 4×3 matrix $\mathbf{M}$ comprises the following individual transformations: translation ($\mathbf{T}$), rotation ($\mathbf{R}$), perspective magnification ($\mathbf{P}$), scaling ($\mathbf{S}$) and cropping ($\mathbf{C}$). $\mathbf{M}$ may be expressed as the matrix resulting from the successive multiplication of each component (Strat 1984):

$$\mathbf{M} = \mathbf{TRPSC}. \qquad (8)$$

Since $\mathbf{M}$ implicitly describes the DSA image acquisition geometry, it provides sufficient information to generate a matching view of the tomographic volume.

The matrix decomposition may be accomplished either analytically (Ganapathy 1984) or

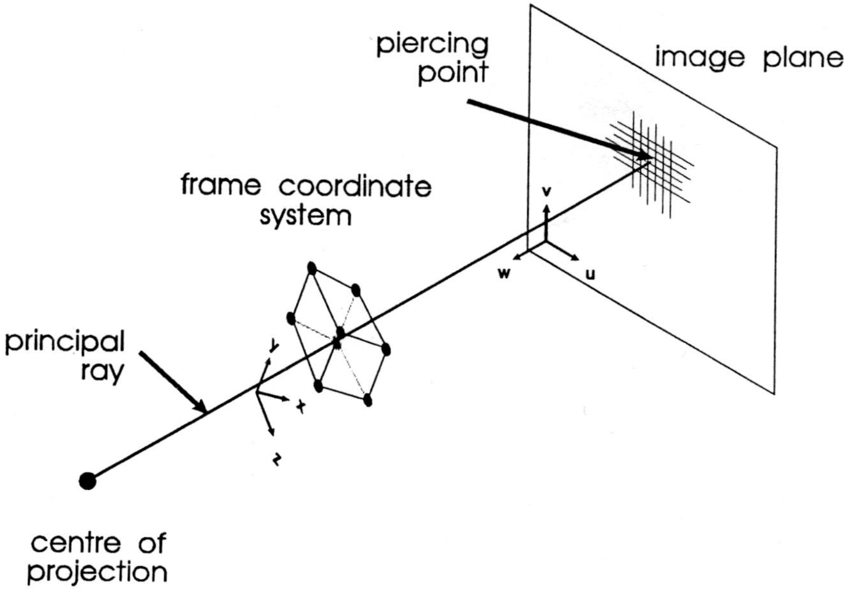

Fig. 12.12 Projection imaging geometry illustrating the coordinate systems of the stereotactic frame and image plane. A mathematical transformation determines where a given 3D point within the frame is projected in the image plane. Note that, by definition, the principal ray is orthogonal to the image plane.

geometrically (Strat 1984). Although it is possible to obtain each component of **M**, only the three rotation angles comprising **R** are required, as well as the *piercing point* from **C** (defined as the point in the image plane intersected by the principal ray (see Fig. 12.12)). Additional information is obtained at later stages in the matching process, as described below.

The tomographic data are loaded into the computer memory such that they comprise a 'volume' in which planes may be accessed perpendicular to any of the three cardinal axes (see Fig. 12.13). A skew correction is performed if necessary, and additional slices are interpolated, according to the imaged slice thickness, to give an isotropically scaled volume (i.e. with cubic voxels). The coordinate systems of the voxel based volume and the stereotactic frame may differ in translations, scaling and rotations. A transformation between the two may be represented as follows:

$$(u\ v\ w) = (x\ y\ z\ 1)\ \mathbf{N}. \qquad (9)$$

The 4×3 homogeneous matrix **N** (not to be confused with the DSA-associated matrix **M**) transforms the stereotactic frame coordinates (x, y, z) into corresponding values (u, v, w) within the voxel based volume (contained in the computer memory).

As described in the previous section, in order to determine **N** at least four points are required* whose corresponding positions (x_i, y_i, z_i) and u_i, v_i, w_i,) are known relative to both the frame and voxel based volume. These points are provided by the fiducial markers on the stereotactic frame and may be determined from at least two of the original (non-interpolated) slices within the volume. Thus, equation (9) expands to give the expression

$$\mathbf{V} = \mathbf{FN}, \qquad (10)$$

where the rows in **V** contain the *volume* coordinates of the fiducial points, and **F** their corresponding stereotactic frame coordinates. The matrix **N** is obtained subsequently via a generalized inverse which provides a least squares solution (Pratt 1978):

$$\mathbf{N} = (\mathbf{F}^T\mathbf{F})^{-1}\mathbf{F}^T\mathbf{V}. \qquad (11)$$

* No more than three may be coplanar.

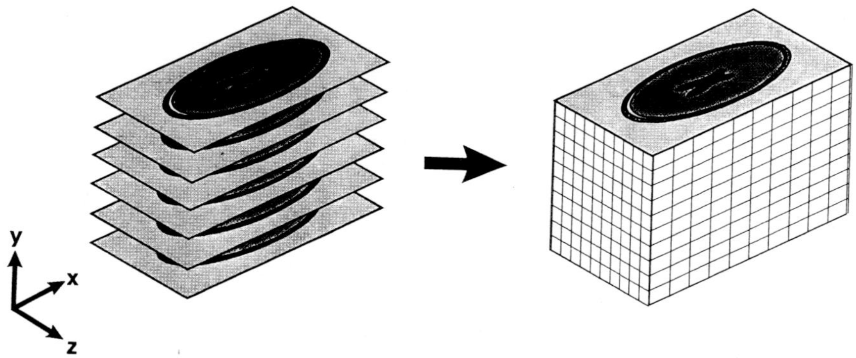

Fig. 12.13 The tomographic data are loaded into computer memory such that they comprise a voxel based volume.

A matrix that performs the reverse transformation of coordinates is also computed (the inverse of **N**). Throughout the matching procedure, each matrix is employed to determine the frame's orientation within the voxel based volume and its position with respect to the intended axis of projection used when creating the rendered image.

The matrix decomposition described earlier provides three angles specifying the orientation of the image plane with respect to the frame in the DSA projection. A separate calculation is performed to determine the frame's orientation in the tomographic volume. The appropriate rotations must now be applied to the data in computer memory to match the DSA projection geometry. These are determined below.

We define the three rotations comprising **R** in equation (8) as follows:

$$\mathbf{R} = R_{proj} = \Theta_{proj}\Phi_{proj}\Psi_{proj} \quad (12)$$

where

$$\Theta_{proj} = \begin{pmatrix} 1 & 0 & 0 \\ 0 & \cos\theta & -\sin\theta \\ 0 & \sin\theta & -\cos\theta \end{pmatrix} \quad (13)$$

$$\Phi_{proj} = \begin{pmatrix} \cos\phi & 0 & \sin\phi \\ 0 & 1 & 0 \\ -\sin\phi & 0 & \cos\phi \end{pmatrix} \quad (14)$$

$$\Psi_{proj} = \begin{pmatrix} \cos\psi & -\sin\psi & 0 \\ \sin\psi & \cos\psi & 0 \\ 0 & 0 & 1 \end{pmatrix} \quad (15)$$

and the angles θ, ϕ and ψ are clockwise rotations, respectively, about the X, Y and Z axes of the image plane. The orientation of the frame within the tomographic volume is represented in a similar fashion:

$$R_{proj} = \Theta_{vol}\Phi_{vol}\Psi_{vol} \,. \quad (16)$$

In order to match the desired orientation specified by R_{proj} we must determine the appropriate rotations to apply to R_{vol}. The desired rotation matrix, R_{align}, is calculated as follows

$$R_{align} = R_{vol}^{-1} R_{proj} \quad (17)$$

The individual angles comprising R_{align} are obtained via its decomposition. These rotations are then performed on the volume contained in the computer memory. Accordingly, the matrix **N** is updated:

$$\mathbf{N}_{new} = \mathbf{N}R_{align} \quad (18)$$

By employing an orthographic projection technique to create the rendered image, a problem arises in creating the perspective view needed to properly match the divergent ray projection of the DSA image. The solution is to scale successive voxel planes, parallel to the image plane, according to the magnification they experience during the radiographic projection (see Figs. 12.14 and 12.15). Since the resizing must be centred along the principal ray, we must first determine where that ray intersects the volume. This is accomplished analytically as follows.

A plane parallel to the front face of the volume is selected, and its orientation with respect to the stereotactic frame is determined. We represent

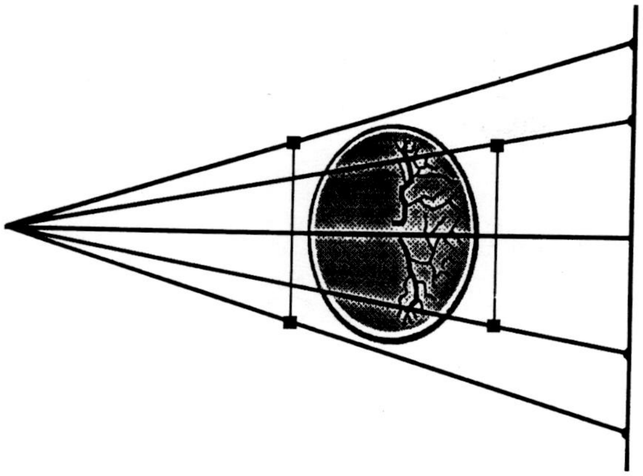

Fig. 12.14 A diverging ray source yields a perspective projection of the imaged object. In order to simulate differential magnification in the rendered image, the volume must be reshaped (see Fig. 12.15).

this mathematically using the standard equation for a plane:

$$ax+by+cz+d = 0. \qquad (19)$$

Having correctly oriented the tomographic data earlier, we are assured that the ray is orthogonal to the front face of the volume and that it intersects each successive plane at the same point.

Equations (2) and (3) together with equation (19) comprise three equations in three unknowns (x, y and z) which, in addition to knowing the piercing point, allow the point of intersection to be calculated in terms of frame coordinates. These coordinates are transformed into the voxel based system via equation (9), and the entire volume is translated by the amounts required to project the point of intersection on to the piercing point in the DSA image. This ensures that the rendered image aligns with the DSA projection when superimposed.

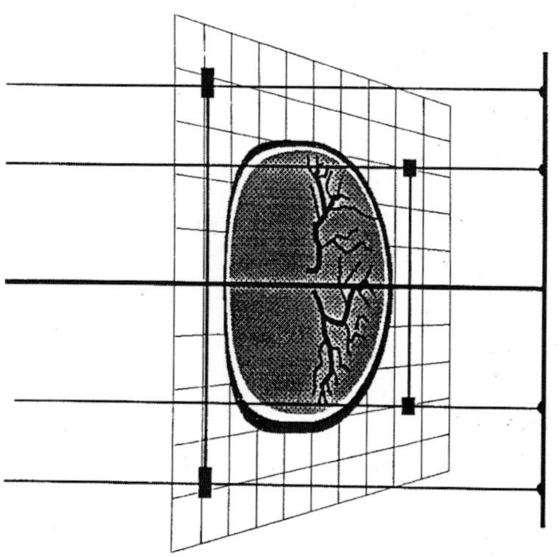

Fig. 12.15 A perspective projection is simulated by resizing successive planes within the tomographic volume prior to rendering the image using an orthographic projection algorithm. This allows 3D points within the volume to be projected to their correct positions in the image plane. Note that the differential magnification, in fact, is not linear as depicted here.

The differential magnification experienced by the volume is simulated as follows. Within each plane of voxels orthogonal to the axis of projection we select a line segment of arbitrary length, centred on the principal ray, and compare the length of its orthographic projection to its actual length in the DSA image. The ratio of the two lengths is the desired resizing factor which is subsequently applied to the selected plane. Alternatively, equation (20) can be used to calculate each resizing factor, R_n directly, given the lengths L_i for the planes in the front and rear of the volume (see Fig. 12.16):

$$R_n = \frac{(N-1)L_{N-1}L_o}{d[(N-1)L_{N-1} + n(L_o-L_{N-1})]} \qquad (20)$$

where R_n is the resizing factor for the plane n, N is the total number of planes in the volume, n is the current plane being processed (0,1,2,3,..N-1), d is the length of a line segment in the volume (in voxels), L_i is the length of a segment in the plane i of the volume when projected in the DSA image (in pixels, i.e. projected voxels); front i=0, rear i=N-1). Note that this resizing operation is a non-linear rescaling from front to back.

At this point, the volume is ready to be rendered. Afterwards, the angiogram is overlaid on the resulting image using a compositing technique (Porter & Duff 1984). It is sometimes useful to vary the transparency between the two images to prevent the vessels from completely occluding the underlying rendered data, or vice versa. A flow-chart summarizing the image matching procedure is provided in Fig. 12.17.

A matched CT–DSA stereo-pair is presented in Fig. 12.18. The CT data were acquired as 5 mm thick, non-overlapping transverse slices. The lateral DSA stereo-pair was acquired using a

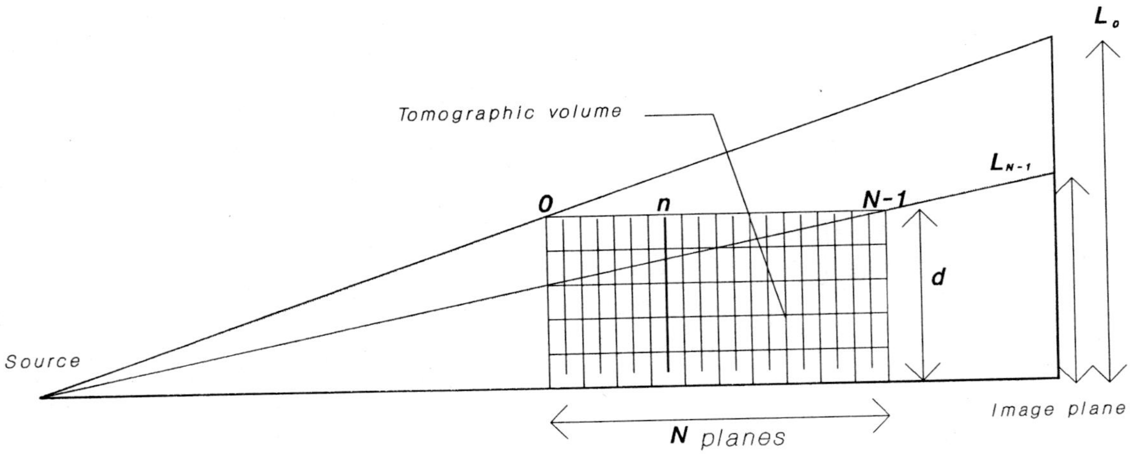

Fig. 12.16 The resizing factor for each plane within the volume is determined using equation (20), which relates the size of a line segment in the current plane to its supposed length when projected in the DSA image.

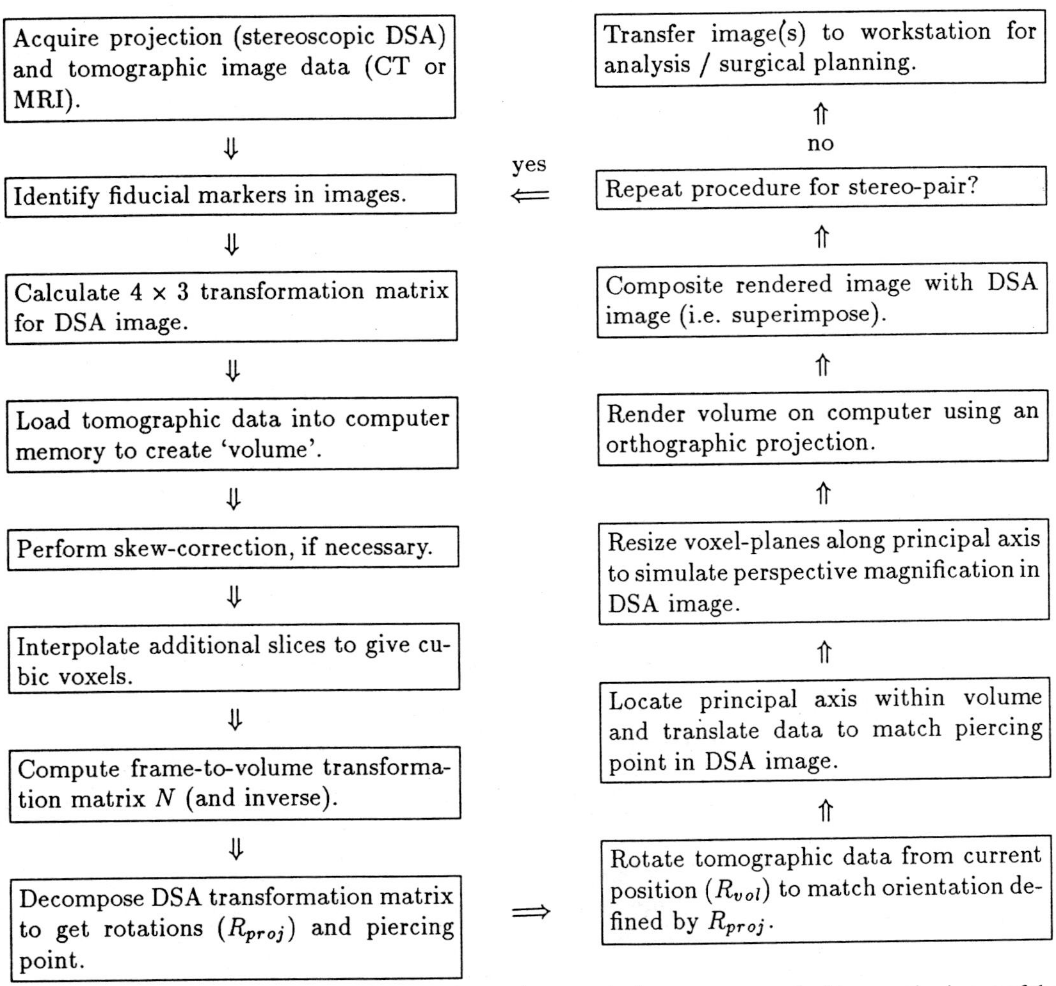

Fig. 12.17 This flow-chart illustrates the sequence of operations required to create a matched perspective image of the tomographic volume for a corresponding DSA projection.

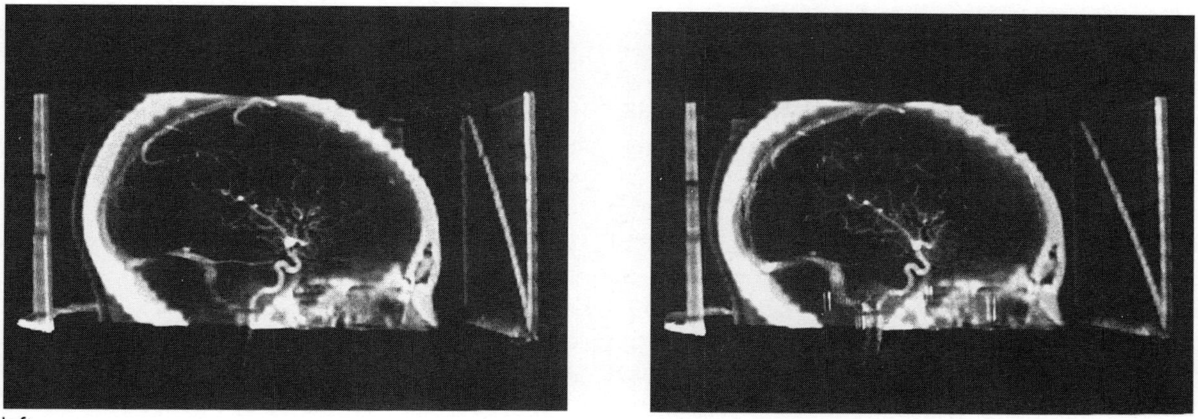

Fig. 12.18 CT–DSA matched stereo-pair. A dual phase angiogram was combined with volumetrically rendered CT data comprised of non-overlapping 5 mm thick slices. The CT fiducial marker plates are seen at the sides.

rotation technique with a 7° angulation and a 270 mm field of view. Prior to rendering, a section of the tomographic volume was removed in order to obtain a better view of the hemisphere of the brain containing the imaged vasculature. A large amount of transparency was applied to the CT data, and a dual phase angiogram was selected in order to observe both arterial and venous phases. The CT fiducial marker plates are seen at the sides.

A matched MRI–DSA stereo-pair is presented in Fig. 12.19. The MRI data were obtained using a T_1 weighted 2D multislice acquisition, giving 64 × 2 mm transverse slices. An arterial phase DSA stereo-pair was selected and overlaid on the rendered volume, which was cut to expose the mid-sagittal anatomy. Note that the vessels follow the appropriate sulcal convolutions in the rendered data.

Methods that attempt to combine the data in three dimensions (by reconstructing the projection data in three dimensions) often encounter difficulties that are dependent upon the quality of the acquired image or peculiarities of the vasculature. It is particularly difficult, for instance, to reconstruct an arteriovenous malformation from a small number of projection images. Similarly, many of the smallest vessels are often neglected or mistaken for artefacts by the reconstruction algorithms. The approach described above relies only on detecting the

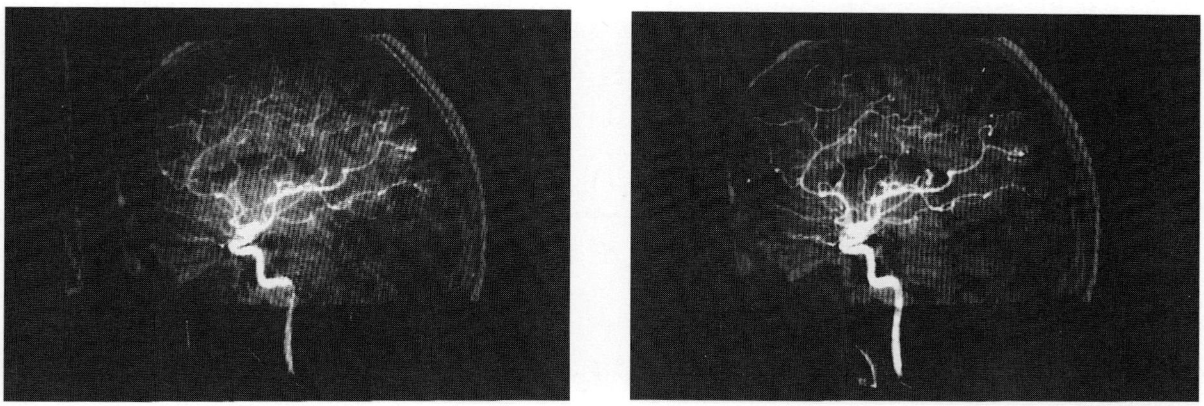

Fig. 12.19 MR–DSA matched stereo-pair. Prior to rendering, the tomographic volume was cut through the mid-sagittal plane. Vessels in the same plane in the arterial phase angiogram are seen to follow the appropriate convolutions.

fiducial markers in the images and is otherwise entirely automated. Since the DSA projection is combined with the rendered image and is not a synthesized representation of the vessels, the observer is responsible for interpreting any ambiguous features.

We note that the matching procedure may also be employed to combine image data that are not acquired under stereotactic conditions. For a single image, a minimum of six points must be identified in the projection whose corresponding positions are known within the tomographic volume. This allows us to calculate a homogeneous transformation matrix that relates the position of the image plane to the coordinate system defined by the tomographic volume. In this case, the matching algorithm is even more straightforward since there are no frame-to-volume transformations required. One must nevertheless accurately identify corresponding points within the projection and tomographic image data. Since there are liable to be appreciable uncertainties, it would be advantageous to identify several additional points in order to minimize errors in the transformation matrix. In this instance, the advantage of a stereoscopic approach is considerable because points are identified simultaneously in each image of the stereopair, so that the observer obtains a better appreciation of the 3D structure, helping to locate the corresponding points in the tomographic data.

REFERENCES

Adams L P 1981 X-ray stereo photogrammetry locating the precise, three-dimensional position of image points. Medical and Biological Engineering and Computing 19: 569–578

Drebin R, Carpenter L, Hanraham P 1988 Volume rendering. ACM Computer Graphics 22(4): 65–74

DuMond J W M 1932 The technic of stereofluoroscopy. Radiology 19: 366–387

Ganapathy S 1984 Decomposition of transformation matrices for robot vision. IEEE Computer Vision and Image Processing 130–139

Haven T J 1987 A liquid-crystal video stereoscope with high extinction ratios, a 28% transmission state, and one-hundred-microsecond switching. True 3D imaging techniques and display technologies, SPIE, pp 23–26

Henri C J, Peters T M 1990 Evaluation of perceived distortions in stereoscopic images. First Conference on Visualization in Biomedical Computing, May, Atlanta, GA, pp 216–222

Henri C J, Peters T M, Lemieux L, Olivier A 1990 Experience with a computerized stereoscopic workstation for neurosurgical planning. First Conference on Visualization in Biomedical Computing, May, Atlanta, GA, pp 450–457

Hodges L F, Peters T M, Wixon S E, Sklebitz H, Henri C J 1990 Workshop on stereoscopic visualization techniques. First Conference on Visualization in Biomedical Computing, May, Atlanta, GA

Jarre H A, Teschendorf O E W 1933 Roentgen-stereoscopy: a review of its present status. Radiology 21: 139–155

Lipton L, Meyer L 1984 A flicker-free field-sequential stereoscopic video system. SMPTE Journal, Nov: 1047–1051

Mannila T 1956 On parallax and variations in the stereoscopic image, with a view to stereofluoroscopy. Acta Radiologica (suppl) 139

Pixar Imaging Computer Chap Tools User's Guide. PIXAR, 2.00 edition, July 1987

Porter T, Duff T 1984 Compositing digital images. ACM Computer Graphics 18(3): 253–259

Pratt W K 1978 Digital image processing. Wiley, New York

Roese J A, Turner A F 1976 Single monitor stereoradiological television system using PLZT electroscopic shutters. Radiology 121: 740–744

Sand R 1984 New aspects and experiences in stereoscopic television. SMPTE Journal, Nov: 1052–1056

Saunders B G 1968 Stereoscopic drawing by computer — is it orthoscopic? Applied Optics 7(8): 1499–1504

Sen Z, King P H, Xiaodong P 1983 Recent progress in X-ray stereoscopes. Medical Physics 10(5): 574–578

Strat T M 1984 Recovering the camera parameters from a transformation matrix. Proceedings DARPA Image Understanding Workshop, 2 October, pp 265–271

Sutherland I E 1974 Three-dimensional data input by tablet. Proceedings of the IEEE 62(4): 453–471

Vogelsang H, Dietz K 1983 Stereoscopic magnification in spinal angiography. American Journal of Neuroradiology 4: 588–589

Worthington C, Peters T M, Ethier R et al 1985 Stereoscopic digital subtraction angiography in neurological assessment. American Journal of Neuroradiology 6: 802–808

13. Robots in neurosurgery

P. A. Finlay

INTRODUCTION

Recent developments in automation technology and medical imaging have opened the way to the effective clinical use of robotic tools. Robots offer the neurosurgeon a number of advantages, including enhanced precision, the facility for minimally invasive surgery and reduced hazard in the case of radiotherapy. However, it should be stressed that not every procedure will benefit from robot assistance, and the surgeon should assess the suitability of robotics on a case-by-case basis at the planning stage.

The principle of image guided robot assisted surgery is simple: three dimensional digital images, reconstructed for example from a computerized tomography (CT) brain scan, are displayed to a surgeon on a computer screen. By pointing to the relevant parts of the screen image with a digitizer, the surgeon indicates a target site within the patient's head and an entry point on the cranium. A simple computer programme then calculates the required initial coordinates and trajectory for a surgical tool such as a biopsy needle to follow. This information is then passed to a robot controller which supervises the joint movements of a robot arm to achieve the required path for a biopsy needle held in the robot gripper.

As with other surgical tools, the surgeon remains in control of the robot at all times. The more advanced surgical robots possess a degree of autonomy, for example enabling them to modify their action in response to signals received from tip mounted sensors, but the surgeon is able to override the robot controller at any point. The design of the surgeon–robot interface is one of the most important features of a surgical robot. A well designed interface presents the surgeon with all the clinically important information in a prioritized and clear format, together with the control options available.

CLINICAL USES OF ROBOTS

What first attracted industrialists to robots in the 1960s was the promise of flexibility, and this remains one of the robot's most valued attributes. The ability to operate on patients of different shapes and sizes, with surgical sites in different places, is of course fundamental. There is, however, an equally important, though more subtle, reason for needing flexibility. This is the rate of change of medical practice. Many examples could be given of conditions which would have been considered inoperable a generation ago until a breakthrough in technique enabled treatment by radical open surgery. Today the same condition is treated by minimally invasive techniques; in a few years time, non-invasive methods may be evolved. Examples range from prostatectomy to cranial lesion resection.

Whilst it would be entirely possible to design an automated system for carrying out a surgical procedure (as the Russians have attempted in radial keratotomy), the danger is that such a machine would be rendered obsolete before it was built by changes in clinical practice. A robot, which falls into the niche of special tools designed to assist in minimally invasive techniques, has the considerable advantage of being reprogrammable and retoolable to suit the next generation of surgical operations; much, in fact, like a human surgeon who witnesses many changes of technique in the course of a career.

Robots have a number of features which enable them to be usefully deployed in the operating theatre. The most self-evident is precision, which when linked to a suitable digital medical image enables a tool to be located to within half a millimetre or less of a given target point. The same accuracy can also be used to enable the robot to insert a tool safely even when it passes close to a critical structure such as the optic nerve. Thus, sites can be accessed with great precision which are impossible to reach at all through manual techniques.

The use of tools with steerable tips enables intracranial volumes to be approached, inspected and, if appropriate, resected using minimally invasive techniques, without the need for a craniotomy. A hole diameter of only a few millimetres in the cranium is all that is necessary. Apart from reducing the complexity of the surgery, this reduces postoperative healing time and complications associated with the cosmetics of postoperative scarring. Duration and extent of anaesthesia is also reduced: a local anaesthetic is often acceptable.

The same workstation which is used by the surgeon for specifying and then monitoring a robot based procedure can also be used pre-operatively for designing and simulating the operation, using computer graphics. This is a most useful aid for planning and optimizing surgery, and also for training purposes.

An obvious indication for using robotics is when the procedure to be carried out involves exposing theatre staff to hazards. Examples of this are surgery or autopsy on highly infectious patients, and radiotherapy. Treatment of intracranial lesions by interstitial radiotherapy is a good example. Accurate positioning of the radioactive pellets within the lesion is important to gain the optimum tumour control combined with minimal damage to surrounding tissue. Under image guidance, a robot can safely position the pellets in the precise spot indicated by the physician.

The steadiness of a robot held tool is another useful feature, and can be a key to successful microsurgery, especially functional neurosurgery.

Looking ahead to the future, the development of telesurgery offers clear benefits to robot users. Telesurgery enables a senior surgeon to supervise a junior colleague at a distant location, using the telecommunication network to transmit medical images to the expert. It is equally possible for the distant surgeon to supervise a robot performing the operation. Indeed, the surgeon need not even be conscious of the fact that the patient is several hundred kilometres away, since the computer interface would be identical to that of the robot in his or her own adjacent theatre suite.

The examples quoted above have all related to the use of robots for carrying out surgical or radiological procedures. But it should not be thought that robots are restricted to this role in the theatre. Robots have been or are being developed for:

- Manoeuvring surgical microscopes (the eyepiece tracks the surgeon's head movements, leaving his or her hands free, whilst the objective stays focused on the surgical site).
- Surgical retraction: the wound is held open at a constant tension which can be varied as required by the surgeon.
- Patient positioning: the robot acts as a programmable jig, which holds the patient's head during surgery. Under voice command of the surgeon, the robot will move the head to a range of prespecified positions.
- Patient handling: this robot physically lifts and transfers patients from trolley to operating table, scanner or bed with considerably less trauma to patients and staff than manual lifts occasion.
- Scrub nurse/fetching and carrying: a number of experimental robots have been developed for this purpose, some with a limited vocabulary for voice control.
- It should not be forgotten that a number of existing clinical tools are essentially robotic in their operation, including external beam radiotherapy accelerators, and tables for CT and magnetic resonance scanning.

The use of robots for image directed surgery, however, remains the application area with the greatest potential and the most interest. Although there are potentially very many opportunities for using robots in different surgical fields, neurosurgery remains one of the most important. This is because the cranium and the spine both

Table 13.1 Typical neurosurgical and radiological procedures for which robots are indicated

Intracranial biopsy
Subdural haematoma drainage
Intracranial cyst drainage
Supratentorial cranial lesion resection
Interstitial radiotherapy
Electrode placement for functional neurosurgery
Insertion of needles into the spine for various purposes

provide a useful rigid datum for the robot, and because the technically complex issues involved in handling soft organs subject to movement through respiration are avoided. In addition, the precision afforded by robotics is often particularly useful in neurosurgery of the head and spine.

An exhaustive listing of neurosurgical operations in which robots are potentially useful would be of only transient value, as the frequent changes in robot technology and clinical practice would combine to make it quickly obsolescent. The list in Table 13.1 is therefore for the sake of example only: additions can readily be made by any surgeon with an eye for synergy.

TERMS IN ROBOTICS

The word 'robot' first appeared in a science fiction work by the Czechoslovak playwright Capek. It means simply 'worker' in Czech. Over the years, many attempts at a formal definition of 'robot' have been made, generally encompassing the idea of a programmable manipulator. None have been entirely satisfactory: perhaps the most acceptable tenet is that of Joseph Engleberger, the American who developed the world's first industrial robot in 1961: 'I know one when I see one!'

Although the definition may be fraught, all robots have characteristics in common, and it is useful to be aware of the following basic glossary.

The space through which a robot arm can move is its *working envelope*. The shape of the working envelope is determined by the geometry and linkages of the arm. This is called the *articulation* of the robot, and a number of classical articulations exist, as shown in Figure 13.1. The three most common in surgical robots are the revolute, the SCARA and the parallel.

The revolute articulation is basically anthropomorphic, and has the great advantage of being able to reach round obstacles. The main disadvantage is a comparatively low precision. SCARA is an acronym of 'selective compliance assembly robot arm', and robots with this articulation have the useful attribute of being stiff in torsion whilst compliant in translation. In simple terms this means that if a probe held by such a robot is pushed sideways, it will tend to move bodily rather than twist. This is helpful if the objective is to insert the probe into a nearby predrilled hole, since twisting would cause it to jam. Parallel robots are oustandingly steady and

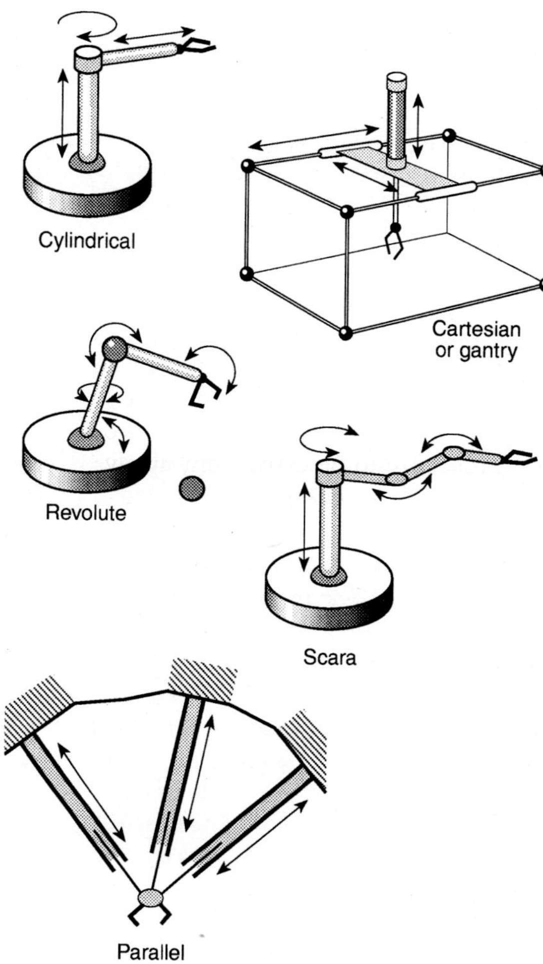

Fig. 13.1 Types of robot articulation.

accurate, and for this reason are preferred for manipulating tools such as surgical microscopes. Their main drawback is a limited working envelope and poor user access.

The different directions of movement of a robot arm are termed its *degrees of freedom.* Usually each joint or *axis* of the robot provides one degree of freedom. There are a total of six independent degrees of freedom which are mathematically possible: three in translation (x, y and z) and three in rotation (roll, pitch and yaw). Most surgical robots will possess at least five. Often one or more axes are duplicated in order to enhance the versatility of the arm. Such robots are termed *kinematically redundant* and are able to reach snake-like into confined spaces.

Another reason for providing kinematic redundancy is to avoid *singularities* in the robot working envelope. A singularity occurs when an axis has reached the limit of its travel. Further motion in the same direction can only be achieved by moving a second axis through a large angle to bring the first back within its range of operation. A human example of this is craning the neck to watch a bird flying directly overhead: at a certain point, further straining of the neck is impossible, and it becomes necessary to twist the torso to compensate. Points of singularity must be avoided in the programming of surgical robots, as they are regions of unpredictable accuracy. A robot without significant singularities is described as 'well conditioned'.

In addition to the arm or manipulator, a robot requires a local computer or *controller* to convert input commands into joint motions. The controller first works out the required motion of each joint in order to move the robot to its specified position whilst avoiding singularities and known obstructions. It then sends appropriate control signals to each joint motor to provide synchronized motion and, whilst the joints are moving, the controller monitors and corrects any incipient positional error.

The tip of a robot arm carries a *tool plate* of some description. This is a simple mounting plate on to which may be fastened various types of *end effectors* — the generic term for toolholders, grippers, probes, etc. Whilst most robots have only a single, fixed, end effector, complex machines may have several automatically changeable units. Some types of end effector serve as holders for an array of surgical tools which are needed sequentially. Other types may possess one or more degrees of freedom of their own, such as in steerable tip endoscopes. In this case, either the robot controller must supervise these additional axes or a separate controller is needed. Not all end effectors hold tools: they may hold cameras, sensors or tissue samples, for example.

One of the more controversial features of a robot is its claimed 'accuracy'. The problem results from the different interpretations put on this term by various suppliers. Because of the confusion, it is better to avoid the word 'accuracy' altogether, and to speak of *repeatability*, which is the precision with which the robot is able to return to a previously visited point, or *absolute accuracy,* which is the precision with which the robot can move from one set of coordinates to another. The second term is more relevant in surgical robotics. In fact, absolute accuracy varies from one notionally identical robot to another, being influenced by the individual engineering tolerances on the robot link lengths and joint angles. There is a procedure for minimizing these errors, and thus maximizing the robot's absolute accuracy, known as characterization, which is an important function considered in more detail below under the heading of 'Calibration'.

When selecting a robot for a particular procedure, it is important to remember that the absolute accuracy and repeatability will both refer to a designated point on the tool plate of the arm. If the surgical procedure requires accurate placement of the tip of a 200 mm long probe extending beyond the toolplate, allowance must be made for the magnification of error resulting from the lever arm effect.

DESIGN AND SELECTION OF ROBOTS

Having determined the working envelope and articulation required, the first consideration in designing or choosing a robot is its power method. Robots may be powered in various ways: the most common method is by electrical motors, but pneumatic and hydraulic systems exist. There are good technical and hygienic reasons for preferring electrical drives unless special requirements dictate otherwise (e.g. pneumatics are useful if deliberate compliance or sponginess is useful). Electric drives may be by stepper motor or servo motor systems. Stepper motors are precise digitally driven actuators which are ideal for discrete indexing of a tool in steps as small as a few micrometres if desired. However, they have comparatively low torque and are thus only suitable for light duties, such as steerable tip tooling or small probe manipulation. Servo drives are faster and more powerful, as well as being more compact, and are the preferred drive for most robot arms. A disadvantage of servo drives is that unless they are carefully shielded they can cause interference with any adjacent medical ultrasonics.

Each axis of the robot requires its own motor, and each motor will have its own drive card in the robot controller. Some designs of robot are effectively modular, enabling additional drive cards to be added to the controller to power extra axes on the robot or end effector.

Feed-back of the position of each axis is provided to the controller by encoders or resolvers at each joint. These generate pulses as the joint is turned (if rotary) or extended (if linear), which are converted by the controller into angles or lengths and compared with the desired position. An average controller will make this comparison about 12 times a second for each axis. Encoders are of two types, absolute and incremental. Absolute encoders indicate a unique position, whereas incremental encoders merely count pulses from some arbitrary datum. For reasons of space and cost, incremental encoders are the norm, and it is thus necessary to define a datum or home position for the robot arm, with reference to which all encoder counts are made. In the event of a power failure, an incremental encoder will lose its pulse count and must be re-datumed by returning the robot to its home position. As this is normally impractical in the middle of a surgical procedure, a battery back-up for the mains power supply is essential.

Encoders are an example of intrinsic robot sensors, that is, internal sensors which monitor the state of the robot. Other examples are microswitches to detect the correct fitting of tools in the end effector and trip sensors to detect failure in the power supply. Surgical robots also feature a range of extrinsic sensors which convey information about the outside world. Examples are force and torque sensors mounted on the end effector to monitor resistance encountered by the tool. Some sensors may be physically separate from the robot, such as cameras to monitor patient position.

An alternative to intrinsic position sensors is the use of an external sensor to monitor the tool tip position directly. This can be achieved, for instance, by using laser triangulation in which a low power laser beam is reflected off a point on the end effector and detected by a fixed photosensor array mounted close to the robot. This technique provides very accurate coordinates of the arm position, and is not affected by internal miscalibration of the robot. It is, however, expensive and not universally effective: problems arise from shadowing by obstructions. Other techniques such as tip mounted accelerometers and external cameras are at an experimental stage. For the moment, therefore, position detection by intrinsic encoders is the norm, but extrinsic sensing will certainly be a future development.

The versatility and sophistication of a robot is largely a function of its controller. The basic function of a controller is path planning, that is, the calculation of the angles or lengths by which each axis must be moved in order for the tool held in the robot end effector to arrive at its target position. Mathematically this involves the solution of a number of inverse kinematic equations, which may have to be modified to take account of obstructions in the robot path. The controller must check not only for collisions between an obstruction and the tool, but for clearance of all parts of the arm as well. Path planning is performed off line, before the robot starts to move. More advanced robot controllers have the ability to effect a plan repair if circumstances change whilst motion is in progress, for example if a new obstruction appears.

ADVANCED ROBOTICS

Some robot controllers under development for neurosurgery have the additional ability to undertake task planning. This involves selecting a suitable path to access a given lesion site, for example. To do this, the controller needs additional knowledge of other intracranial structures, including the positions of blood vessels, nerves and eloquent regions of brain. The controller assigns a cost to each such structure, and then calculates the least cost entry point and trajectory. This is displayed to the surgeon for approval or editing before being passed to the path planner for implementation.

Robots and controllers of this sophistication fall into a new category — so called advanced or third generation robots. The distinctive feature of an advanced robot is its ability to work at least semiautonomously in an unstructured environment. Advanced robots are thus necessarily intelligent and sensor rich systems. Surgical versions are currently at the development stage but are likely to supplant second generation robots once they become commercially available, due to their greatly enhanced versatility and ease of use.

The components of a typical advanced surgical robot are shown in Figure 13.2. The essential starting point is a computer model of the patient derived from medical images. In its simplest form this may be a reconstructed three dimensional CT image, but more information can be added by fusing images of more than one modality, and by superimposing a digitized brain atlas on to the image in order to indicate functional regions. This latter operation requires a standard brain atlas to be 'warped' to suit the topography of the

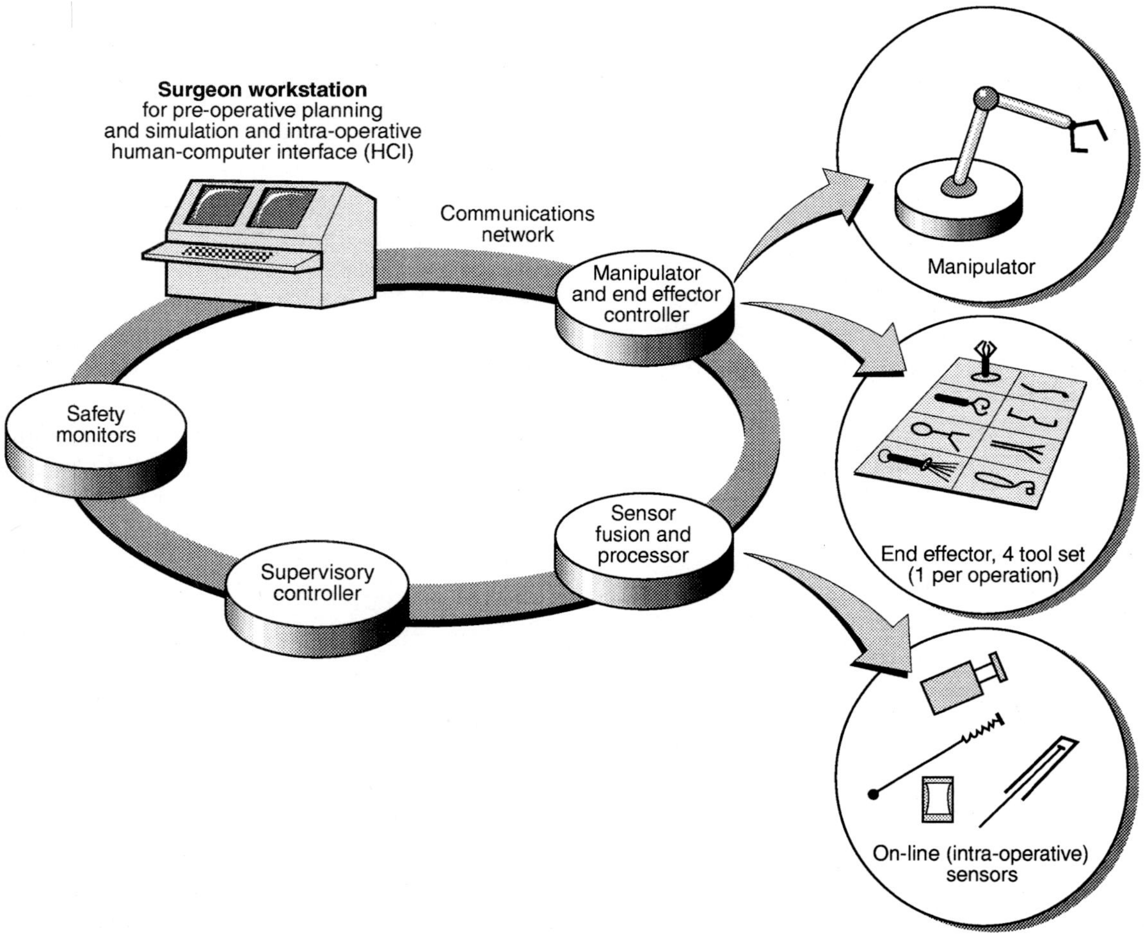

Fig. 13.2 Physical components of an advanced surgical robot.

particular patient. A final feature of the model, to be added by the surgeon, is the location of the target site or volume which the robot held tool must access.

The patient model can then be added to the computer's 'world' model, which includes a representation of the robot and the relevant parts of the operating theatre. This representation then contains all the geometric data needed for task and path planning.

Additional non-image information is also needed to complete the world model. This includes a description of the procedure to be carried out, which may be specified by the surgeon or be previously known to the computer in the form of a rule based expert system. Depending on the procedure, other patient data are also required, including details such as age, sex and history.

During the time that the robot is in use, a range of extrinsic sensors provides a continuous stream of information which is used to update the world model, and possibly to activate safety trips causing the robot to stop or withdraw. This sensor information is processed by the controller, which uses a series of rules to determine the importance of a given combination of signals. A separate safety monitor is normal, which independently monitors the procedure and can initiate alarms and priority actions.

A key feature of an advanced surgical robot is its method of communicating with the surgeon, usually referred to as the human computer interface or HCI. In a well designed system, the surgeon is able to control and monitor every aspect of the procedure through the HCI, which will display to him or her both a real time video image of the procedure and, on a separate screen, a computer simulation of the procedure as it progresses, based on the world model. Any urgent information, such as an unexpected sensor reading, is displayed concurrently, together with a list of over-ride options.

ROBOT ASSISTED AND ROBOT CONDUCTED SURGERY

The level of autonomy accorded to a surgical robot is limited more by medical ethics and the confidence of the surgeon than by robot technology. It is ethically necessary for the surgeon to be in control of the operation, but this does not mean that he or she is required to approve every single movement of the robot arm in a sequence.

It is possible to distinguish between invasive and non-invasive surgical robots. Non-invasive versions do not make physical contact with the patient but rather act as intelligent positioning aids by holding a guide tube at the correct position and angle over the patient's head. The surgeon manually inserts biopsy probes, for example, using the guide tube to set the trajectory. They are thus the robotic equivalent of the stereotactic frame, with the advantage of avoiding both the invasive step of frame fitting and the error prone setting up of frame coordinates.

One of the main reasons for the development of non-invasive robots has been concern about product liability legislation, especially in the USA. Recent advances in the technology of safety critical systems enable invasive robots to be deployed without unacceptable risks.

Nevertheless, safety is still a matter of concern to robot suppliers and surgeon users. The field of surgical robots is too new to have official standards, but a consensus among developers has led to a number of features being incorporated into invasive robots to minimize the risks of error. These features include:

- Physical stops to prevent the robot moving outside its permitted zone and light barriers to shut down the robot if an unauthorized person penetrates the robot working area
- High ratio gearboxes between each motor and its joint to limit the speed of the robot and prevent the arm being back-driven by an external force
- Force and torque sensors to limit the forces which the robot can exert
- Duplication of critical sensors and mechanical components
- Use of safety critical software techniques in writing code
- Separate safety monitor or 'watchdog' to ensure correct control and monitoring functions.

There remain a number of issues about which a consensus has yet to emerge — how should the robot respond, for example, to obviously wrong instructions from the surgeon? Is the robot ever to over-rule the surgeon? And there is the vexed question of expert systems, widely available as diagnostic aids but never allowed to respond to that diagnosis without confirmation from a physician. At some point in the development of medicine, it will become appropriate to 'close the loop' and allow the expert system not only to diagnose but also initiate treatment based on the diagnosis. This is of relevance to surgical robots, which are well suited to linking with expert systems. The analogy of autopilots in airliners is a powerful one. In the early days, the human pilot used the autopilot as a tool, with little decision making power. Current fly-by-wire aircraft give precedence to the autopilot over the human. This change has resulted in greater air safety and, significantly, no diminution of the role of the aircraft captain.

Calibration

In the practical use of surgical robots, the calibration of a number of different components is essential in order for the expected absolute accuracy to be achieved. Firstly, the robot has to be calibrated internally or characterized so that the kinematic equations used by the controller in calculating joint motion have the correct parameters. Secondly, the images which produce the patient model must be referenced to a common datum or matched and registered to the robot, Finally, the robot must be externally calibrated by being registered to the patient.

The purpose of internal calibration, or characterization, of the robot, it will be recalled, is to correct any small errors resulting from manufacturing tolerance in link lengths and joint angles, and to compensate for small deflections in the arm caused by the weight of the payload and the self-weight of the robot.

Characterization of the robot is often performed by the manufacturer, but is best carried out in situ when the robot is first set up. The end effector should be carrying an average payload. This is because both the attitude of the robot and its payload can affect the characterization process. There have been cases of robots being characterized for normal use which have subsequently been suspended inverted from the ceiling. Errors due to the effect of gravity, which had been compensated for in the initial calibration, became double their precharacterization value!

Characterization is effected by driving the robot to a number of points in an accurate grid pattern spaced over the working area. The errors between instructed and achieved positions are recorded and are mathematically combined to form a difference matrix. This is then loaded into the controller and modifies the kinematic equations of motion.

It is to be expected that future generations of robot will feature direct monitoring of tool tip position using extrinsic sensing techniques such as laser triangulation. When that breakthrough occurs, characterization will no longer be necessary, but until then it remains a tedious essential.

Matching of images from different modalities, the second category of calibration, is dealt with in Chapter 12. In order to match these to the patient, some form of reference point is needed. This may be provided by the fiducials of a stereotactic frame, but of course an advantage of robotics is that an invasively fitted frame is unnecessary. Other types of reference points may be provided by anatomical landmarks, or by non-invasively fitted fiducial systems such as dental brace supported frames. So long as a feature can be nominated which is common to the patient model and real patient, matching can be achieved by a simple coordinate transformation matrix.

The final necessary calibration is to reference the robot to the patient. If the patient is fitted with a stereotactic frame, calibration is conveniently achieved by physically connecting the base of the robot to a point on the frame. Some light robots can even be mounted on the frame. The robot must then be driven to a fixed zero point which corresponds to the zero point of the world model. This is most easily effected by requiring the robot to drive a pyramid shaped pin held in its end effector into a matching hole on the frame: this particular geometry of pin-in-hole will only fit at a single unique position and angle, thus determining all six degrees of freedom.

If a stereotactic frame is not fitted, the robot can be physically secured to the operating table and the patient's head placed in a convenient clamp. A special head cap can then be held by the robot end effector and placed over the patient's head. The cap contains a number of displacement transducers which detect the skull position and register the offset of the robot in six degrees of freedom. This is then converted to an error matrix and used to modify the robot's coordinates in the conventional way. The cap can then be removed from the patient and the robot and effector, and the robot will remain calibrated to the patient so long as the latter is not moved.

As well as the robot arm, it is necessary to ensure that each tool used by the robot is calibrated. This can be achieved by causing the robot to place each tool it picks up in a calibration station before attempting anything else. The calibration station measures the tool tip position relative to the tool plate (known as the tool offset), and as a by-product confirms that the tool is the correct one for this stage of the procedure, and that it is correctly fitted to the end effector. Details of the tool offset are needed by the robot controller in order to ensure accurate placement of the tip.

The robot in use: an example

As an example of the level of robot surgery which will soon be possible, the progress of a typical (but fictitious) intracranial tumour resection will be considered. Some of the techniques which will be described are still at an experimental stage, but all will be available in the near future.

Initial CT scanning indicating the probable presence of a single supratentorial lesion has taken place, and the surgeon opts for a robot assisted biopsy and resection. An angiogram is performed to delineate the position of blood vessels, and this information, together with the CT scan data, is provided to the robot workstation, where a reconstructed three dimensional patient model is set up and displayed on a screen

The surgeon, using a digitizer, indicates the volume of the suspected lesion and also nominates three points for biopsy sampling. The robot workstation then accesses its rule base and proposes an entry point and trajectory for a biopsy probe. This is shown to the surgeon as a line superimposed on the patient model. The proposed design seems satisfactory to the surgeon. He next asks the workstation to simulate a resection of the tumour, using a steerable tip ultrasonic knife and suction unit. The workstation shows, using computer graphics, the insertion of the resecting tool and the removal of the tumour volume. The surgeon checks that all is well with this strategy, and when he is satisfied types in a command to load this sequence to the robot.

The sedated patient is now brought into the theatre and the entry point chosen by the robot is prepared. A tray containing a set of robot end effectors and tools appropriate for this procedure is opened and fitted to its slot on the robot base. The robot is secured to the operating table and calibrated to the patient using the head cap technique. A local anaesthetic is administered to the entry point, and the robot then makes an opening in the skin, exposing the cranium, and then pauses while the surgeon performs diathermy and satisfies himself that all is well. The robot changes tools, and drills through the cranium. It changes tools again and opens the dura and pia, exposing the brain. The surgeon orders the robot to pause while he checks the site once more.

Next the robot picks up a biopsy probe and slowly inserts it down the planned trajectory. The surgeon is now monitoring the operation from his HCI console. He sees the progress of the probe plotted on the patient model. A sensor mounted at the probe tip measures tissue hardness, and a sudden change in reading indicates the lesion boundary. This is notified to the surgeon who compares it with his own earlier delineation of the tumour volume. Probe insertion continues to the first of the three biopsy sites, where samples are taken using the inner cannula of the probe and withdrawn for analysis. This process is repeated at the other two sites. The robot then withdraws the probe and returns to its rest position.

Pathology confirms the presence of a lesion, and the surgeon decides to proceed with the resection. The robot picks up a guide cannula and slowly inserts this down the path followed by the biopsy probe until the lesion boundary is sensed. The resecting tool is then inserted down the guide cannula, and resection then commences, with the surgeon monitoring the removal of successive layers of tumour on his screen. When the entire volume has been removed, the resecting tool is withdrawn, leaving the guide cannula in place. The surgeon commands the robot to pick up an endoscopic camera, and the robot inserts this down the guide cannula and manoeuvres it under control of the surgeon. Images from the camera are displayed directly on to a screen at the HCI console, and the surgeon satisfies himself that no visible trace of lesion remains. The endoscope is then withdrawn and the cannula removed. The surgeon closes the wound and the patient is taken to recovery.

After the operation, the toolset is taken for autoclaving. The robot, which was draped up to its end effector, is immediately ready for the next procedure.

CONCLUSIONS

It will have been recognized that surgical robotics is a field currently in its infancy. There is little doubt, however, that, linked to image processing facilities, surgical robots offer a significant improvement in the quality of treatment which can be provided in certain common neurosurgical procedures. Their precision, dexterity, reliability and flexibility combine to present the physician with an invaluable tool for advancing the progress of neurosurgery.

14. Future developments in stereotaxy

M. F. Pell D. G. T. Thomas

INTRODUCTION

With the rapid and dramatic improvement in neuroradiological imaging and current technology assisted by the increasing use of computer hardware and related software, modern stereotactic neurosurgery has become an important part of mainstream neurosurgery, and is now available throughout the world. Future developments will be involved with image integration and further computer software developments, new instrumentation with a trend towards frameless and open stereotaxy and relocatable frames and the increasing use of stereotaxy in therapy.

FRAMELESS AND OPEN STEREOTAXY

Conventional stereotactic frame systems allow precise spatial information from computerized tomography (CT), magnetic resonance imaging (MRI) and angiography to be used for operative procedures such as biopsy, excision or aspiration of various intracranial lesions (Apuzzo et al 1987, Bradford et al 1987, Thomas et al 1988, Thomas & Nouby 1989, Pell & Thomas 1991). A variety of stereotactic systems with these head frames are in commercial use. Target localization with these head frames has been shown to be accurate, but its use in open craniotomy has been limited by the presence of the frame during the procedure and the need for the frame to remain fixed in the same position to allow reproduction of information from different imaging modalities. These limitations have been somewhat overcome by the development of modern target centred arc-quadrant stereotactic systems such as the Cosman–Roberts–Wells (CRW) system, which may be rotated out of the operative field with no loss of spatial coordinates (Apuzzo et al 1984), and the relocatable stereotactic frame such as the Gill–Thomas–Cosman localizer (Thomas et al 1990).

More recent developments have evolved in stereotactic technique that require no mechanical linkage with a frame. Reference points on a patient's skull can be identified on imaging studies, and touching these points (three or more) with a digitizer at the time of the actual surgical procedure defines a plane which allows construction of a stereotactic coordinate system.

Modern developments in computer interaction with imaging techniques allow intraoperative imaging of intracranial lesions from external cranial landmarks, such as the external auditory meatus, bridge of the nasion, inion, or junction of coronal and squamosal sutures. Intracranial structures and lesions as shown on preoperative imaging may be assigned stereotactic coordinates that can be reproduced during operation using the combination of a digitizer in the operating suite and computer interaction with the preoperative images.

Several systems based on this method have been developed that incorporate frameless stereotactic coordinates, including the neurosurgical stereotactic operating arm developed by Guthrie et al (1990) and the so called 'neuronavigator' system by Watanabe with the University of Tokyo Group (Watanabe et al 1987, 1990, 1991) and the University of Osaka Group (Kato et al 1991).

The stereotactic operating arm as designed by Guthrie and colleagues at the George

Washington University (1989, 1990) involves a five jointed arm where the angle at each joint is measured with a small rotary optical encoder which is coupled to a computer. The Cartesian coordinates of the tip of the arm are calculated using arm dimensions and encoder input. The arm is calibrated between the patient's head and points on a preoperative CT scan obtained with three radiopaque markers placed on the calvarium at the time of the initial imaging and present on the skull at the time of surgery. The inherent error of the initial prototype of the Guthrie system is between 2 and 4 mm.

Similarly, the multijoint arm guided navigational system of Watanabe and his coworkers at the University of Tokyo, the neuronavigator, has eliminated the need for a head frame by using head markers for reference frame transformation. One end of the multijoint arm is fixed to a skull clamp on the surgical table and the free end of the arm is used as a pointing device which is introduced into the surgical field when required to correlate the surgical field with preoperative CT images. The limitations of the system are the inconvenience of the large articulated arm and the 5 mm error of the system (Watanabe et al 1987, 1990).

The computer assisted neurosurgical navigational system (CANS navigator) (Kato et al 1991) uses a magnetic field instead of a frame or arm for spatial position determination in order to display dynamically surgical manipulation on the preoperative CT or MRI scans. The three dimensional digitizer utilizes a low frequency magnetic field to detect the three dimensional coordinates and the three orientational angles of the small magnetic field sensor with respect to the magnetic field source reference frame. The CANS navigator has been reported in use with 10 patients undergoing open surgery (Gybels et al 1990) with reference frame calibration adding only several minutes to the surgical procedures, including total removal of olfactory groove meningiomas, metastatic brain tumours and arteriovenous malformations. The error within the CANS navigational system is presently 4 mm and is affected by drift of the three dimensional digitizer, electromagnetic noise surrounding the magnetic field source and sensor, and poor spatial position of the scalp marker in calibrations. Brain distortion during surgery still remains a problem with the interpretation of the probe position during brain retraction, release of cerebrospinal fluid during operation or when a large mass of tumour is being removed.

Future developments may include the development of specially designed operating rooms to provide the stereotactic coordinate matrix (Kelly 1991) whereby laser scanning of the patient's head will record its position within the coordinate system. The operating microscope will be robotically controlled and positioned within this coordinate matrix.

IMAGE INTEGRATION

Computer reconstruction of imaged data (CT, MRI and digital subtraction angiography) allows three dimensional and two dimensional multiplanar representation of target position and volume in stereotactic space (Kelly et al 1986). The development of CT guided stereotactic techniques and three dimensional computer graphics allows the simulation of stereotactic surgery as well as obtaining qualitative target data and spatial relationships between the target and adjacent structures (Kim et al 1990).

The diffusion of high resolution imaging devices (MRI, CT) together with the rapid development of computer graphics makes it possible to utilize the principles of stereotaxy in the field of microneurosurgery (Giorgi et al 1990). This technique for combining data and computer imaging into a three dimensional workstation for the planning of stereotactic surgical procedures is under development at several centres (Leksell 1951, Kobayashi et al 1989, Kenny et al 1990, Kim et al 1990) and uses a number of commercially available computer systems such as the Sun workstation (Zamorano et al 1990).

Computerized image processing under stereotactic conditions is similar for all available systems and involves data acquisition, three dimensional/two dimensional computerized stereotactic preplanning and, finally, the stereotactic surgical procedure.

Data acquisition involves the use of MRI, CT and angiographic examinations performed under stereotactic conditions using various commercially available stereotactic frames — including the CRW, Leksell and Reichert–Mundinger frames involving pin fixation to the skull, or the more recently available relocatable frame system (Gill–Thomas–Cosman (GTC) localizer, Radionics, Burlington, Massuchusetts, USA). Images from the various modalities acquired under stereotactic conditions are then analysed in a common environment by digitizing into a computer system. The system allows for the neurosurgeon to determine the stereotactic coordinates of any target he or she identifies with the cursor. By superimposing the images, the exact anatomical confines of the target can be determined. Targets can be reached safely using approaches which avoid areas of high functional relevance and with integration of digital subtraction angiography, the exact position of the cerebral blood vessels in relationship to the lesion and to the probe can be ascertained in order to avoid the accidental puncture of a blood vessel.

Future developments in computer integration with stereotactic images include the display of the whole time sequence of digital subtraction angiography images (instead of a single exposure) and the integration of three dimensional MRI angiographic images (Gybels et al 1990). Trends in computer development are towards increased speed and storage capabilities, further miniaturization, greater reliability and decreased cost. User friendly software is being made available for the use of the neurosurgeon in the operating suite.

With the advent of two of the newer imaging techniques, positron emission tomography and magnetic resonance spectroscopy, an ever increasing number of metabolic and functional parameters within the brain may now be accurately measured in three dimensional space. Integration of this functional data with the structural and functional information provided by CT is an essential step to the better understanding of pathological processes in the brain and in effectively planning and monitoring treatment (Thomas et al 1990).

The current limitations of viewing three dimensional objects in anatomical detail on a two dimensional screen could be overcome by the development of holography in neurosurgical practice. A projection holographic display of the combined imaging data would provide a true three dimensional picture of the lesion and the surrounding anatomical structures. Further refinement would include the use of vascular holography where blood vessels could be suspended in a three dimensional computer imaged matrix. The limitation to the use of holography at present is the time taken to produce a quality projection holograph, which currently is days, but if this were reduced to minutes or hours for completion then holography could be incorporated into stereotactic practice (Kelly 1991).

ENDOSCOPIC SURGERY AND ULTRASOUND

The use of endoscopic neurosurgery with or without stereotactic guidance has been in use for some years, especially in regard to tumours and colloid cysts of the third ventricle (Powell et al 1983, Apuzzo et al 1984, Ostertag 1990).

With the development of finer endoscopes, coupled with stereotactic instrumentation and intraoperative laser surgery, there will be an increasing use of endoscopy in the future in neurosurgical procedures. Early prototypes incorporating these ideas have already been developed (Otsuki et al 1990).

In order to remove deep seated brain tumours with minimum insult to surrounding brain, Otsuki and coworkers have developed a stereotactic endoscopic system consisting of a guiding tube with a side window for the use of various microsurgical instruments and fine endoscopes for the visualization of operative procedures. The stereotactically inserted guiding tube acts like a brain retractor, and the endoscope, which can be manipulated independently from the guiding tube, acts as a microscope for viewing the deep and confined operative field. This open system endoscopy has been used to remove 15 intraxial lesions in conjunction with neodymium–yttrium aluminium garnet (Nd–YAG) and carbon dioxide laser vaporization (Otsuki et al 1990).

The development of smaller ultrasound probes also increases the possibility of direct intraoperative control of image directed neurosurgical procedures.

USE OF STEREOTACTIC INSTRUMENTATION IN THERAPEUTICS

Radiosurgery

Stereotactic radiosurgery is not a new concept, having been described by Leksell in 1951 (Leksell 1983).

Radiosurgery has developed by increasing the sophistication of machinery such as the gamma knife (Leksell 1971, 1983) or the less expensive linear accelerator (Lunsford et al 1991). Initially used for functional neurosurgery and to treat certain tumours and inoperable arteriovenous malformations, radiosurgery is now used to treat a variety of lesions, including arteriovenous malformations, pituitary lesions, caroticocavernous fistulas, acoustic neurinomas, Cushing's disease and craniopharyngiomas.

Future developments of radiosurgery will see an increase in the use of the various systems with regard to the types of lesion treated. More sophisticated computer software with greater precision in planning will be introduced.

The goal of stereotactic radiosurgery is to deliver a carefully controlled quantity of energy from an external source to the restricted volume of an intracranial lesion for the purpose of its elimination, with a minimal degree of radiation to the surrounding site. Optimal stereotactic radiosurgery would utilize the most therapeutic irradiation dose associated with the lowest incidence of complications (Lunsford et al 1991).

Currently under investigation is the use of three dimensional dose/volume histograms to create treatment plans that will reduce the dose received by the surrounding brain (Lunsford et al 1991).

Improvements in computer dose planning would allow a computer and an artificial intelligence programme to try to fit combinations of various shot locations, collimator sizes, weighting factors and blocking patterns in order to determine the best possible options to provide the closest fit of the isodose envelope to the defined lesional volume and to output the final number of shots, collimator sizes, coordinates of each shot and weighting and blocking patterns (Kelly 1991).

Another area of development is the use and efficacy of radiation sensitizers in radiosurgery. If an agent could be found to sensitize a tumour but not the surrounding brain then the therapeutic dose required to cause obliteration could be reduced, thereby reducing the incidence of complications (Lunsford et al 1991).

Fractionated radiotherapy

Standard external beam radiotherapy provides maximal irradiation to the known tumour mass and lower levels of radiation to the known tumour infiltration around the margins of the lesions. The limitations of this conventional form of treatment include damage to vulnerable areas of the brain and the area of maximal irradiation is not calculated by stereotactic coordinates (Kenny et al 1990).

Whilst stereotactic radiosurgery provides precise spatial coordinates for the delivery of high dose radiation, treatment of tumours such as malignant glioma is best performed by fractionated radiotherapy for radiobiological reasons (Kenny et al 1990). A number of centres are currently investigating the role of fractionated radiation by stereotactic means. This has been made more simple by the use of the recently developed relocatable stereotactic frames. One such is the GTC localizer, which is accurately relocatable over an extended period and is both non-invasive and yet rigidly fixed relative to the skull. It uses the patient's upper dentition and/or hard palate as the prime site for locating the frame on the head. The frame acts as a platform upon which the stereotactic apparatus may be mounted. Any region of interest chosen within the head, such as the tumour mass, for focal irradiation is defined in terms of the stereotactic coordinates of the chosen equipment (Thomas et al 1990).

Brachytherapy

Interstitial brachytherapy with radioactive sources implanted under stereotactic control is currently available for malignant intra-axial brain tumours and recurrent gliomas (Bernstein & Gutin 1981, Mundinger & Weigel 1984, Coffey & Friedman 1987, Gutin et al 1987). Intracavity irradiation of cystic craniopharyngioma is also performed in many centres (Julow et al 1988, Pan et al 1990).

Increasing interest in brachytherapy in the near future may be coupled with an expansion of antitumour agents delivered to the tumour bed by stereotactic means. As well as radioisotopes, chemotherapeutic agents may be delivered by stereotactic means to specific locations within the CT–MRI defined volume of tumour infiltration. Such an interstitial implant of chemodes should allow an even distribution of chemotherapeutic agents but tissue culture studies would have to be undertaken to assess the short and long term neural toxicity and dose requirements (Kelly 1991). Biological response modifiers, modulating the immune system or local growth factor response, might also be implanted intralesionally in a similar way.

Hyperthermia

Nd–YAG laser energy can be transmitted through quartz fibres and can be inserted into deep seated tumours under stereotactic control. Interstitial hyperthermia using a controlled Nd–YAG laser has been used in experimental and clinical studies (Sugiyama et al 1990, Salcman & Samaris 1981) but still has the limitations of maintaining a stable temperature and may leave intact tumour cells at the periphery of the irradiated areas.

These problems may be overcome with further research into combining laser hyperthermia with systemic chemotherapy and photodynamic therapy (Sakai et al 1987). Other methods of stereotactic hyperthermia for brain tumours under investigation are the use of radio frequency (Yoketa et al 1990) and stereotactically implanted heating systems (Kobayashi et al 1989).

EXTRACRANIAL STEREOTAXY

Whilst much progress has been made in the use of stereotactic instrumentation for intracranial lesions, little attention up to now has been paid to the use of stereotaxy for lesions within the body cavities and spinal canal. Heikkinen (1990) has reported the use of a modification of a standard Laitinen stereotactic device for use in three dimensional localization of a herniated lumbar disc and percutaneous discectomy. He concluded that stereotactic devices could be used for endoscopic operations of the lumbar spine if the frame includes a semicircular arc with a radius of 15 cm or more. The future may see advances in stereotactic instrumentation for use in extracranial stereotactic surgery.

CONCLUSION

Present day image directed surgery of brain tumours has improved over classical neurosurgical techniques, mainly by making formerly inaccessible lesions operable and by lessening the risks of surgical intervention. All neurosurgeons and oncologists who treat patients with brain tumours can use currently available instrumentation to their patients' benefit. Research is day by day advancing the frontiers of what is practicable and of use in the management of these patients.

REFERENCES

Apuzzo M J, Chandrasoma P T, Zelman V, Gianotta S L, Weiss M H 1984 Computed tomographic guidance stereotaxis in the management of lesions of the third ventricular region. Neurosurgery 15: 502–508

Apuzzo M L J, Chandrasoma P T, Cohen D et al 1987 Computer imaging stereotaxy: experience and perspective related to 500 procedures applied to brain masses. Neurosurgery 20: 930–937

Bernstein M, Gutin P H 1981 Interstitial irradiation of brain tumours: a review. Neurosurgery 741–750

Bradford R, Thomas D G T, Bydder G M 1987 MRI directed stereotactic biopsy of cerebral lesions. Acta Neurochirurgica (suppl) 39: 25–27

Coffey R J, Friedman W A 1987 Interstitial brachytherapy of management of brain tumours using computed tomography —guided stereotaxis and available imaging software: technical report. Neurosurgery 20: 4–7

Giorgi C, Casolino D S, Franzini A, Servello D, Passerini A, Broggi G, Pluchino F 1989 Computer assisted planning of stereotactic neurosurgical procedures. Child Nervous System 5: 299–302

Giorgi C, Casolino D S, Ongania E, Franzini A, Broggi G,

Pluchino F 1990 Guided microsurgery by computer assisted three dimensional analysis of neuro anatomical data stereotactically acquired. Stereotactic and Functional Neurosurgery 54/55: 482–487

Guthrie B L, Kaplan R, Kelly P J 1989 Freehand stereotaxy: neurosurgical stereotactic operating arm. Proceedings of the Neurosurgical Society of America 59–61 (abstract)

Guthrie B L, Kaplan R, Kelly P J 1990 Neurosurgical stereotactic operating arm. Stereotactic and Functional Neurosurgery 54/55: 497

Gutin P H, Leibel S A, Wara W M et al 1987 Recurrent malignant gliomas: survival following interstitial brachytherapy with high-activity iodine - 125 Sources. Journal of Neurosurgery 67: 864–873

Gybels J, Vandermeulen D, Suetens P, Marchal G, Wilms G 1990 A prototype medical workstation for computer-assisted stereotactic neurosurgery. Stereotactic and Functional Neurosurgery 54/55: 493–496

Heikkinen E R 1990 Stereotactic endoscopy applied to operations of herniated lumbar discs: technical note. Stereotactic and Functional Neurosurgery 54/55: 413–417

Julow J, Lanyi F, Hajda M, Szeifert G, Simkovic M, Toth S Z, Pasztor E 1988 Further experiences in the treatment of cystic craniopharyngiomas with yttrium GO silicate colloid. Acta Neurochirurgica (Wien) 42(Suppl): 113–119

Kato A, Yoshimura T, Hayakawa T, Tomita Y, Ikeda T, Mitomo M, Harada K, Mogami M 1991 A frameless, armless navigational system for computer-assisted neurosurgery: technical note. Journal of Neurosurgery 74: 845–849

Kelly P, Kall B, Goerss S 1986 Results of computer-assisted stereotactic laser resection of deep seated intracranial lesions. Mayo Clinic Proceedings 61: 20–27

Kelly P J 1991 Future possibilities in tumour stereotaxis. W B Saunders, Philadelphia, pp 387–400

Kenny B G, Hitchcock E R, Kitchen G, Dalton E 1990 Stereotactic fractionated irradiation. Stereotactic and Functional Neurosurgery 54/55: 547–548

Kim S H, Chung S S, Yoo S K, Kim W K 1990 Three dimensional computer simulation of stereotactic surgery. Stereotactic and Functional Neurosurgery 54/55: 488–492

Kobayashi T, Tanaka T, Kida Y et al 1989 Interstitial hyperthermia of experimental brain tumour using implant heating system. Journal of Neuro-oncology 7: 201–208

Leksell L 1951 The stereotaxic method and radiosurgery of the brain. Acta Chirurgica Scandinavica 102: 316–319

Leksell L 1971 Stereotaxis and neurosurgery: an operative system. Charles C Thomas, Springfield, IL

Leksell L 1983 Stereotactic radiosurgery. Journal of Neurology, Neurosurgery and Psychiatry 46: 797–803

Lunsford L D, Kondziolka D, Flickinger J C et al 1991 Stereotactic radiosurgery for arteriovenous malformations of the brain. Journal of neurosurgery 75: 512–524

Mundinger F, Weigel K 1984 Long-term results of stereotactic interstitial curietherapy. Acta Neurochirurgica (Suppl) 33: 367–371

Ostertag Ch H 1990 The stereotaxic endoscopic approach in surgical techniques in the management of colloid cysts of the third ventricle. In: Symon L (ed) Advances and technical standards in neurosurgery, Vol 17. Springer-Verlag, Wien, pp 143–148

Otsuki T, Yoshimoto T, Jokura H, Katakura R 1990 Stereotactic laser surgery for deep-seated brain tumours by open-system endoscopy. Stereotactic and Functional Neurosurgery 54/55: 404–408

Pan D H, Lee L S, Huang C H, Wang T T 1990 Stereotactic internal irradiation for cystic craniopharyngiomas: a 6-year experience. Stereotactic and Functional Neurosurgery 54/55: 525–530

Pell M F, Thomas D G T 1991 The initial experience with the Cosman-Roberts-Wells stereotactic system. British Journal of Neurosurgery 5: 123–128

Peters T M, Clark J A, Pike G B, Henry C, Collins L, Leksell D, Jeppsson O 1989 Stereotactic neurosurgery planning on a personal-computer based workstation. Journal of Digital Imaging 2: 75–81

Peters T M, Henri C, Pike G B, Clark J A, Collins L, Olivier A 1990 Integration of stereoscopic DSA with three-dimensional image reconstruction for stereotactic planning. Stereotactic and Functional Neurosurgery 54/55: 471–476

Powell M P, Torrens M J, Thomson J L G et al 1983 Isodense colloid cysts of the third ventricle: a diagnosis and therapeutic problem resolved by ventriculoscopy. Neurosurgery 13: 234–237

Sakai T, Fujishima L, Tanaka T et al 1987 Laser hyperthermia for deep seated brain tumour using Nd–Yag laser. Journal of the Japanese Society for Lasers in Medicine 8: 75–76

Salcman M, Samaras G M 1981 Hyperthermia for brain tumours: biophysical rationale. Neurosurgery 9: 327–335

Sugiyama K, Jakai T, Fujishima I, Ryu H, Uemura K, Yokoyama T 1990 Stereotactic interstitial laser hyperthermia using Nd-Yag laser. Stereotactic and Functional Neurosurgery 54/55: 501–505

Thomas D G T, Nouby R M 1989 Experiences in 300 cases of CT directed stereotactic surgery for lesion biopsy and aspiration of haematoma. British Journal of Neurosurgery 3: 321–326

Thomas D G T, Bradford R, Gill S et al 1988 Computer directed stereotaxic biopsy of intrinsic brain stem lesions. British Journal of Neurosurgery 2: 235–240

Thomas D G T, Gill S S, Wilson C B, Darling S L, Parkins C S 1990 Use of relocatable stereotactic frame to integrate positron emission tomography and computed tomography images: application in human malignant brain tumours. Stereotactic and Functional Neurosurgery 54/55: 388–392

Watanabe E, Watanabe T, Manaka S, Mayanagi Y, Takakura K 1987 Three dimensional digitiser (neuro-navigator): a new equipment for CT guided stereotaxic surgery. Surgical Neurology 27: 543–547

Watanabe E, Mayanagi Y, Hanamura T, Manaka S, Yoshimoto S, Takakura K 1990 Multi modality stereotactic guiding system (neuronavigator). Stereotactic and Functional Neurosurgery 54/55: 497–498

Watanabe E, Mayanagi Y, Kosugi Y, Manaka S, Takakura K 1991 Open surgery assisted by the neuronavigator, a stereotactic articulated sensitive arm. Neurosurgery 28: 792–800

Winston K R, Lutz W 1988 Linear accelerator as a neurosurgical tool for stereotactic radiosurgery. Neurosurgery 22: 454–464

Yoketa H, Komai N, Nakai E, Hakvra T, Hayashi S 1990 Stereotactic hyperthermia for brain tumours. Stereotactic and Functional Neurosurgery 54/55: 506–513

Zamorano Lucia, Dugovny M, Chavantes C, Malik G, Husman J 1990 Image - guided stereotactic centred craniotomy and laser resection of solid intracranial lesions. Stereotactic and Functional Neurosurgery 54/55: 398–403

Index